Traumatic Disorders of the Ankle

Traumatic Disorders of the Ankle

Edited by
William C. Hamilton, M.D.
Clinical Assistant Professor of Orthopaedic Surgery
Jefferson Medical College
of Thomas Jefferson University

With 293 Figures in 498 Parts

Springer-Verlag
New York Berlin Heidelberg Tokyo

WILLIAM C. HAMILTON, M.D., Clinical Assistant Professor of Orthopaedic Surgery, Jefferson Medical College of Thomas Jefferson University, 342 Lankenau Medical Building, Philadelphia, PA19151, U.S.A.

Medical Illustrator:
Steve P. Gigliotti, P.O. Box 67, Broomall, PA 19008, U.S.A.

X-ray Conversions:
Carlin Medical Photography, Westwood, NJ 07675, U.S.A.

Library of Congress Cataloging in Publication Data
Main entry under title:

Traumatic disorders of the ankle.

Bibliography: p.
Includes index.
1. Ankle—Wounds and injuries. I. Hamilton,
William C. [DNLM: 1. Ankle—Injuries. WE 880 T777]
RD562.T7 1983   617′.584044   83–10610

Typeset by Kingsport Press, Kingsport, Tennessee
Printed and bound by Halliday Lithograph, West Hanover, Massachusetts
Printed in the United States of America.

9 8 7 6 5 4 3 2 1

ISBN 0–387–90831–5 Springer-Verlag   New York   Berlin   Heidelberg   Tokyo
ISBN 3–540–90831–5 Springer-Verlag   Berlin   Heidelberg   New York   Tokyo

To
Carole, Wendy, Amy, and Craig

Contents

Contributors

James H. Beaty, M.D., Clinical Instructor of Orthopaedics, University of Tennessee Center for the Health Sciences, Memphis, Tennessee; Staff, The Campbell Clinic, LaBonheur Children's Medical Center, and Tennessee Crippled Children's Services, Memphis, Tennessee 38104

S. Terry Canale, M.D., Clinical Assistant Professor of Orthopaedics, University of Tennessee Center for the Health Sciences, Memphis, Tennessee; Chief of Orthopaedics and Chief of Surgery, LeBonheur Children's Medical Center; Staff, the Campbell Clinic, Memphis, Tennessee 38104

Jerome M. Cotler, M.D., Clinical Professor, Department of Orthopaedic Surgery, Jefferson Medical College of Thomas Jefferson University, Philadelphia, Pennsylvania; Attending Physician, Thomas Jefferson University Hospital, Philadelphia, Pennsylvania 19151

Robert P. Good, M.D., Instructor, Department of Orthopaedic Surgery, Jefferson Medical College of Thomas Jefferson University, Philadelphia, Pennsylvania 19151; Attending Physician, The Bryn Mawr Hospital, Bryn Mawr, Pennsylvania 19010

William C. Hamilton, M.D., Clinical Assistant Professor, Department of Orthopaedic Surgery, Jefferson Medical College of Thomas Jefferson University, Philadelphia, Pennsylvania; Attending Physician, The Lankenau Hospital, Philadelphia, Pennsylvania 19151

J. David Hoffman, M.D., Clinical Assistant Professor, Department of Orthopaedic Surgery, Jefferson Medical College of Thomas Jefferson University, Philadelphia, Pennsylvania; Attending Physician, Thomas Jefferson University Hospital, Philadelphia, Pennsylvania 19151

Eric L. Hume, M.D., Assistant Professor, Department of Orthopaedic Surgery, Jefferson Medical College of Thomas Jefferson University, Philadelphia, Pennsylvania; Attending Physician, Thomas Jefferson University Hospital, Philadelphia, Pennsylvania 19151.

Peter D. Pizzutillo, M.D., Director of Medical Education, Alfred I. duPont Institute, Wilmington, Delaware/19899, and Clinical Assistant Professor, Department of Orthopaedic Surgery, Thomas Jefferson University, Philadelphia, Pennsylvania 19151

Kent M. Samuelson, M.D., Clinical Associate Professor, Division of Orthopaedic Surgery, University of Utah School of Medicine, Salt Lake City, Utah; Attending Staff Surgeon, LDS Hospital, Director, Intermountain Orthopaedic Research Institute, Salt Lake City, Utah 84132

Preface

The management of ankle injuries has long been a stumbling block for orthopaedists in training. As a first year resident, I was fortunate to encounter the series of articles by N. Lauge-Hansen and T. Baek Kristensen that classified ankle injuries according to their mechanism. I found this information quite helpful throughout my residency and early years of practice.

Several years ago, an attempt was made to summarize this material for the benefit of the orthopaedic house staff of Thomas Jefferson University. It quickly become obvious that such a "manual" would require a great deal of professional illustration and editorial assistance in order to be effective. Almost simultaneously, a fortuitous encounter with Ms. Marie Low (at that time Medical Editor of Springer-Verlag New York Incorporated) provided both the stimulus and the means to present this information in the manner and detail which it deserved.

Contributors were carefully selected for their knowledge and experience in particular areas and for their willingness to cooperate in providing a smooth-flowing manuscript.

This text contains little new material. Rather, it represents an attempt to bring together, under one cover, the wealth of extant information on this subject. Wherever a consensus could not be perceived, conflicting views have been summarized as objectively as possible. Unfortunately, there are still many aspects of ankle injury for which we have more questions than answers.

Acknowledgements

Although a proper list of acknowledgements would require many pages (to the chagrin of our editors), this text would not be complete without formally mentioning at least the following:

The many patients with both simple and complex ankle injuries who daily entrust themselves to our care and without whom this text would have little merit.

The library staffs of the Thomas Jefferson University and the Lankenau Hospital, who were always willing and able to locate old and sometimes obscure reference material. Special thanks are due to Mrs. Loann Scarpato in this regard.

The secretaries, Jane Malone and Ann Louise Smith, who worked tirelessly to type and retype the many versions of this book.

Marie Norton, of the Lankenau Hospital Medical Records Department, and Mary Cozzo, of my office, who so promptly and successfully located the radiographic examples.

Photographers, Larry Kradel and Doug Thayer, for their excellent reproductions.

The operating room personnel: Eileen Fetzer, Lynn Larkin, Michele LeMarbre, Muffy Montgomery, and Molly Putnam for their invaluable assistance obtaining photographs.

Our illustrator, Steve Gigliotti, who willingly and enthusiastically met with me every Thursday night for almost 2 years and was always agreeable to one more "small change."

Anna Deus and the other members of the Springer-Verlag editorial staff who were so patient with us amateurs.

Very special thanks to Administrative Assistant, Louise Lang, who insisted that we "could" complete this book and to Marie Low, formerly of Springer-Verlag, who insisted that we "would" complete it.

And last but not least, a special debt of gratitude to my wife, who, over the past few years, learned how to do most home repairs herself—and to my young children who learned how to function and play without making noise.

WILLIAM C. HAMILTON

Chapter 1 Anatomy

William C. Hamilton

In order to understand the complex injury patterns encountered about the ankle and to discuss their etiology and treatment, it is necessary to review briefly the gross anatomy of this region with particular emphasis on bone and ligament relationships.

The distal tibia and fibula are intimately bound together in an amphiarthrodial relationship by the short, firm tibiofibular ligaments. Together, the distal tibia and fibula form a concave mortise [18] in which the talus (tenon) is firmly held by the medial (deltoid) and lateral collateral ligaments (Fig. 1.1). Dyssymmetry between the bone and soft tissue of the medial and lateral sides of the ankle is an early indication that the ankle does not function as a true hinge.

Osteology

Tibia

The tibia in its distal one-third gradually becomes quadrilateral in cross-section and flares immediately proximal to its articular surface or plafond [22,23]. This plafond is wider anteriorly than posteriorly (Fig. 1.2) [10]. Medially, the distal tibia is prolonged in a slight varus direction to form the medial malleolus, whose concave inner surface is lined with articular cartilage continuous with that of the tibial plafond (Fig. 1.3A) [1]. As pointed out by Bonnin [3], and recently emphasized by Pankovich and Shivaram [24], the medial malleolus is composed of an anterior and posterior colliculus, separated from each other on the inner side by the intercollicular groove. The anterior colliculus extends further distally than the posterior colliculus. The articular facet of the posterior colliculus is smaller than that of the anterior colliculus. The external aspect of the posterior colliculus is grooved for the posterior tibial and flexor digitorum longus tendons (Fig. 1.3A).

The distal tibia provides an articular surface that is concave from front to back and from side to side. The side-to-side concavity, however, is divided in the midline by a slight convex ridge which runs sagitally and corresponds to a compa-

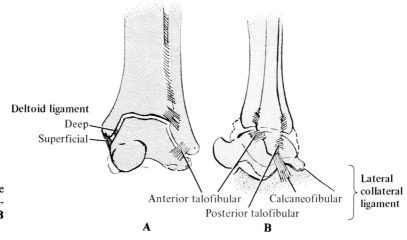

Fig. 1.1. Ankle joint: mortise and tenon with collateral ligaments. **A** Frontal view. **B** Lateral view.

Deltoid ligament
Deep
Superficial

Anterior talofibular
Posterior talofibular
Calcaneofibular

Lateral collateral ligament

A **B**

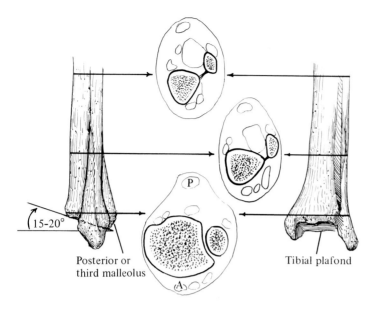

Fig. 1.2. Tibial plafond and distal tibiofibular relationships.

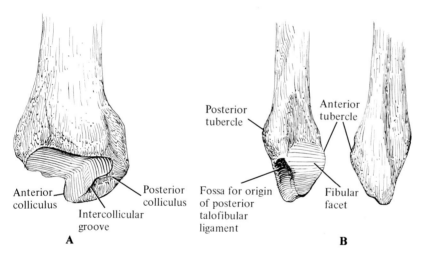

Fig. 1.3 The malleoli. **A** Medial. **B** Lateral.

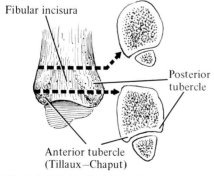

Fig. 1.4. Fibular incisura of the distal tibia.

rable depression in the weight-bearing surface of the talus (Fig. 1.1A) [14]. The posterior edge of the distal tibia extends further distally than the anterior edge, such that the articular surface faces anteriorly 15–20° (Fig. 1.2) [22]. The prominent posterior margin of the distal tibia has been termed the "posterior malleolus" by Destot [7] and the "third malleolus" by Trethowan [29].

Along the lateral aspect of the distal tibia (Fig. 1.4), there is a groove or depression of variable depth (fibular groove, peroneal groove, fibular incisura, tibiofibular incisura) that accommo-

Fig. 1.5. The talus. **A** Superior view. **B** Frontal view. **C** Lateral view. **D** Posterolateral view. **E** Inferior view.

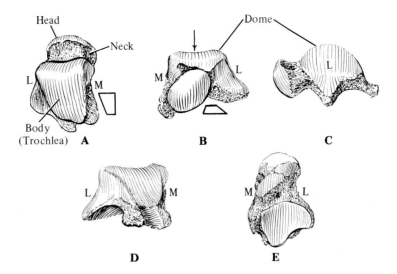

dates the distal fibula and becomes more prominent distally due to the emergence of tubercles at its anterior and posterior borders [30]. The anterior tubercle of the distal tibia (tubercle of Tillaux-Chaput) is consistently more prominent than the posterior tubercle.

Fibula

The fibula enlarges distally to form the bulbous lateral malleolus whose tip is located posterior and approximately 1 cm distal to the medial malleolus (Fig. 1.2). The inner surface of the lateral malleolus provides a triangular facet that articulates with the lateral aspect of the talus (Fig. 1.3B) [2]. Immediately posterior to this facet is a fossa that serves as origin for the posterior talofibular ligament (Fig. 1.10E). Corresponding to the tubercles of the distal tibia, the lateral malleolus displays subtle prominences or tubercles anteriorly and posteriorly; the posterior tubercle is consistently more proximal than the anterior tubercle. The posterior border of the distal fibula is grooved to accommodate the peroneal tendons.

Talus

The talus (Fig. 1.5) is composed of three parts: the head, neck (collum), and the body (trochlea). The talus has no muscle attachments and is covered by articular cartilage on most of its surface [14]. The trochlea of the talus is wider anteriorly than posteriorly by approximately 25% [8,10,

14,21] and the superior surface is wider below than above, so that it resembles a wedge in both a horizontal and a vertical plane (Fig. 1.5A,B) [6].

The articular surface of the talar dome is convex from front to back (Fig. 1.5C) and from side to side except for a slight sagittal depression (Fig. 1.5B) which mates with the distal tibia and provides for an intimate fit between these two bones [13]. The articular cartilage of the talar dome continues medially and laterally to form relatively vertical facets that articulate with the malleoli (Fig. 1.5B). The fibular facet is larger, deeper, more vertical, and faces more posteriorly than the inner (tibial) facet (Fig. 1.5B–D) [6,8].

Whereas the medial edge of the talus is relatively straight, running in an anteroposterior direction, the lateral border is oblique (Fig. 1.5A). This divergence contributes to the wider anterior dimension of the talus. The talar neck is broad and short (Fig. 1.5A,C). The head of the talus is convex and articulates with the concave surface of the navicular. The under surface of the talus is occupied by three facets for articulation with the calcaneus (Fig. 1.5E) [12].

Ligamentous Anatomy

Tibiofibular Syndesmosis

The distal tibiofibular articulation is not a true synovial joint but rather a syndesmosis (Fig. 1.6).

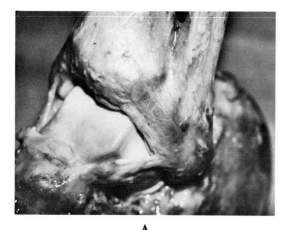

A

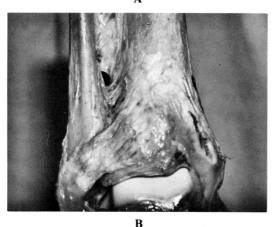

B

Fig. 1.6. Tibiofibular syndesmosis. **A** Anterior view. **B** Posterior view.

The convex medial aspect of the distal fibula is stabilized in the shallow peroneal groove of the distal tibia by five distinct ligamentous structures.

The Anterior Inferior Tibiofibular Ligament (AITFL)

The AITFL (anterior lateral malleolar ligament) [7,17] binds the anterior margins of the tibia and fibula (Fig. 1.7A,C) [10]. It is a well-developed, stout structure approximately 2 cm wide, 2 cm long, and 0.5 cm thick, extending from the anterior tubercle of the tibia in a distal, lateral, and posterior direction to insert on a roughened tubercle on the anterior aspect of the lateral malleolus [15,19,13].

The Posterior Inferior Tibiofibular Ligament (PITFL)

The PITFL (posterior lateral malleolar ligament) [7,17] binds the posterior margin of the crural bones. It extends from the posterior tubercle of the tibia to a tubercle on the posterior border of the fibula just behind and above the fibular facet (Fig. 1.7B,C). Since this tubercle is proximal to that on which the AITFL inserts, the course of the PITFL is less vertical than that of the ATIFL [25].

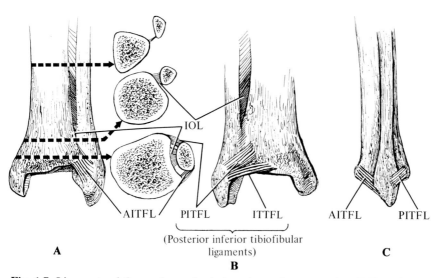

Fig. 1.7. Ligaments of the syndesmosis, **A** Anterior and cross section. **B** Posterior and **C** Lateral views.

The Inferior Transverse Tibiofibular Ligament (ITTFL)

The ITTFL [5,20] is situated distal and deep to the posterior inferior tibiofibular ligament (Fig. 1.7B). It originates along the posterior edge of the tibia, adjacent to the articular surface, and courses laterally and relatively transversely to insert on the inner aspect of the lateral malleolus behind the fibular facet, adjacent to the fibers of the PITFL. This tough, fibrocartilaginous structure extends below the posterior edge of the tibia and bridges the angle formed by the intersection of these bones, such that it reinforces and deepens the posterior aspect of the ankle joint, much like a labrum. Some authors consider this structure as part of the posterior inferior tibiofibular ligament [9,20].

Interosseous Membrane and Ligament

The crural **interosseous membrane** (IOM) consists of thin aponeurotic fibers that extend from the posterior tibial margin in an oblique direction, downward and laterally, to insert along the medial aspect of the fibula (Fig. 1.7A,B) [30]. Distally, at a variable distance above the ankle, the interosseous membrane condenses to become the **interosseous ligament** (IOL) (Fig. 1.7A,B) [30]. The fibers of this ligament are short and thick and extend only a short distance between the peroneal groove of the tibia and the medial aspect of the fibula, just behind and above the lateral malleolus facet, posterior to the mid-axis of the fibula. The interosseous ligament is continuous with the posterior inferior tibiofibular ligament and distinction between the two can sometimes be difficult [25]. Some authors believe that this structure represents the strongest link between the tibia and fibula [10,30]; others do not even mention this ligament [4,11]. It is noteworthy that the strength and length of the interosseous ligament varies greatly in different individuals [20,24].

Between the distal tibia and fibula, there is a sagittal recess of variable height that communicates with the ankle joint. Viewing the medial aspect of the distal fibula, one notes that between the anterior and posterior groups of tibiofibular ligaments (Fig. 1.8) there is an area oriented obliquely in a distal and anterior direction, which is devoid of ligamentous attachment and therefore relatively unprotected [25].

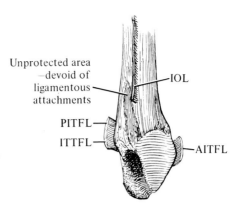

Fig. 1.8. Medial aspect of the distal fibula.

Capsule

The capsule (Fig. 1.1B) of the ankle joint originates from the bone-cartilage border of the tibia, fibula, and talus. It is thin and redundant anteriorly and posteriorly [16,23], but is reinforced medially and laterally to form specialized collateral ligaments [23].

Deltoid Ligament

The medial collateral or deltoid ligament (Fig. 1.9) has been accurately described by Pankovich and Shivaram [24]. It is composed of superficial and deep portions. The fan-shaped **superficial** portion (Fig. 1.9A) consists of long fibers, originating in continuity with the tibial periosteum from the anterior colliculus and the anterior aspect of the posterior colliculus of the medial malleolus. Three distinct bands can be identified within the superficial deltoid ligament: the *naviculotibial* band inserts into the medial aspect of the navicular and the adjacent calcaneonavicular ligament; the *calcaneotibial* band inserts into the sustentaculum tali of the calcaneus; the *superficial talotibial* band travels posteriorly and inferiorly to insert on the anterior aspect of the medial tubercle of the talus.

The functionally more important **deep deltoid ligament** (Fig. 1.9B,C) is short and occupies a relatively transverse plane between the medial malleolus and the talus. The deep deltoid ligament originates primarily from the posterior colliculus and the intercollicular groove and inserts along the medial surface of the talus. Two distinct elements can be identified within the deep deltoid ligament. The *deep anterior talotibial* portion lies

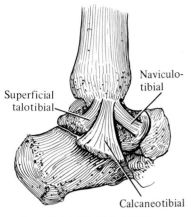

Superficial
talotibial

Naviculo-
tibial

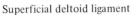

Calcaneotibial

Superficial deltoid ligament

A

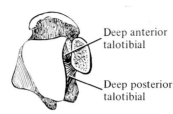

Deep anterior
talotibial

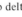

Deep posterior
talotibial

Deep deltoid ligament

B

Fig. 1.9. The deltoid ligament. **A** Superficial deltoid ligament. **B** Deep deltoid ligament. **C** Horizontal cross-section through the ankle joint, just below the dome of the talus, demonstrating the deep deltoid ligament medially as well as the anterior and posterior talofibular ligaments laterally.

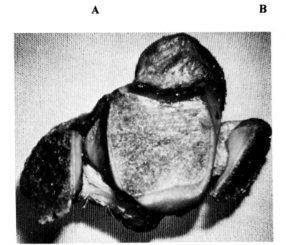

C

under the calcaneotibial ligament and courses laterally and slightly anteriorly to insert on the talus near its neck; the *deep posterior talotibial* ligament courses laterally and slightly posteriorly to insert in the vicinity of the tubercle of the talus.

Lateral Collateral Ligament

The lateral collateral ligament complex (Fig. 1.10) is composed of three distinct structures [18]. The *anterior talofibular ligament* (Figs. 1.9C and 1.10A,D,E) originates from the anterior aspect of the lateral malleolus, just below the insertion of the anterior inferior tibiofibular ligament and just anterior to the fibular facet; it courses distally and medially to insert on the neck of the talus [10,28]. This ligament is a well-

defined, flat, capsular condensation measuring approximately 6–8 mm in width and 2 cm in length.

The triangular *posterior talofibular ligament* (Figs. 1.9C and 1.10) originates from the fossa behind and below the lateral malleolar facet and courses medially and posteriorly to a broad insertion along the posterior articular margin of the trochlea talus [26,28], immediately lateral to the groove for the flexor hallucis longus [10]. When viewed in its entirety, the posterior talofibular ligament is obviously the largest component of the lateral ligament complex [12].

Unlike the anterior and posterior talofibular ligaments, the *calcaneofibular* (Fig. 1.10A–C) component or middle fasciculus of the lateral collateral ligament is an extracapsular structure. It arises from the anterior tip of the lateral malleolus and extends distally, medially, and approximately 30° posteriorly across the talofibular and talocalcaneal joints to insert on the lateral aspect of the calcaneus just above and behind the peroneal tubercle. This ligament is partially obscured by the overlying peroneal tendons, with which it is in intimate contact [10,18].

Fig. 1.10. The three fasciculi of the lateral collateral ligament. **A** Lateral schematic. **B** and **C** Schematic and photograph of dissected specimen (posterior view). **D** Schematic (cross-section). **E** Radiograph of cross-section obtained through the talus at the inferior limit of the medial malleolus, demonstrating the size and orientation of the posterior talofibular ligament as well as its origin from the posterior fossa of the lateral malleolus. Note also the distal and especially medial inclination of the anterior talofibular ligament.

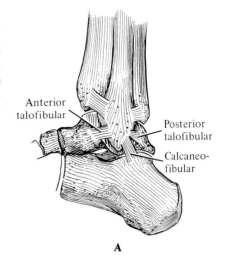

A

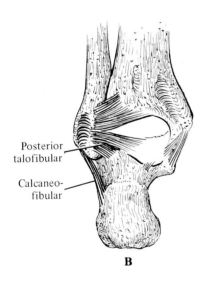

B

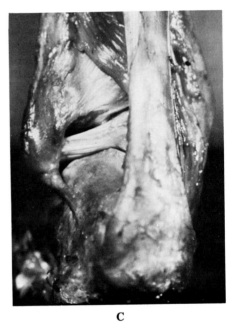

C

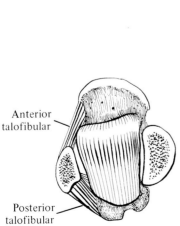

D

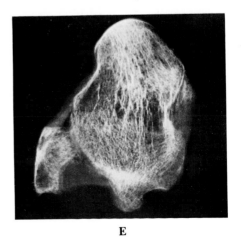

E

Muscle Groups and Retinacula

Muscle groups cross the ankle on its anterior, posteromedial, and posterolateral aspects (Fig. 1.11). Because the tendons observe a sudden change in direction at the ankle, they rely upon fascial bands for their stability.

Tendons of the anterior compartment (Fig. 1.12) are stabilized by the overlying superior (transverse crural ligament) and inferior (cruciate crural ligament) extensor retinacula, which send perpendicular septa that define specific tendon compartments. From medial to lateral, the anterior tibial, extensor hallucis longus, and extensor digitorum longus (with peroneus tertius) tendons cross the anterior aspect of the ankle in individual compartments [31].

The flexor retinaculum (laciniate ligament) and its fibrous connections with the posteromedial tibia and ankle joint capsule define four compartments behind the medial malleolus (Fig. 1.11). From front to back, these compartments transmit the posterior tibial tendon, flexor digitorum longus tendon, posterior tibial neurovascular bundle, and the flexor hallucis longus tendon en route to the foot [31]. The posterior tibial and flexor digitorum longus sheaths groove the posterior and middle parts of the superficial deltoid ligament, as they make their turn into the foot (Fig. 1.13) [24].

Posterolaterally, the superior peroneal retinaculum anchors the tendons of the peroneus brevis and longus above and behind the lateral malleolus; the inferior peroneal retinaculum anchors these structures to the calcaneus distal to the lateral malleolus (Fig. 1.14). Under the superior peroneal retinaculum, these tendons are enclosed within a common sheath which then bifurcates, so that under the inferior peroneal retinaculum the tendons are separate [31].

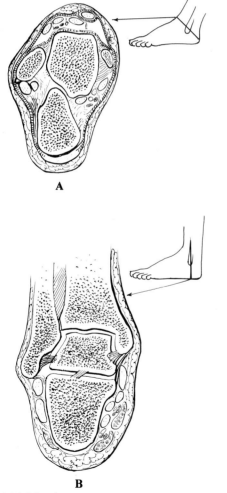

A

B

Fig. 1.11. Muscle groups and retinacula about the ankle.

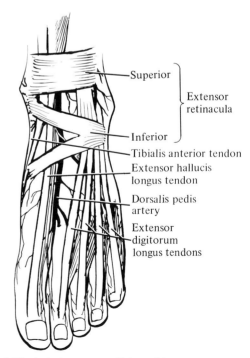

Superior
Extensor retinacula
Inferior
Tibialis anterior tendon
Extensor hallucis longus tendon
Dorsalis pedis artery
Extensor digitorum longus tendons

Fig. 1.12. Anterior aspect of the ankle.

Fig. 1.13. Medial aspect of the ankle and hindfoot.

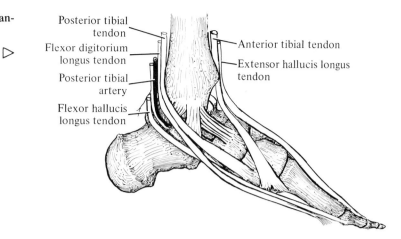

Posterior tibial tendon

Flexor digitorium longus tendon

Posterior tibial artery

Flexor hallucis longus tendon

Anterior tibial tendon

Extensor hallucis longus tendon

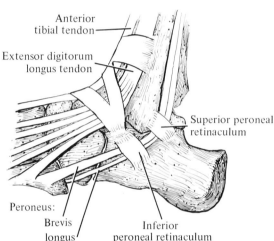

Anterior tibial tendon

Extensor digitorum longus tendon

Superior peroneal retinaculum

Peroneus:
Brevis
longus

Inferior peroneal retinaculum

Fig. 1.14. Lateral aspect of the ankle and hindfoot.

Vascular Anatomy

The ankle is well vascularized by both the anterior and posterior tibial arterial systems which anastomose freely in this area [31].

In the lower third of the leg, the **anterior tibial artery** with its venae comitantes and the deep branch of the peroneal nerve occupy the interval between the anterior tibial and extensor hallucis longus muscles (Fig. 1.16). This neurovascular bundle crosses the ankle midway between the malleoli beneath the tendon of the extensor hallucis longus (Fig. 1.15). Proximal to the ankle, the bundle is situated medial to the extensor hallucis longus; distal to the ankle, it is situated lateral

to this tendon. At the level of the ankle, the anterior tibial artery gives off *anterior medial and anterior lateral malleolar branches,* and then continues into the foot as the dorsalis pedis artery.

The *anterior lateral malleolar artery* passes beneath the extensor digitorum longus and peroneus tertius tendons to ramify over the lateral malleolus and anastomose with malleolar branches of the posterior tibial artery and with the perforating branch of the peroneal artery. The *anterior medial malleolar artery* arises oppo-

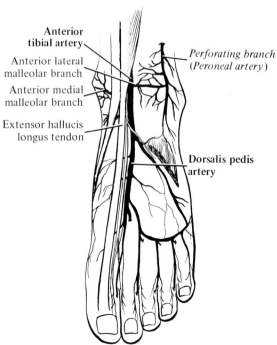

Anterior tibial artery

Anterior lateral malleolar branch

Anterior medial malleolar branch

Extensor hallucis longus tendon

Perforating branch (Peroneal artery)

Dorsalis pedis artery

Fig. 1.15. Anterior tibial arterial system.

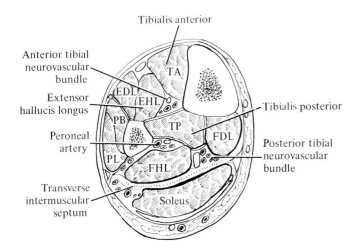

Fig. 1.16. Cross-section of lower limb at the level of mid-calf.

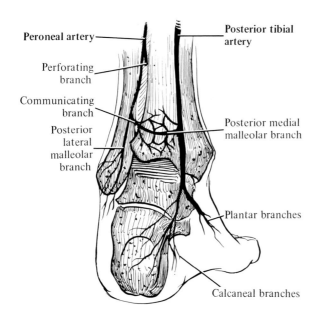

Fig. 1.17. Peroneal and posterior tibial arterial systems.

site the anterior lateral malleolar artery and courses between the anterior tibial tendon and joint capsule to ramify over the medial ankle and anastomose with malleolar branches of the posterior tibial artery.

The **posterior tibial artery,** after giving rise to the peroneal artery below the lower border of the popliteus muscle, descends through the calf immediately deep to the transverse intermuscular septum (Fig. 1.16). In the lower third of the leg, the artery becomes superficial and passes behind the medial malleolus in the third compartment of the flexor retinaculum between the flexor digitorum longus and the flexor hallucis longus

tendons (Fig. 1.13). Throughout its course in the lower leg and at the ankle, the posterior tibial artery is accompanied by the tibial nerve and usually two venae comitantes. At the level of the ankle, the posterior tibial artery provides the *posterior medial malleolar branch* (Fig. 1.17).

The **peroneal artery,** the largest branch of the posterior tibial, descends through the deep compartment of the calf in close proximity to the posteromedial border of the fibula (Fig. 1.16) and provides three important branches in the vicinity of the ankle (Fig. 1.17): the *perforating branch* enters the anterior compartment of the leg at the upper border of the interosseous ligament, supplies the syndesmosis, and anastomoses with the anterior tibial system; the *communicating branch* anastomoses with the posterior tibial system across the back of the ankle; the terminal branch or *posterior lateral malleolar artery* anastomoses over the lateral ankle with the anterior lateral malleolar branch of the anterior tibial artery.

The deep venous system essentially parallels the arterial tree. Significant superficial veins include the great and the small saphenous veins. The *great (long) saphenous vein* crosses the ankle joint just anterior to the medial malleolus and should be protected during surgical exposures in this area (Fig. 1.18). The *lesser (short) saphenous vein* is formed by a confluence of tributaries posterior to the lateral malleolus; it courses proximally in subcutaneous tissues immediately lateral to the Achilles tendon (Fig. 1.19).

Cutaneous Nerves

The **sural** (calf) nerve is formed at a variable distance above the ankle by the merging of the medial sural (tibial) and a communicating branch of the lateral sural (peroneal) cutaneous nerves. It accompanies the lesser saphenous vein in the calf and at the level of the ankle it occupies a superficial position parallel and posterior to the

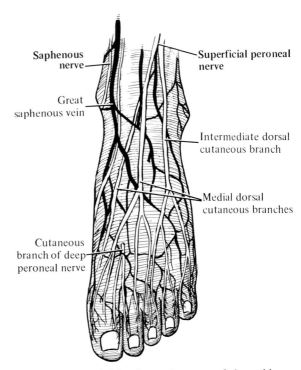

Fig. 1.18. Superficial veins and nerves of the ankle and foot (anterior view).

peroneal tendons (Fig. 1.19). The sural nerve terminates as the *dorsal lateral cutaneous nerve* of the foot [12].

The **saphenous** nerve accompanies the great saphenous vein and arborizes just below the me-

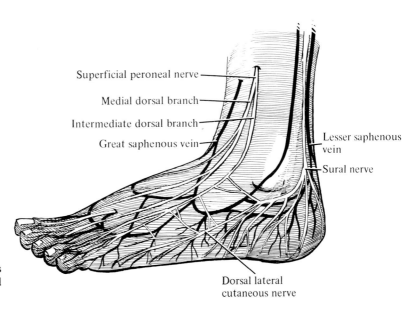

Fig. 1.19. Superficial veins and nerves of the ankle and foot (lateral view).

dial malleolus to supply sensation to the medial
aspect of the ankle and hindfoot (Fig. 1.18). It
has little surgical significance at this level.

The **superficial peroneal** nerve, a branch of
the common peroneal nerve, pierces the deep fascia to become subcutaneous in the distal third
of the leg and almost immediately divides into
two branches, the *medial dorsal cutaneous nerve*
and the *intermediate dorsal cutaneous nerve.*
These branches cross the ankle superficial to the
extensor retinacula and supply sensation to the
dorsum of the foot (Fig. 1.18). The medial dorsal
cutaneous nerve innervates primarily the dorsum
and sides of the medial two and the medial half
of the third toes. The intermediate dorsal cutaneous branch supplies sensation to the lateral foot
and toes and communicates with the terminal
twigs of the dorsal lateral cutaneous branch of
the sural nerve. The web space and opposing
sides of the first and second toes comprise the
autonomous zone of the deep peroneal nerve via
its dorsal digital branches.

References

1. Bohler L: The Treatment of Fractures, 5th ed. New York, Grune & Stratton, 1956.
2. Bolin H: The fibula and its relationship to the tibia and talus in injuries due to forced external rotation. Acta Radiol 56:439, 1961.
3. Bonnin J: Injuries to the Ankle. New York, Grune & Stratton, 1950.
4. Bonnin J: A Complete Outline of Fractures. London, Heinemann, 1951.
5. Broström L: Sprained ankles. I. Anatomic lesions in recent sprains. Acta Chir Scand 128:483, 1964.
6. Cave EF: Ankle injuries. In: Fractures and Other Injuries. Chicago, Year Book Medical, 1958.
7. Cedell C-A: Rupture of the posterior talotibial ligament with avulsion of a bone fragment from talus. Acta Orthop Scand 45:454, 1974.
8. Close JR, Inman VD: The Action of the Ankle Joint. Prosthetic Devices Research Project, Institute of Engineering Research, University of California, Berkeley. Advisory Committee on Artificial Limbs, National Research Council, Series II, Issue 22, April 1952.
9. Colonna PC, Ralston EL: Operative approaches to the ankle joint. Am J Surg 82:44, 1951.
10. Dabezies E, D'Ambrosia RD, Shoji H: Classification and treatment of ankle fractures. Orthopedics 1:365, 1978.
11. Golterman AFL: Diagnosis and treatment of tibiofibular diastasis. Arch Chir Neerl 16:185, 1964.
12. Goss CM: Anatomy of the Human Body by Henry Gray, 28th ed. Philadelphia, Lea & Febiger, 1966.
13. Grath G: Widening of the ankle mortise. A clinical and experimental study. Acta Chir Scand (Suppl) 263:1, 1960.
14. Henderson MS: Fractures of the ankle. Wisc Med 31:684, 1932.
15. Kaye JJ, Bohne, WHO: A radiographic study of the ligamentous anatomy of the ankle. Radiology 125:659, 1977.
16. Lauge-Hansen N: Fractures of the ankle. II. Combined experimental-surgical and experimental-roentgenologic investigations. Arch Surg 60:957, 1950.
17. Lauge-Hansen N: Fractures of the ankle. V. Pronation-dorsiflexion fracture. Arch Surg 67:813, 1953.
18. McLaughlin HL: Trauma. Philadelphia, Saunders, 1960.
19. Menelaus MB: Injuries of the anterior inferior tibiofibular ligament. Aust NZ J Surg 30:279, 1960.
20. Monk CJE: Injuries of the tibiofibular ligaments. J Bone Joint Surg 56B:263, 1974.
21. Mukherjee SK, Pringle RM, Baxter AD: Fractures of the lateral process of the talus. A report of 13 cases. J Bone Joint Surg 56B:263, 1974.
22. Neufeld AJ: Ankle joint fractures and their treatment. Clin Orthop Rel Res 42:91, 1965.
23. Nyström G: A contribution to the treatment of fractures of the posterior border of the tibia by malleolar fractures. Acta Radiol 25:672, 1944.
24. Pankovich AM, Shivaram MS: Anatomical basis of variability in injuries of medial malleolus and the deltoid ligament. I. Anatomical studies. Acta Orthop Scand 50:217, 1979.
25. Patrick J: Direct approach to trimalleolar fractures. J Bone Joint Surg 47:236, 1965.
26. Pennal GF: Subluxation of the ankle. Can Med Assoc J 49:92, 1943.
27. Pott P: Remarks on fractures and dislocations. In: Chirurgical Works of Pott. London, Wood & Innes, 1808.
28. Robichon J, Pegington J, Moonje VB, DesJardins JP: The functional anatomy of the ankle joint and its relationship to ankle injuries. Can J Surg 15:145, 1972.
29. Trethowan WH: Fractures in the neighborhood of the ankle joint. II. The operative treatment of ankle fractures. Lancet 1:90, 1926.
30. Vasli S: Operative treatment of ankle fractures. Acta Chir Scand (Suppl) 226:1, 1957.
31. Woodburne RT: Essentials of Human Anatomy, 3rd ed. New York, Oxford University Press, 1965.

Chapter 2   Functional Anatomy

KENT M. SAMUELSON

> When in a state of integrity, the ankle joint is kept in a condition of equilibrium by the antagonizing muscles and malleoli with their ligaments.
>
> Dupuytren [9]

Definitions

The study of ankle fractures has unfortunately been complicated at times by lack of standardized terminology to describe ankle and foot motion. In an effort to obviate this problem, the following scheme will be adopted and utilized throughout this book.

Dorsiflexion/plantarflexion: motion of the talus in a cephalad/caudad direction about a transverse axis through the talus, i.e., movement in the sagittal plane [22,24,26]. This provides approximately 50–60° of motion (Fig. 2.1) [3,17,28].

Internal/external rotation: medial/lateral rotation of the talus about a vertical axis through the tibia, i.e., movement in the horizontal plane [22,35,36]. Experimentally, this amounts to 5–6° [5]. Clinically this motion can be perceived but it cannot be effectively measured (Fig. 2.2) [17].

Adduction/abduction: medial/lateral rotation of the talus about its longitudinal axis, i.e., motion in the coronal plane (Fig. 2.3) [10,35,36]. These motions in the past have sometimes been referred to as tibial flexion (adduction) and fibular flexion (abduction) [10]. Adduction/abduction are sometimes used in another sense to describe medial/lateral deviation of the forefoot in the horizontal plane around a vertical axis through the midfoot [22,24]; adduction/abduction of the foot under these circumstances produces internal/external rotation at the tibiotalar joint (Fig. 2.4). Unless specified

▷

Fig. 2.3. Adduction/abduction of the *hindfoot* occurs in the frontal plane, i.e., about a longitudinal axis.

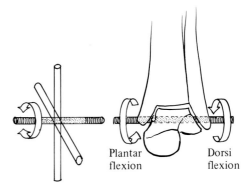

Plantar flexion   Dorsi flexion

Fig. 2.1. Dorsiflexion/plantarflexion occurs in the sagittal plane, i.e., about a transverse axis.

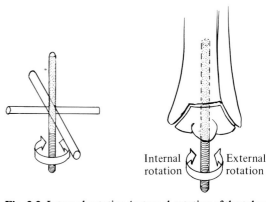

Internal rotation   External rotation

Fig. 2.2. Internal rotation/external rotation of the talus occurs in a horizontal plane, i.e., about a vertical axis.

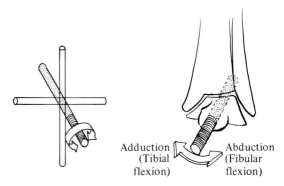

Adduction (Tibial flexion)   Abduction (Fibular flexion)

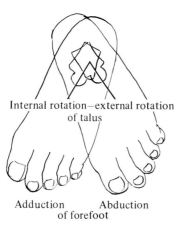

Internal rotation—external rotation
of talus

Adduction   Abduction
of forefoot

Fig. 2.4. Adduction/abduction of the *forefoot* occurs in a horizontal plane, i.e., about a vertical axis. Adduction/abduction of the forefoot with the ankle in neutral position is transmitted to the talus as internal/external rotation.

nation refers to the opposite motion and is characterized by movement of the foot about its longitudinal axis, such that the first metatarsal moves in a caudad direction and the fifth metatarsal moves in a cephalad direction [10,51]. Pronation implies eversion (subtalar joint), external rotation (tibiotalar joint), and abduction of the forefoot [22,24,26]. Supination is generally, but not always, associated with plantarflexion at the ankle; similarly, pronation is usually accompanied by dorsiflexion [10]. In maximal supination or pronation, the foot forms a rigid lever and resists further motion in that direction. This explains how rather trivial rotational forces can produce significant ankle injury [27].

Motion at the Ankle Joint

otherwise, adduction/abduction in this book will refer to rotation of the talus about its longitudinal axis, i.e., tibial flexion/fibular flexion.

Inversion/eversion: medial/lateral rotation of the heel on an oblique axis through the subtalar joint [14,24].

Supination/pronation: complex motions involving the entire ankle and foot (Fig. 2.5). Supination is characterized by movement of the foot about a longitudinal axis, such that the first metatarsal moves in a cranial direction and the fifth metatarsal moves in a caudad direction [10,51]. Supination implies inversion (subtalar joint), medial rotation (tibiotalar joint), and adduction of the forefoot [22,24,26]. Pro-

There has been considerable discussion and disagreement in the literature regarding the type of motion that occurs at the ankle joint. Clinically, the situation is complicated by the fact that the joints of the hindfoot normally act in concert with the ankle joint to produce relatively complex motions. The subtalar and talonavicular joints function together as the peritalar joint and the talonavicular and calcaneocuboid joints form a functional unit called the mid-tarsal joint [45]. Because of the close proximity of these joints to the ankle, it is difficult to clinically isolate ankle motion from peritalar and/or mid-tarsal motion. However, for the purposes of this discus-

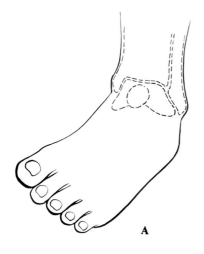

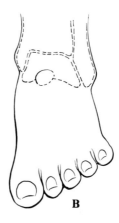

A   B   **Fig. 2.5. A** Supination. **B** Pronation.

sion, we will concern ourselves only with the motion that occurs at the tibiotalar joint.

The ankle is a remarkable example of the functional interplay of bone and ligamentous structures and their protective action upon one another [39]. The ankle has been described as a ginglymus or hinge joint [16,28]; this represents an oversimplification, however [4,6,48]. In a true hinge, the center of rotation is fixed and motion occurs in a single plane. In the ankle, however, plantar- and dorsiflexion are associated with forward and backward gliding of the trochlea of the talus within the tibiofibular mortise, such that the center of rotation changes [24]. Also, the anteroposterior glide of the trochlea tali occurs to a greater extent on the lateral than the medial side (note that the lateral edge of the trochlea has a larger radius than the medial edge [Fig. 1.5A]), resulting in rotation of the talus in the horizontal plane of approximately 5–6° [5]. Normally, plantarflexion of the ankle is accompanied by internal rotation and dorsiflexion by external rotation of the talus within the tibiofibular mortise [18].

Barnett and Napier [2] described two axes of rotation. One exists when the ankle moves from neutral to plantarflexion and the other exists for motion from neutral to dorsiflexion. Close [5] observed that with dorsiflexion of the ankle, "the tibia rotates a few degrees medially about its long axis on the talus." Wyller [55] stated that the ankle behaves like a poorly mounted wheel and swerves slightly from side to side with dorsi- and plantarflexion.

Inman [19] has presented an excellent review and discussion of the literature on this subject in addition to a summary of his own findings relative to ankle motion. He observed that, although motion may not be exactly around a single axis, for practical purposes, ankle motion can be considered to be uniaxial in 80% of specimens; in the other 20%, the axis changes not more than 10° when viewed in the transverse plane. Inman concluded that, as an approximation, the axis can be considered to pass slightly distal to the tips of the medial and lateral malleoli. Thus, the axis is slightly oblique when viewed in the lateral and frontal projections with the lateral end of the axis more distal and posterior than the medial end (Fig. 2.6).

From the literature, it is clear that actual ankle motion combines dorsi- and plantarflexion with

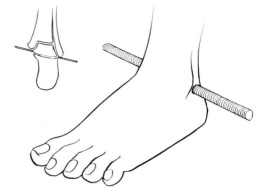

Fig. 2.6. The axis of the ankle joint can be approximated by a line drawn just distal to the tips of the medial and lateral malleoli.

slight internal and external rotation and some gliding of the talus on the tibia. However, the major components of ankle motion are dorsi- and plantarflexion; thus from a practical standpoint, the ankle can be considered to rotate approximately around a single oblique axis that passes slightly distal to the tips of the malleoli. Various ranges have been given for normal passive ankle motion; 15–20° dorsiflexion and 40–50° plantarflexion are considered average [1,-17,29]. Ankle motion occurring during normal gait has been reported to range from 14 to 35° [34,49,54].

Active Control of Ankle Motion

Active motion of the ankle is controlled by the motor units that cross the joint. There are no muscles or tendons that attach directly to the talus; therefore, all motor units acting on the talus do so indirectly through at least one of the tarsal joints.

In general, the functional strength of a motor unit is determined by the power of the muscle and the length of the lever arm from the muscle to the axis of rotation of the joint. The lever arm is a line which is constructed perpendicular to the long axis of the motor unit, intersecting the axis of rotation. From this, it is obvious that the most powerful motor unit acting upon the ankle is the tendo Achilles (Fig. 2.7A). It has the largest muscle mass and the longest lever arm. The posterior tibial tendon is a weak plan-

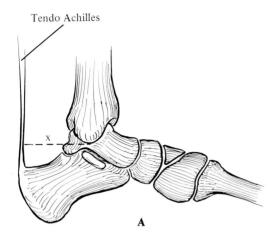

Tendo Achilles

A

Fig. 2.7. Plantar flexors of the ankle. The tendo Achilles has a long lever arm. The posterior tibial tendon, toe flexors and peroneal tendons have a short lever arm, since they cross the ankle joint near the axis of dorsi/plantarflexion.

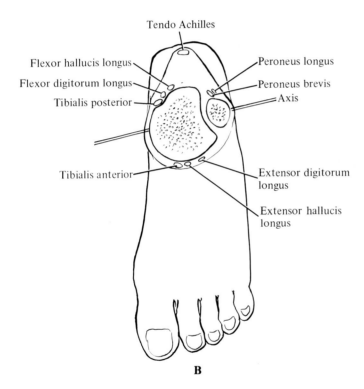

Tendo Achilles

Flexor hallucis longus

Flexor digitorum longus

Tibialis posterior

Peroneus longus

Peroneus brevis

Axis

Tibialis anterior

Extensor digitorum longus

Extensor hallucis longus

B

tarflexor, since it crosses the ankle joint near the axis of rotation, and thus has a short lever arm (Fig. 2.7B). The lever arms of the flexor digitorum longus and flexor hallucis longus are slightly longer; however, they insert much further distally than the posterior tibial tendon, and thus are not effective plantarflexors of the ankle either. A similar situation exists on the lateral side where the peroneal tendons cross the ankle close to the axis of rotation, and thus have minimal, if any, active effect on plantarflexion. Anteri-orly, the lever arms of the tibialis anterior, extensor hallucis longus, and extensor digitorum longus tendons are roughly comparable. The anterior tibialis, however, is the most effective dorsiflexor because it inserts closest to the talus. The long toe extensors cross all of the midfoot joints and insert distal to the metatarsophalangeal joints, and thus are not especially effective as dorsiflexors of the ankle. In pathologic conditions, resulting in weakness of the tibialis anterior, the long toe extensors will dorsiflex the ankle; this frequently results in clawing deformity of the toes.

Ankle Stability

Motion and stability are interconnected since both are determined, to a great extent, by the interrelationship of the individual bones and articular surfaces, as well as by the size, configuration, and orientation of the ligamentous structures.

With weight bearing, there is a certain degree of stability provided solely by the shapes of the articular surfaces. The generally concave shape of the tibial plafond, articulating with the convex body of the talus, provides some anteroposterior stability. This is enhanced posteriorly by the posterior malleolus, which extends further distally than does the anterior malleolus.

The mortise configuration of the distal tibia and fibula provides most of the medial-lateral and torsional stability. The tibiofibular mortise is oriented in an externally rotated position 15–20° relative to the axis of the knee and approximately 96° relative to the midline of the foot (Fig. 2.8) [20]. This is easy to appreciate clinically since the ankle axis of rotation passes approximately through the tips of the malleoli, and the lateral malleolus lies slightly posterior to the medial malleolus. This can also be demonstrated roentgenographically since, to obtain a true lateral view of the body of the talus, it is necessary to internally rotate the foot until the malleoli are superimposed [8].

When viewed from above, the medial and lateral articular facets of the talus appear to converge posteriorly. Measurements of the width of the trochlea tali, anteriorly and posteriorly, show a difference of 0–6 mm with the anterior dimension being the greater [2,19]. In less than 5% of cases, the sides are essentially parallel without significant wedging. This apparent narrowing of the posterior trochlea originally led to the idea that the ankle was rendered unstable in extreme plantarflexion, since the narrower posterior part of the talus occupied the wider mortise in this position. This concept, however, has been refuted. Actually, the malleoli closely approximate the sides of the talus in all positions throughout the normal range of motion [5,19]. If then, the

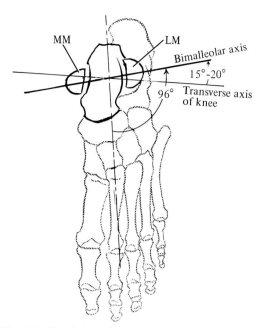

Fig. 2.8. The tibiofibular mortise is externally rotated 15–20° relative to the transverse axis of the knee and approximately 96° relative to the midline of the foot.

ankle joint is to be stable throughout the range of motion, there must either be widening and narrowing of the mortise with motion and/or a type of complex motion of the talus on the tibia, such that the width of the mortise remains appropriate throughout the physiologic range of ankle motion.

It has been demonstrated that, as dorsiflexion occurs, the malleoli separate up to 1.5 mm, in regular increments, and the lateral malleolus rotates externally as much as 5–6° [2,5]. The reverse occurs in plantarflexion. Barnett and Napier [2] did not find a good correlation between the degree of wedging of the trochlear surface of the talus and the mobility of the fibula. Inman described the trochlea as being a segment of a cone which confers stability to the ankle in all positions with a need for only minimal separation of the malleoli [19]. There is some controversy as to how much separation actually occurs with motion.

It has been shown that during gait the fibula moves proximally and distally [43,53]; this motion is associated with external rotation of the lateral malleolus and widening of the mortise. Clinically, it is difficult to measure accurately the relative motion of the two bones and a number of artifacts are introduced in cadaver studies. It is clear, however, that at least some motion does occur under normal circumstances.

The Tibiofibular Syndesmosis

In addition to ankle dorsiflexion [7,24,30,46], both weight bearing [7,26] and posterior translation of the talus [30] serve to wedge the distal or anterior trochlea into the mortise; these functions are similarly associated with proximal-lateral translation [3,30,51] as well as external rotation of the fibula with respect to the tibia [1, 4,5,48]. This motion is permitted and controlled by the tibiofibular ligaments which absorb stress and decelerate the talus during ordinary activities. This stress-absorbing mechanism is important to ankle function [5].

Although all four tibiofibular ligaments serve to prevent excessive lateral displacement of the fibula with resultant widening of the mortise, only the anterior inferior tibiofibular ligament is in a good position to limit external rotation of the fibula with respect to the tibia. The other tibiofibular ligaments are located too close to the vertical axis of rotation of the fibula to provide much, if any, constraint in this direction (Fig. 2.9). In cadaver studies, when the anterior inferior tibiofibular ligament alone is sectioned and the talus is rotated externally, the anterior tibiofibular interval can be increased approximately 4–10 mm, as the fibula rotates externally and translates posteriorly [31]. This occurs without any substantial increase in the intermalleolar distance [5]. Exaggerated external rotation of the fibula following loss of the anterior inferior tibiofibular ligament has been referred to clinically as "anterior diastasis" [13,33]. Progressive sectioning of the remaining tibiofibular ligaments permits further external rotation and posterior displacement of the fibula, but the greatest single increment results from division of the anterior inferior tibiofibular ligament [5].

Although the anterior and posterior inferior tibiofibular ligaments are consistently large and strong, the strength of the interosseous ligament varies considerably from person to person [33]. In certain patients the ligament is virtually nonexistent, and rupture or section of the anterior

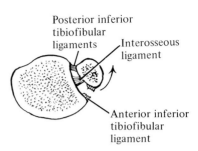

Fig. 2.9. All the tibiofibular ligaments serve to prevent lateral displacement of the distal fibula: The anterior inferior tibiofibular ligament is in the best position to control external rotation and posterior displacement of the fibula.

and posterior ligaments in these cases will render the tibiofibular mortise quite unstable.

Even when all of the tibiofibular ligaments have been sectioned, widening of the mortise beyond 2 mm is prevented by the intact deltoid ligament [5,12,18,23,48,57]. Therefore, both the deltoid and tibiofibular ligaments contribute to the integrity of the tibiofibular syndesmosis [39].

The Collateral Ligaments

Deltoid Ligament

The three superficial bands of the deltoid ligament are positioned primarily in the sagittal plane and are far removed from the longitudinal axis of the talus [5]. They are generally well suited to resist abduction of the talus [28], but are poorly positioned to prevent lateral displacement or external rotation of the talus in the horizontal plane (Fig. 2.10). Isolated section of one or all of the components of the superficial deltoid ligament, with all other structures intact, has little effect on ankle stability [37,39].

Resistance to lateral translation and external rotation of the talus is provided primarily by the deep deltoid ligament [24], whose anterior and posterior talotibial components travel relatively horizontally from the medial malleolus to the medial aspect of the talus (Fig. 2.10) [5,52]. Even so, experimental section of the deep fibers of the deltoid ligament will permit only minimal lateral talar displacement or talar external rota-

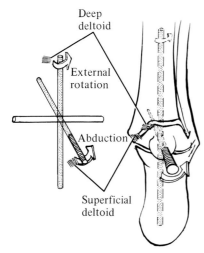

Fig. 2.10. The superficial fibers of the deltoid ligament are well situated to control abduction of the talus. The deep fibers of the deltoid ligament control external rotation of the talus.

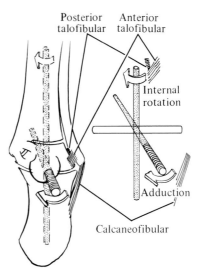

Fig. 2.11. The posterior talofibular and calcaneofibular ligaments control adduction of the talus and hindfoot. The anterior and posterior talofibular ligaments control internal rotation of the talus.

tion, provided the distal fibula and tibiofibular syndesmosis are intact [48,56].

Fibers of the superficial and deep deltoid ligament that lie anterior and posterior to the transverse axis of talar rotation are effective in limiting ankle plantarflexion and dorsiflexion, respectively [28,37].

Lateral Ligaments—Lateral Ligamentous Complex

The anterior talofibular ligament is taut in all ankle positions, but by virtue of its distal and medial course from the fibula to the talus, it is best suited to restrict internal rotation and plantarflexion of the ankle (Fig. 2.11) [38,42]. Anatomically, it is poorly situated to prevent adduction of the talus within the ankle mortise. The calcaneofibular ligament, on the other hand, courses posteriorly and distally from the fibula to the calcaneus. It bridges the extreme lateral aspect of the ankle and talocalcaneal joints [11]; in this position, it is sufficiently removed from the longitudinal axis of talar rotation that it effectively limits talar "tilt" or adduction (Fig. 2.11) [28]. This is especially true in maximal dorsiflexion when the ligament becomes very taut and pursues a near vertical course from the fibula to the calcaneus [11,38].

Although the large size of the posterior talofibular ligament suggests that it has an important role in ankle stability [52], little is known about its specific function [11]. Located behind the transverse axis of ankle motion, it seems to serve as a check to dorsiflexion of the ankle [11,28,38]. Also, the anterior fibers of this triangular structure are short and pursue a relatively horizontal course to the talus (Fig. 1.10); they are, therefore, well designed to restrict adduction, medial translation, and internal rotation of the talus within the mortise. This ligament provides a firm bond between the distal fibula and talus, such that these bones move together in the production and reduction of external rotation/abduction fractures of the lateral malleolus (Fig. 10.19) [21,-40,47].

Hamilton et al. [15], in the course of cadaver dissections of the lateral ligamentous complex, observed the following: Isolated section of the anterior talofibular ligament and adjacent anterolateral capsule permitted exaggerated plantarflexion/internal rotation of the talus within the ankle mortise. This permitted a modest degree of adduction tilt of the talus. Subsequent section of the calcaneofibular ligament resulted in significant adduction instability, and if the posterior talofibular ligament was also severed, gross instability or dislocation ensued. On the other hand, if the calcaneofibular and/or posterior talofibular ligaments were sectioned with the anterior talo-fibular ligament intact, only minimal talar instability could be demonstrated.

It appeared as though rupture or violation of the anterior talofibular ligament was necessary, but not sufficient, to produce significant adduction instability of the talus. The talus, when concentrically reduced within the tibiofibular mortise, was prevented from undergoing significant adduction tilt by the bony wall of the lateral malleolus. With excessive plantarflexion/internal rotation of the talus, as permitted by rupture of the anterior talofibular ligament, the lateral corner of the talus was able to subluxate anteriorly out of the mortise (Fig. 9.2). The talus was then only constrained by the calcaneofibular and posterior talofibular ligaments. When one or both of these ligaments were also violated, significant instability ensued.

It appears that the prime function of the anterior talofibular ligament is to limit internal rotation/plantarflexion of the talus within the ankle mortise. By maintaining the talus concentrically reduced within the mortise, maximal advantage of fibular restraint is realized.

Forces Across the Ankle

The actual forces across the ankle with ambulation have not been directly measured. On the basis of a mathematical model, Seirge and Arvikar [44] estimated the maximum force across the ankle to be 5.2 times the body weight. Stauffer et al. [49] performed a two-dimensional force analysis of the ankle. They found that the maximum compressive force across the ankle with gait was 4.5–5.5 times the body weight (mean, 4.73). Anteroposterior shear forces of the talus on the distal tibia varied with gait and were approximately 35% of body weight in the anterior direction and 70% of body weight in the posterior direction. Forces in the medial-lateral direction with gait have not yet been determined. With normal gait on level ground, such forces are probably less than body weight. However, on uneven ground or with turning, running, or other athletic activities, the forces probably are at least several times body weight.

Fibula

Normally, there is constant contact between the articular surfaces of the talus and the lateral malleolus during the entire range of ankle motion [25,32]. Although the exact configuration of the talofibular joint varies from person to person, the joint is always oriented obliquely (Fig. 2.12A). Forces generated between the distal fibula and the talus must be perpendicular to the joint surfaces, and therefore can be broken down into horizontal and vertical components. The forces acting in a horizontal direction relate to the buttressing effect of the fibula, and the forces operating in a vertical direction relate to the weight-bearing function of the fibula (Fig. 2.12B)

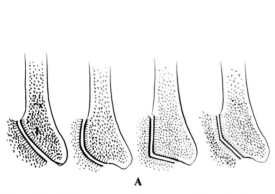

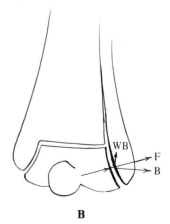

A   **B**

Fig. 2.12. A The exact configuration of the talofibular joint varies from individual to individual. **B** Forces acting across the talofibular joint can be analyzed in terms of vertical/weight-bearing (WB) and horizontal/buttressing (B) components.

[25]. As demonstrated by Lambert [25], the fibula is responsible for transmitting one-sixth of the static body weight across the ankle joint.

Distortion or displacement of the distal fibula, besides affecting the load carried through the talofibular joint, is liable to permit lateral translation or external rotation of the talus with respect to the distal tibial articular surface. Breitenfelder (1957) and Willenegger (1960) have shown that even minimal lateral rotation or displacement of the lateral malleolus significantly alters the contact area between the tibia and talus [50]. Ramsey and Hamilton [41] have demonstrated that as little as 1 mm of lateral talar shift can effect a 42% reduction of the tibiotalar contact surface. Such a disturbance may predispose to joint incongruity and eventual arthrosis.

References

1. American Medical Association: Guide to the Evaluation of Permanent Impairment. 1977.
2. Barnett CH, Napier JR: The axis of rotation at the ankle joint in man. Its influence upon the form of the talus and the morbidity of the fibula. J Anat 86:1, 1952.
3. Cave EF (ed): Fractures and Other Injuries. Chicago, Year Book Medical, 1958.
4. Cedell C-A: Ankle lesions. Acta Orthop Scand 46:425, 1975.
5. Close J: Some applications of the functional anatomy of the ankle joint. J Bone Joint Surg 38A:761, 1956.
6. Close JR, Inman VD: The Action of the Ankle Joint. Prosthetic Devices Research Project, Institute of Engineering Research, University of California, Berkeley. Advisory Committee on Artificial Limbs, National Research Council, Series II, Issue 22, 1952.
7. Dabezies E, D'Ambrosia RD, Shoji H: Classification and treatment of ankle fractures. Orthopaedics 1:365, 1978.
8. Dunn HK, Samuelson KM: Flat-top talus. A long-term report of 20 club feet. J Bone Joint Surg 56A:57, 1974.
9. Dupuytren BG: On the Injuries and Diseases of Bones. Translated by LeGros Clark. London, New Syndenham Society, 1847.
10. Ferreira AP, DeWet IS, Dommisse GF: Fractures and dislocations of the ankle joint. S Afr Med J 54:1095, 1978.
11. Fowler PJ: Ligamentous anatomy and physical examinations. Am J Sports Med 5:229, 1977.
12. Gaston SR, McLaughlin HL: Complex fracture of the lateral malleolus. J Trauma 1:69, 1961.
13. Golterman AFL: Diagnosis and treatment of tibiofibular diastasis. Arch Chir Neerl 16:185, 1964.
14. Goss CM: Anatomy of the Human Body by Henry Gray, 28th ed. Philadelphia, Lea & Febiger, 1966.
15. Hamilton WC, Good RP, Cotler JM: Personal communication.
16. Harvey JP Jr: Fractures of the ankle. A clinical survey of 181 cases. Clin Orthop 42:57, 1965.
17. Heck CV, Hendryson IE, Rowe CR: Joint Motion: Method of Measuring and Recording. Chicago American Academy of Orthopaedic Surgeons, 1965.
18. Hughes SPF: External rotational injury of the ankle joint with displacement of the talus. Ann Roy Coll Surg 59:61, 1977.
19. Inman VT: The Joints of the Ankle, 1st ed. Baltimore, Williams & Wilkins, 1976.
20. Isman RE, Inman VT: Anthropometric Studies of the Human Foot and Ankle. Biomechanics Laboratory, University of California, San Francisco and Berkeley. Technical Report 58. San Francisco, The Laboratory, 1968.
21. Jergesen F: Open reduction of fractures and dislocations of the ankle. Am J Surg 98:136, 1959.
22. Kleiger B: The mechanism of ankle injuries. J Bone Joint Surg 38A:59, 1956.
23. Kleiger B: Treatment of oblique fractures of the fibula. J Bone Joint Surg 43:969, 1961.
24. Kleiger B: Mechanisms of ankle injury. Orthop Clin North Am 5:127, 1974.
25. Lambert KL: The weight-bearing function of the fibula. A strain gauge study. J Bone Joint Surg 53A:507, 1971.
26. Lauge-Hansen N: Fractures of the ankle. II. Combined experimental-surgical and experimental-roentgenologic investigations. Arch Surg 60:957, 1950.
27. Lewis JL: The effect of ankle-injury forces. J Bone Joint Surg 46A:1380, 1964.
28. Magnusson R: On the late results in non-operated cases of malleolar fractures. Acta Chir Scand (Suppl) 84:1, 1944.
29. Mann RA: Biomechanics of the Foot. American Academy of Orthopaedic Surgeons, Atlas of Orthotics: Biomechanical Principles and Application. St. Louis, Mosby, 1975.
30. McLaughlin HL: Trauma. Philadelphia, Saunders, 1960.
31. Menelaus MB: Injuries of the anterior inferior tibio-fibular ligament. Aust NZ J Surg 30:279, 1960.
32. Mitchell WG, Shafton GW, Sclafani SJ: Mandatory open reduction. Its role in displaced ankle fractures. J Trauma 19:602, 1979.
33. Monk CJE: Injuries of the tibio-fibular ligaments. J Bone Joint Surg 51:330, 1969.
34. Murray MP, Drought AB, Kory RC: Walking patterns of normal men. J Bone Joint Surg 46A:335, 1964.
35. Pankovich AM: Fractures of the fibula proximal to the distal tibiofibular syndesmosis. J Bone Joint Surg 60A:221, 1978.
36. Pankovich, AM: Fractures of the fibula at the

distal tibio-fibular syndesmosis. Clin Orthop Rel Res 143:138, 1979.

37. Pankovich AM, Shivaram MS: Anatomical basis of variability in injuries of medial malleolus and the deltoid ligament. I. Anatomical studies. Acta Orthop Scand 50:217, 1979.

38. Percy EC, Hill RO, Callaghan JE: The "sprained" ankle. J Trauma 9:972, 1969.

39. Phillips RS, Balmer GA, Monk CJE: The external rotation fracture of the fibular malleolus. Br J Surg 56:55, 1969.

40. Platt H: Introduction to a discussion on fractures in the neighborhood of the ankle-joint. Lancet 1:33, 1926.

41. Ramsey P, Hamilton W: Changes in tibiotalar area of contact caused by lateral talar shift. J Bone Joint Surg 58A:356, 1976.

42. Robichon J, Desjardins P, Pegington J, Moonje VB: Functional anatomy of the ankle joint and its relationship to ankle injuries. J Bone Joint Surg 55B:662, 1973.

43. Scranton PE Jr, McMaster JG, Kelly E: Dynamic fibular function. A new concept. Clin Orthop 118:76, 1976.

44. Seirge A, Arvikar RJ: The prediction of muscular load sharing and joint forces in the lower extremities during walking. J Biomech 8:89, 1975.

45. Shephard E: Tarsal movements. J Bone Joint Surg 33B:258, 1951.

46. Smith MGH: Inferior tibio-fibular diastasis treated by cross screwing. J Bone Joint Surg 45B:737, 1963.

47. Speed JS, Boyd HB: Operative reconstruction of malunited fractures about the ankle. J Bone Joint Surg 18:270, 1936.

48. Staples OS: Ligamentous injuries of the ankle joint. Clin Orthop 42:21, 1965.

49. Stauffer RN, Chao EYS, Brewster RC: Force and motion analysis of the normal, diseased, and prosthetic ankle joint. Clin Orthop Rel Res 127:189, 1977.

50. Svend-Hansen H, Bremerskov U, Baekgaard N: Ankle fractures treated by fixation of medial malleolus alone. Late results in 29 patients. Acta Orthop Scand 49:211, 1978.

51. Vasli S: Operative treatment of ankle fractures. Acta Chir Scand (Suppl) 226:1, 1957.

52. Walsh WM, Hughston JC: Unstable ankle fractures in athletes. Am J Sports Med 4:173, 1976.

53. Weinert CR Jr, McMaster JH, Scranton PE Jr, Ferguson RJ: Human Fibular Dynamics in Foot Science. American Orthopaedic Foot Society. Philadelphia, Saunders, 1976.

54. Wright DG, Desai SM, Henderson WH: Action of the subtalar and ankle-joint complex during the stance phase of walking. J Bone Joint Surg 46A:361, 1964.

55. Wyller T: The axis of the ankle joint and its importance in subtalar arthrodesis. Acta Orthop Scand 33:320, 1963.

56. Yablon IG, Heller FG, Shouse L: The key role of the lateral malleolus in displaced fractures of the ankle. J Bone Joint Surg 59A:169, 1977.

57. Yadav SS: Ankle stability after resection of the distal third of the fibula for giant-cell lesions. Report of two cases. Clin Orthop 155:105, 1981.

Chapter 3   Surgical Anatomy

WILLIAM C. HAMILTON

In selecting the appropriate surgical approach to the ankle for treatment of fractures and ligamentous lesions, many important factors need to be taken into consideration, not the least of which is the nature and location of the injury or combination of injuries. The soft tissues about the ankle are relatively intolerant of excessive retraction, so that an improperly placed incision may jeopardize accurate repair and/or compromise the integrity of the skin and other important soft tissue structures [13].

As a general rule, straight incisions are less likely to be complicated by healing problems than curved incisions, since tension is more evenly distributed [3,10]. As always, skin incisions should not be placed directly over bony prominences where subcutaneous tissue is sparse, since formation of a painful scar is likely. A small skin incision frequently proves to be false economy [17,18].

Where multiple incisions are necessary, care should be taken to maintain an adequate bridge of intervening skin (7 cm or more) [20]. This can be difficult to judge when the skin is stretched due to swelling or deformity, and it is better, under these circumstances, to leave too large rather than too small a bridge of intact tissue.

Although considerable innovation is sometimes necessary due to peculiar injury combinations or local skin conditions, the more standard surgical approaches will be summarized here.

Anterolateral Approach

The skin incision begins over the anterolateral leg, approximately 2 in. proximal to the tibial plafond, and extends over the anterolateral aspect of the ankle toward the base of the fourth metatarsal (Fig. 3.1) [8]. Part or all of the incision may be employed. No cutaneous nerves are encountered if the incision is properly placed, but care should be taken not to damage, by retraction, the intermediate dorsal cutaneous branch of the superficial peroneal nerve, which lies in subcutaneous tissues of the medial flap.

The superior and inferior extensor retinacula are encountered in the proximal and distal one-third of the incision, respectively, and must be divided unless a very limited exposure will suffice. Proximally, the perforating branch of the peroneal artery can usually be spared, but the lateral malleolar artery is encountered directly over the ankle joint and usually must be sacrificed. Similarly, the lateral tarsal artery is encountered if dissection is carried out distal to the talonavicular joint.

By retracting the extensor tendons medially, the ankle joint capsule is easily identified and incised. If necessary, the extensor digitorum brevis can be re-

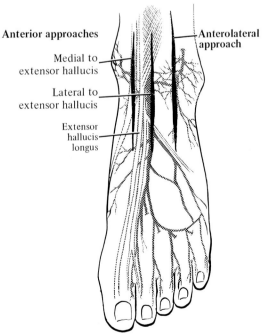

Fig. 3.1. Anterior and anterolateral approaches to the ankle.

flected from its origin on the calcaneus. With distal dissection, the subtalar, talonavicular, calcaneocuboid, and lateral metatarsal joints can be exposed through this incision.

This approach in its entirety provides excellent visualization of the anterior tibiofibular syndesmosis and the tibiotalar joint as well as the articular surface of the talus for fixation of fractures of the talar dome and neck or for excision of the talus. The middle one-third of the incision usually suffices to remove osteocartilaginous loose bodies from the ankle joint. This approach does not provide for easy access to the medial tibiotalar space and is, therefore, not especially well-suited for ankle arthrodesis.

Anterior Approaches

The ankle can be approached anteriorly either lateral or medial to the extensor hallucis longus tendon (Fig. 3.1). Both alternatives provide visualization of the entire anterior ankle.

Anterior Approach Lateral to the Extensor Hallucis Longus—Between the Extensor Digitorum Longus and Extensor Hallucis Longus

An anterior longitudinal incision is placed midway between the malleoli with care to protect the medial dorsal cutaneous branch of the superficial peroneal nerve. The superior and inferior extensor retinacula are incised in line with the skin incision, directly over the dorsalis pedis artery. After identifying, ligating, and dividing the lateral malleolar and lateral tarsal branches, the dorsalis pedis artery and accompanying deep peroneal nerve can be retracted medially with the extensor hallucis longus tendon. The extensor digitorum longus tendon is retracted laterally to expose the anterior capsule of the ankle joint [5].

Anterior Approach Medial to the Extensor Hallucis Longus—Between the Extensor Hallucis Longus and Anterior Tibial Tendon

The skin and extensor retinaculum are divided over the interval between the extensor hallucis longus and the anterior tibial tendons. After ligating and dividing the medial malleolar artery, the neurovascular bundle

is retracted laterally with the extensor hallucis longus tendon, and the anterior tibial tendon is retracted medially, exposing the ankle capsule. The medial tarsal artery originates further distally than the lateral tarsal artery, and therefore can be spared in all but the most extensive exposures in this area. Exposure is comparable to that obtained through the interval lateral to the extensor hallucis longus with the added advantage that the vascular supply is less disturbed [21].

Medial Approaches

Medial approaches (Fig. 3.2) are usually employed for injuries of the medial malleolus or deltoid ligament, although certain posterior tibial lip fractures are best approached from the medial side. Although transverse approaches have been described [25], longitudinal incisions are preferred, since they permit more extensive exposure.

Generally, an anteromedial incision is preferred for fixation of medial malleolar fractures since this approach permits optimal visualization of the tibial plafond–medial malleolus articular surface (mortise angle) [13,14,20]. On the other hand, exposure of the deep deltoid ligament requires a posteromedial approach with mobilization of the flexor tendons [14,20].

Anteromedial Approach

A "J"-shaped incision is begun 2 in. proximal to the tibial plafond, extended anterior to the medial malleolus, and then curved distally and posteriorly to end

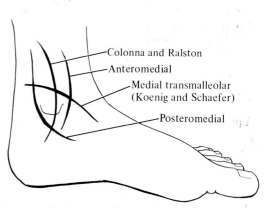

Fig. 3.2. Medial approaches to the ankle.

just below the tip of the malleolus. Care should be taken to avoid damaging the posterior tibial tendon which can be surprisingly superficial below the tip of the medial malleolus. The saphenous vein and terminal branches of the saphenous nerve should be avoided in the anterior limb of the exposure [2,14,19].

The medial tibiotalar space is well visualized with this approach, and fractures of the medial malleolus can be held reduced with the articular surface under direct vision as screws are inserted from the tip of the malleolus, through a small vertical incision in the calcaneotibial portion of the superficial deltoid ligament. Direct visualization of the joint surface improves perception and makes joint violation by screws or wires less likely.

Posteromedial Approach (Medial Inferior Approach)

A posterior "J"-shaped incision is centered behind the medial malleolus and extended distally to just beyond the tip of the malleolus. After division of the laciniate ligament, the posterior tibial tendon is mobilized and retracted anteriorly, exposing the deep deltoid ligament [4,14]. If necessary to facilitate exposure, the flexor digitorum longus tendon can also be mobilized and retracted anteriorly [1,9,20,22].

Broomhead has described a similar incision to approach the posterior lip of the tibia [1]. For this purpose, however, the vertical limb of the incision should be placed further posteriorly, midway between the posterior border of the tibia and the tendo Achilles. The posterior tibial and flexor tendons as well as the neurovascular bundle are retracted posteriorly and medially to expose the back of the distal tibia and ankle joint.

Colonna and Ralston described an approach for reduction of medial and/or posterior malleolar fractures that employs a medial incision gently curved with the apex anteriorly [5]. In order to expose the posterior malleolus, the posterior tibial and flexor digitorum longus tendons are mobilized anteriorly, while the neurovascular bundle and flexor hallucis longus are retracted posteriorly and laterally.

Medial Transmalleolar Approach

This approach was initially described in association with osteotomy of the medial malleolus [16]. The incision is relatively transverse just above the medial malleolus and curved slightly, convex proximally. Osteotomy of the medial malleolus is rarely indicated to expose the posterotibial margin, but occasionally, with large basal medial malleolar fractures, the malleolar fragment can be reflected distally to expose the tibial articular surface from front to back [16,18,23].

Lateral Approaches

Lateral approaches (Fig. 3.3) are generally utilized for tibiofibular ligament injuries or fractures of the lateral malleolus or anterolateral tibial lip.

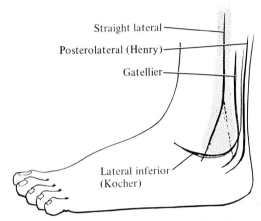

Fig. 3.3. Lateral approaches to the ankle region.

Straight Lateral Approach

A straight lateral incision (Fig. 3.3) is ideally suited for fractures of the distal fibula [3,18,19,25]. In its distal extent, however, it should be curved gently anteriorly [18] or posteriorly [9] to facilitate exposure of the fibular borders and simultaneously avoid placing the scar directly over the prominent malleolus. The proximal straight limb of the incision is situated posterior to the extensor structures and anterior to the peroneal tendons, lesser saphenous vein, and sural nerve. Therefore, the incision can be made direct to the bone with a minimum of soft tissue dissection. Occasionally, it is advisable to move the upper longitudinal limb of the incision anteriorly [14] or posteriorly [9] to the fibular border. The distal fibula once exposed can be stripped subperiosteally on its anterior, posterior, and lateral surfaces as far distally as the lateral malleolus. Medially, the dissection is limited if the interosseous membrane and interosseous ligament are intact; these structures should be carefully preserved. Distally, at the level of the lateral malleolus, stripping becomes difficult at the insertion of the anterior and posterior inferior tibiofibular ligaments, but the interval between these structures and the overlying tissue can be easily identified and developed.

Posterolateral (Henry) Approach

The posterolateral (Henry) approach provides access to the posterior border of the tibia as well as the distal fibula (Fig. 3.3) [12]. It is especially well suited for fractures of the posterolateral tibial lip associated with fractures of the lateral malleolus [7,14,20,24,25]. Henry emphasized that the lateral edge of the Achilles tendon is free of soleus fibers, and therefore medial mobilization of the tendon is less traumatic than lateral retraction.

The patient should be positioned prone with the foot in plantarflexion. The skin incision is placed at the outer edge of the Achilles tendon, posterior to the sural nerve and short saphenous vein, and extends distally below the lateral malleolus. The flexor hallucis longus muscle is stripped from its origin on the fibula and retracted medially. The distal tibia and tibiofibular syndesmosis are approached between the flexor hallucis longus and distal fibula through what Henry described as the "strategic interval" (Fig. 3.4).

Lateral Inferior (Kocher) Approach

The skin incision extends from the head-neck of the talus posteriorly in a gentle curve under the lateral malleolus, paralleling the peroneal tendons for a variable distance proximally (Fig. 3.3) [15]. The sural nerve and lesser saphenous vein lie posterior to the incision. The intermediate dorsal cutaneous branch of the peroneal nerve crosses the anterior extent of the incision and should be handled carefully. This approach affords excellent visualization of the anterior talofibular ligament and anterolateral capsule. By incising the inferior peroneal retinaculum, the peroneal tendons can be mobilized to expose the entire calcaneofibular ligament [14].

Transfibular (Gatellier) Approach

The skin incision is placed along the posterior border of the fibula and extends distally and anteriorly under the lateral malleolus (Figs. 3.3 and 3.5) [6,11,23]. The peroneal tendons are carefully mobilized and retracted anteriorly. This necessitates detachment of the lowest

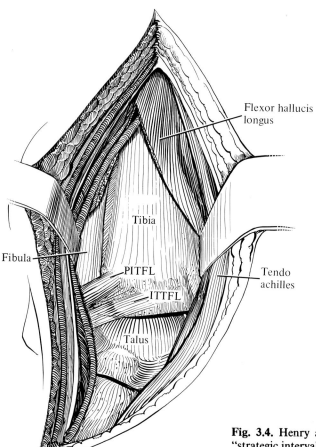

Fig. 3.4. Henry approach to the posterior ankle through the "strategic interval" between the flexor hallucis longus and distal fibula.

fibers of the peroneus brevis from the fibula. The fracture line of the fibula is used for dissecting the fibula from the tibia, by sectioning the tibiofibular ligaments. The distal fibular fragment is then easily mobilized, being attached only by the three fasciculi of the lateral collateral ligament distally (Fig. 3.5). This exposure provides excellent visualization of the posterior and lateral aspects of the distal tibia. At the completion of the procedure, the fibular fracture is reduced and fixed; frequently, a distal tibiofibular transfixion screw is required to stabilize the syndesmosis.

This approach is well suited for ankle arthrodesis and also for internal fixation of posterior malleolar lip fractures, where the tibiofibular ligaments have already been ruptured as part of the injury complex. Intentional violation of these ligaments should be avoided if at all possible.

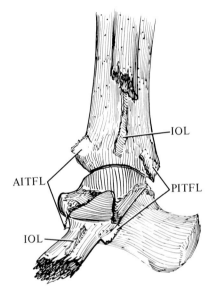

Fig. 3.5. Lateral transmalleolar (Gatellier) approach.

Posterior Approaches

Exploration and repair of the tendo Achilles or posterior tibial margin is best accomplished through the posterolateral incision of Henry, described above. Straight posterior approaches to the ankle joint via Achilles tenotomy (Picot) [11,21] or osteotomy of the calcaneus (Alglave) [11] are rarely indicated, except possibly for difficult reconstructive procedures.

References

1. Broomhead R: Discussion on fractures in the region of ankle-joint. Proc Roy Soc Med 25:1082, 1932.
2. Burgess E: Fractures of the ankle, J Bone Joint Surg 26:721, 1944.
3. Burwell HN, Charnley AD: Treatment of displaced fractures at the ankle by rigid internal fixation and early joint movement. J Bone Joint Surg 47B:634, 1965.
4. Close R: Some application of the functional anatomy of the ankle joint. J Bone Joint Surg 38A:761, 1956.
5. Colonna PC, Ralston EL: Operative approaches to the ankle joint. Am J Surg 82:44, 1951.
6. Coonrad RW: Fracture-dislocations of the ankle joint with impaction injury of the lateral weight-bearing surface of the tibia. J Bone Joint Surg 52A:1337, 1970.
7. Cox FJ, Laxson WW: Fractures about the ankle joint. Am J Surg 83:674, 1952.
8. Crenshaw AH: Campbell's Operative Orthopaedics, 5th ed. St. Louis, Mosby, 1971.
9. Dabezies E, D'Ambrosia RD, Shoji H: Classification and treatment of ankle fractures. Orthopedics 1:365, 1978.
10. Denham RA: Internal fixation for unstable ankle fractures. J Bone Joint Surg 46B:206, 1964.
11. Gatellier J: The juxtaretroperoneal route in the operative treatment of fractures of the malleolus with posterior marginal fragment. Surg Gynecol Obstet 52:67, 1931.
12. Henry AK: Extensile Exposure. Edinburgh, Churchill Livingstone, 1973.
13. Hughes J: The medial malleolus in ankle fractures. Orthop Clin North Am 11:649, 1980.
14. Jergeson F: Open reduction of fractures and dislocations of the ankle. Am J Surg 98:136, 1959.
15. Kocher T: Textbook of Operative Surgery, 3rd ed. London, Adam and Charles Black, 1911.
16. König F, Schäfer P: Osteoplastic surgical exposures of the ankle joint. Dtsch Z Chir 215:196, 1929.
17. Lane WA: Method of procedure in operations on simple fractures. Br Med J 4:1452, 1912.
18. McLaughlin HL, Ryder CT Jr: Open reduction and internal fixation for fractures of the tibia and ankle. Surg Clin North Am 29:1523, 1949.
19. Mitchell WG, Shafton GW, Sclafani JA: Mandatory open reduction. Its role in displaced ankle fractures. J Trauma 19:602, 1979.
20. Müller ME, Allgöwer M, Schneider R, Willenegger H: Manual of Internal Fixation. New York, Springer-Verlag, 1979.
21. Nicola T: Atlas of Surgical Approaches to Bones and Joints. New York, Macmillan, 1945.
22. Nyström G: The contribution to the treatment of fractures of the posterior border of the tibia by malleolar fractures. Acta Radiol 25:672, 1944.
23. Patrick J: Direct approach to trimalleolar fractures. J Bone Joint Surg 47B:236, 1965.
24. Solonen KA, Lauttamus L: Operative treatment of ankle fractures. Acta Orthop Scand 39:223, 1968.
25. Wade PA, Lance EM: The operative treatment of fracture-dislocation of the ankle joint. Clin Orthop Rel Res 42:37, 1965.

Chapter 4   Radiography of the Ankle

J. DAVID HOFFMAN

One cannot properly separate the issues of patient presentation, clinical history, mechanism of injury, and positive physical findings from the more technical imperatives of radiologic technique. The actual image is valuable when its salient features are perceived by the observer, and this is only possible after appropriate clinical evaluation. The perception of diagnostic information from these images, in conjunction with integration of other information, should help the practitioner to arrive at a decision concerning the patient's management.

Radiographs often give a false sense of security, and there are many compelling reasons for being wary. For example, rotational deformities are often missed because of failure to appreciate the three dimensions. The many borderlands of normal, variants, artifacts, Mach bands, and optical illusions abound and must be recognized as such [35,37,46,58,83]. Shadows comprising the bone and soft tissues capriciously conspire to distort, conceal, and mystify. It is an unfortunate truth that our very sensitive advanced imaging technology often deceives and misleads; one must be on guard so as not to be "disadvantaged" by technologic advancement [78].

One must also be skeptical and critical so as not to be trapped into responding impetuously—impelled by the seemingly abnormal criterion or criteria. Overresponse to X-ray disclosures exclusively and alone is a pitfall to be avoided. The clinical picture must support the radiographic conclusion, and vice versa. A scrupulously careful and exhaustive search must continue, so as to avoid the wrong response. This may include comparative radiographs, stress and strain films under anesthesia, and/or arthrography [8,13,14,15].

Moreover, one must be alert to the fact that because of spontaneous repositioning of joint dissociations and their attendant fractures, a "normal" radiographic appearance following acute and severe traumatic dislocation can be a commonplace manifestation. The fracture and dislocation dynamically self-correct, or are reduced by some proper emergency splinting or other fortuitous positioning. It is obvious that such repositioning is deceptive, but it is certainly not a fortunate correction if the injury remains undetected and is improperly treated. In such situations, critical analysis and intuition are crucial: priority for a high index of suspicion is paramount in these occult cases.

It is also important to remember that the detection of ankle injury requires a careful determination of all parameters of concern. This may extend both above and below the ankle joint, to include the proximal knee joint and the long bones of the lower extremity. Both clinical and radiographic study must proceed along the entire length of the extremity from the knee and tibiofibular joint above, to those articulations below the ankle, including the hindfoot and its "supinator line" [25,32].

Before discussing the views per se and what they may reveal, it is essential to emphasize that properly positioned, projected, exposed, and processed screen films be obtained in the first place. Properly positioned, well-defined projections are crucial. Whenever a simultaneous examination of the opposite, uninjured extremity is involved, it must be obtained in "exactly accordant projections" [10,24]. The production of a radiograph with optimal detail takes into account many factors, beginning with screen films and consideration of subject and film density, plus contrast techniques. A simplified and lucid discussion of these technical imaging considerations can be obtained by referring to Pennocks's "Radiologic Interpretation of Bone" [154]. No known modification or sophistication of viewing conditions can possibly help when using underexposed films. It is equally important that the radiographic films, when obtained, be viewed in a manner most conducive to revelation of that which is contained. Variable luminance from the viewbox and high intensity illumination systems, plus a magnifier and acute angle approaches to the projecting image, are essentials [35].

Routine Projections

Discussions as to what constitutes routine radiographic projections, as well as the techniques employed, vary considerably from text to text. It is interesting to note how little standardization or agreement there is on just how to best obtain even the most routine of views.

All authorities will agree, however, that the ankle joint must be projected according to what is being sought in the way of general and specific information. The differing anterior or frontal positionings must take into account the amount of external and internal tibial torsion and the position of the fibula relative to the tibia, which usually varies from case to case and even from one ankle to the other in the same individual.

Immediate and overriding problems of the patient's intense pain, the acuteness and fragility of the parts and their associated lesions, plus the encumbrances of potentially bulky and partially opacifying splints, are some of the variables, and these become the complicating issues in positioning, projection, and imaging. The positioning of parts, the distances between the object and the X-ray source, and projections of the central ray, with its angles of inclination, are most obviously some of the important variables.

The anatomic planes of the projected surfaces and the plane of the X-ray beam are always contingent upon one another. The projecting central X ray and the inclination of the beam at straight and oblique angles, with centering to a particular part, will change appearances dramatically. Sometimes the obscure and occult become obvious by a relatively minimal maneuvering of the anatomy and the X-ray relative to one another. It cannot be overemphasized that positioning techniques can act as a source of both discovery and occlusion [10,52,57,62,85,94,97,136,160].

The Standard Anterioposterior View

The ankle is vertical or at right angles to the central X-ray beam for this particular evaluation of the mortise (Fig. 4.1). The lateral border of the foot, or the fifth metatarsal, lies perpendicular to the table. The ankle at all times is flexed enough and the foot is pronated enough to place its long axis in the vertical position relative to the X-ray and screen. Some elevation of the foot and dorsiflexion, with maximal pronation, have been recommended [85]. But, the degree of plantar- or dorsiflexion of the ankle does not appear to matter much, provided the leg is not allowed to rotate in or out. Most projections of the ankle in the anteroposterior (AP) plane allow that the sole of the foot will be at right angles to the leg and to the plate.

Attention to the articulating relationships between the trochlea of the talus and the tibial plafond is preeminent. This projection is essential for careful discovery of the congruence, or lack thereof, between the superior weight-bearing surface of the talus and the horizontal plate of the distal tibia. The complex juxtaposed concavoconvex talar and tibial surfaces are expected to be perfectly congruent in this particular frontal view. The slightest incongruence should be scrutinized, and the reasons sought.

The medial space between the tibial malleolus and the talus is of paramount importance and may be the only clue to deltoid ligament attenuation and rupture. This space can be initially discriminated in the standard AP view, and more particularly in the mortise view to be discussed below. There is some dispute as to what this space should normally be and what it represents when thought to be abnormally large. The space, when properly projected, is most usually nearly equal to the space above—that between the tibial plafond and the trochlea of the talus [94]. In general, the space between the lateral border of the medial malleolus and the medial border of the talus very seldom properly exceeds 3 mm. Any measurement of more than 3 mm is considered presumptive evidence of deltoid disruption.

▷

Fig. 4.4. Internal oblique view (45°). Since the bimalleolar axis is externally rotated approximately 20° in the neutral projection, the 45° internal rotation view is performed by placing the bimalleolar axis into 25° of internal rotation.

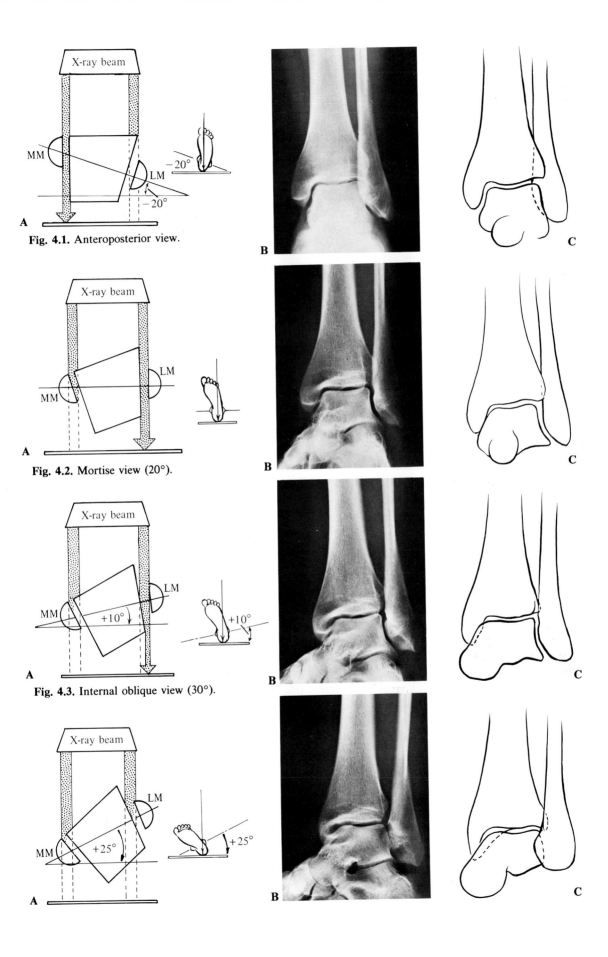

Fig. 4.1. Anteroposterior view.

Fig. 4.2. Mortise view (20°).

Fig. 4.3. Internal oblique view (30°).

Measurements exceeding 4 mm must be considered indicative of a serious breach in the integrity of the deltoid ligament [48,94].

In the straight AP radiograph, since the malleoli are not parallel to each other, the mortise is in part always obscured. The important relationships between the talus and the tibia and the tibia and fibula cannot all be assessed optimally in this projection. This is due to natural overlap of projecting bony opacities [52]. The distal overlapping of the usually contiguous tibia and fibula almost invariably disallows any observation of the so-called syndesmotic clear space. When the great toe is perpendicular to the plane of the table top and to the plain film or intensifying screen, the ankle joint will automatically project an image in a slightly externally rotated plane in the routine AP view.

Best clarification of the medial, lateral, and superior spaces in an AP projection of the tibiotalar joint and mortise, usually requires further internal rotation. However it is impossible to critically examine the lateral and medial clear spaces simultaneously in any single projection. In such situations, combined imaging techniques and special views become imperative. The search must then proceed to other views, seeking more supportive evidence, for or against disorder.

The Mortise View

The so-called mortise view (Fig. 4.2) cannot be properly achieved in every case by resorting to any set recipe of rotations, and never by utilizing an empiric and doctrinaire angle of internal rotation of the leg, ankle, and foot. As previously discussed, the medial joint space and the distal tibiofibular joint syndesmosis can only be best appreciated in a somewhat internally rotated projection of the ankle. In this projection, the mortise is more completely visualized and the distal tibiofibular joint is opened [61]. Usually 15–20° of internal rotation will allow the malleoli to parallel the table top and film, thus providing a mortise view [52].

In order to obtain a mortise view, the patient remains in the supine position previously employed in the standard AP view. The back of the heel remains in contact with the film. The ankle is supported in flexion, and the limb is rotated medially until the medial and lateral malleoli are equidistant from the film. In this position, the axis of the fourth metatarsal shaft is, in general, at right angles to the film [109]. The tube should be centered straight, 1 cm proximal to the tip of the medial malleolus, or 2 cm proximal to the tip of the lateral malleolus.

Obviously, overt fractures of the medial and lateral malleolus are usually, but not invariably, projected in the frontal AP and mortise views. In both of these views, the lateral malleolus is in some 15° of valgus normally, and if not rotated and displaced by fracture, it is concave on its lateral surface at the level of the ankle joint [9]. The articular surface of the medial malleolus normally projects in a varus direction relative to the long axis of the tibial shaft. The mortise view "places the medial articular surface of the talus tangent to the X-ray beam, and the short concave line representing the posteromedial surface of the talus falls slightly lateral to the medial articular surface [133]." This position also assures that the clear space between the fibula and talus can be properly visualized simultaneously with the other spaces. The more subtle aspects of the study of the lateral fibulotalar joint have been discussed by Bolin [10]. In addition, limb rotation must be sufficient enough to minimize the usual overshadowing of the tibiofibular joint. At times, the overshadowing can be more completely eliminated due to an excessively shallow tibiofibular groove [8,10,23,24,85].

In the mortise view, as in the standard AP view, a careful scrutiny for small flakes of bone may be rewarded; these are indicative of important ligamentous avulsions. At times, subtle fractures of the incisura fibularis, representing the third fragment of Tillaux, may be projected. As an evident fracture, however, its position and size can be even better confirmed by oblique projections at greater angles of internal and external rotation.

The Oblique View

Transverse and oblique malleolar fractures and their relative positions usually should be revealed in the AP and mortise views; however, best discernment of malleolar fractures rests upon oblique views [61,89], and these must always be included in proper projectioning of ankle injuries. The oblique views are obtained with the patient supine, usually at angles of 45° in both internal and external rotation. Internally rotated projections are usually the more useful [89]. (Fig. 4.4)

With the patient recumbent, the ipsilateral hip is supported and lifted enough to assist the leg and foot in internal posturing. The leg and foot are rotated medially, as a unit, to 45°, in order to accomplish the internally rotated oblique view. When the ankle is the subject of study, the foot is dorsiflexed to a neutral position so as to avoid superimposition of the calcaneus and the lateral malleolus. The central ray is directed to the midpoint of the ankle, perpendicular and exactly halfway between the tips of the medial and lateral malleoli.

This view will reveal the lateral side of the mortise, and especially the tibiofibular syndesmosis and the talofibular joint. The distal ends of the tibia and fibula, and especially the lateral malleolus, are also well projected in this view. Plantar- and dorsiflexion of the foot relative to the ankle predict whether the talus and talocalcaneal articulation are represented.

In internal oblique views encompassing the calcaneus and talus, one can see to better advantage the neck of the talus, the posterior subtalar joint, and the sustentaculum tali. These are complemented by lateral views, to be described below.

A 30° internally rotated oblique (Fig. 4.3), or bimalleolar, view is the recommended posturing for best visualization of the lateral joint space and the syndesmosis. This is an especially important dimension of examination, especially when the talus reveals itself to have subluxated laterally in other frontal views. When there is an isolated fibular fracture due to supination and outward rotation injury, the precise fit of the distal tibia and the articular facet of the talus may be vitiated as the result of outward-, proximal-, and dorsal-directed movement of the distal fibular fragment. It subtly, but importantly, opens up the lateral clear space and widens the mortise sufficiently to invite the talus to escape (Fig. 4.5). At the same time, this results in an increase in the medial clear space, which might be misinterpreted as a deltoid ligament tear [23].

According to Berridge and Bonnin [8], exactly comparable films taken in 30° of internal rotation should be obtained in doubtful cases, where one suspects a tibiofibular diastasis. They recommend other studies in addition, including external rota-

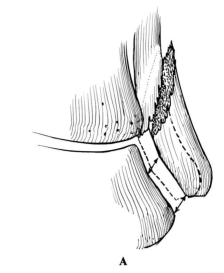

A

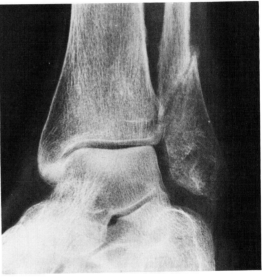

B

Fig. 4.5. Illustration (**A**) and radiograph (**B**) of a displaced lateral malleolar fracture "inviting" the talus to escape laterally.

tion and dorsiflexion stress, to further attempt to force open the joint in diastasis. Lauge-Hansen [85] considers any measurements in this area as giving unreliable results in regard to the width of the syndesmotic space. Bolin [10] has concluded that no matter how the so-called clear space or "la ligne claire" is projected, it can never be projected free under normal circumstances, since there are neither flat nor parallel areas between the overlapping surfaces [23,24].

External oblique films (Fig. 4.6), usually projected at 45–55°, are used to identify subtle frac-

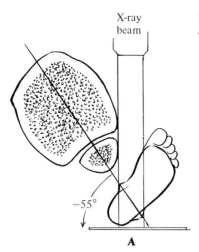

X-ray
beam

−55°

A

Fig. 4.6. External oblique view—taken with the limb externally rotated 45–55°.

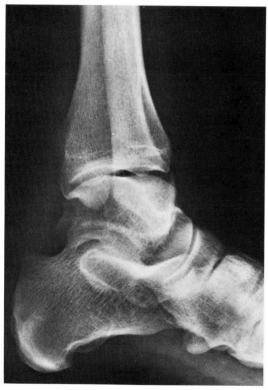

B

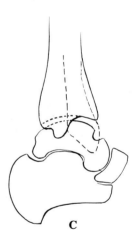

C

tures of the distal articulating surfaces of the tibia, the anterior syndesmotic area, and the posterior tibial lip. They are always adjunctive to the standard AP and mortise views, and to the lateral views described below. In the analysis of isolated rupture of the anterior tibiofibular ligament, which is a rare lesion, it is important to recognize fractures at the syndesmosis when they exist. Anterior syndesmotic fractures are usually

obscured unless the ankle is projected at 55° of external rotation of the leg (Fig. 10.5C) [23].

The Lateral View

Since the congruent positioning of the talus relative to the tibia is as crucial as its AP congruence, lateral projections are essential elements of the

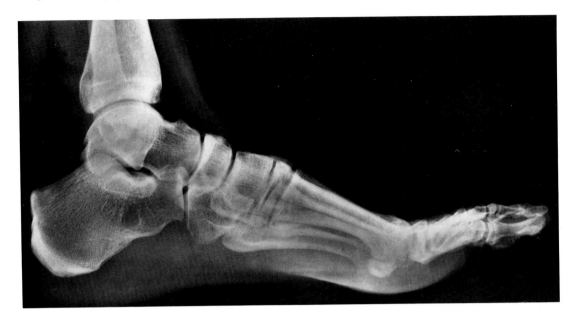

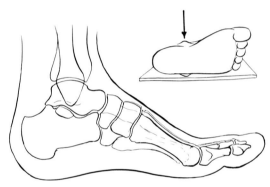

Fig. 4.7. True lateral view.

ankle study (Fig. 4.7). The lateral projection can be obtained with either the medial or lateral malleolus against the cassette. It is believed that the projected image is better with the medial malleolus in contact with the film holder. Exact positioning is believed to be easier since this is the flat side of the foot and ankle, and the joint per se is closer to the film [105]. Obviously, this may not be possible in the presence of acute injury.

In either of the foregoing positions, it is essential that the axis of the malleoli be perpendicular to the cassette. The malleoli must be superimposed upon each other, and this projection should include the entire os calcis and the bones of the midfoot, including the base of the fifth metatarsal [61]. The central ray is projected perpendicular to the medial malleolus, with the foot in neutral position. The X-ray tube should be centered straight, 2 cm above the tip of the lateral malleolus (lateromedial position), or 1 cm above the tip of the medial malleolus (mediolateral position). It is important to place the medial and lateral margins of the trochlea tali in coincidence in order to maintain a congruent surface projection that is parallel to the distal articular surface of the tibia [9]. Obviously, internal or external rotation will distort the projected tibiotalar articulation.

The lateral projection is important for discovery of the respective congruence of the distal talus and tibia—and also for discovery of the integrity of the anterior and posterior malleolar buttress. If the styloid processes of the medial and lateral malleoli are superimposed, the contiguous surfaces of the dome of the talus and the distal tibia should be smooth and symmetric. Any anterior or posterior irregularity, and any subluxation or dislocation of the talus in relation to the tibial plafond, should be appreciated.

The lateral projection usually reveals the anterior tibia and its entire anterior lip. The shadow of the dorsal distal part of the tibia is seen dorsal to the posterior contour of the fibula. The distal fibula and the lateral malleolus are seen distinctly on well-exposed films in spite of the fact that they are obscured by other bone: the anterior contour of the lateral malleolus lies somewhat in front of the anterior contour of the distal end of the fibula. This fact plays a significant role in appreciation of the oblique spiral fracture of the lateral malleolus. Frequently, this lesion will be represented by posterior displacement of the lateral malleolus with respect to the fibula on the lateral projection, despite relatively normal frontal views. If the entire fibula is projected posterior to the tibia in a true lateral projection, then a dislocation of the fibula (Bosworth lesion) must exist (Figs. 4.14 and 4.15) [11,42,95,98,-107,136] (See Chapter 6).

In the normal foot and ankle, both the calcaneus and talus should be well seen in the lateral projection. The neck of the talus should be critically scrutinized in this projection [20,21]. A relatively nondisplaced fracture of the neck of the talus is not at all rare [88,126]. In addition, the lateral view allows the best discrimination of the os trigonum [70].

The subtalar joints can be appreciated as to the posterior and anterior facets in the routine lateral projection [105]. Care should be taken so as not to overlook a subtalar dislocation; the observer often fails to see this obvious dissociation—his attention riveted elsewhere [82, 134,170].

Although the lateral projection invariably reveals the posterior lip of the tibia, it may fail to reveal the full extent of a nondisplaced or minimally displaced fracture, even if it is of considerable size. Fractures of the distal fibula and posterior aspect of the tibia tend to obfuscate each other. Fractures of the posterior and anterior colliculus of the medial malleolus may coexist with slices of bone from the adjacent posteromedial surface of the tibia (Fig. 13.2). In order to differentiate them and to discriminate between fracture lines of the fibula, posterior tubercle, and posterior colliculus, specialized lateral views and lateral tomography may be necessary.

Hendelberg [62] has discussed the problem of projecting fractures involving the posterior lip of the tibia and the posterior aspect of the tibia. He recommends that the foot should be rotated so that the posterior aspect of the fibula and the posterior margin of the tibia coincide exactly. The goal of obtaining the plane of the fracture coincident to the plane of the X-ray and vice versa may be better achieved in this way. This "poor lateral" view is obtained with the ankle and foot in slight external rotation (Fig. 4.8) [97]. The X-ray beam should be directed laterally and slightly from the back. In addition to offering other subtle guidelines for discriminating these often occult lesions, Hendelberg [62] discusses their appearance in frontal views; thus vital clues are offered as to the shape and size of posterior tibial fractures. Described in AP and mortise views are typical inverted U- and V-shaped opacities peculiar to fractures of the posterior tibial lip (Fig. 4.9). Furthermore, this type of fracture may be better observed in external oblique projections of 45–55° [61].

A superior inferior oblique lateral view (Fig. 4.10) has also been described, wherein the extremity is placed with the lateral aspect of the ankle against the cassette. The central ray is directed to the ankle, with the tube tilted 25–30° cephalad and 5° dorsally, along with a decrease in the focus distance to 30–40 cm [105]. This projection is virtually identical to the oblique lateral views illustrated by Lauge-Hansen [85]. This view is frequently required to differentiate an oblique spiral fracture of the distal end of the fibula from a fracture of the dorsal part of the tibia, which often runs parallel with the former, causing occlusion in standard lateral projections. This projection also demonstrates well the sinus tarsi as well as the middle and posterior facets of the subtalar joint.

The Oblique Dorsiplantar View

The oblique dorsiplantar view (lateromedial oblique projection; Feist-Mankin position) [105] of the foot (Fig. 4.11) is taken with the patient supine and the knees flexed. The plantar aspect of the foot is placed on a wedge (the angle of the block at 45°), and the foot and ankle are pronated. The central ray is in the mid-plane of the dorsal aspect of the foot, with the tube straight [109].

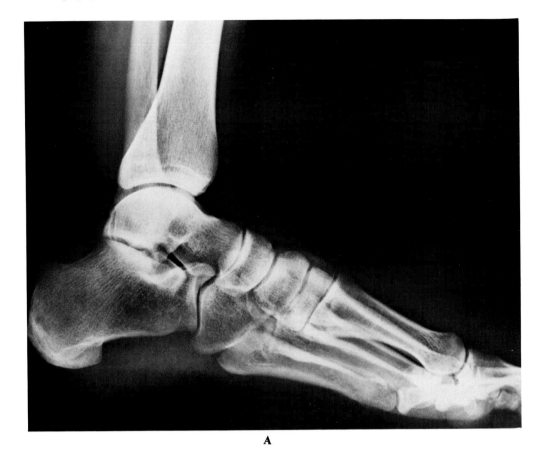

A

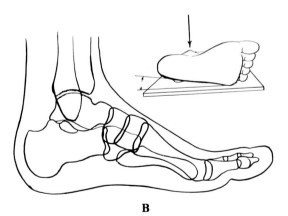

B

Fig. 4.8. "Poor lateral" view.

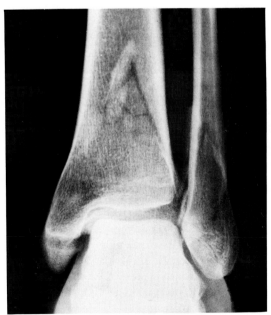

Fig. 4.9. Anteroposterior radiograph of a large displaced posterior tibial fracture. Note the inverted V-shaped metaphyseal density.

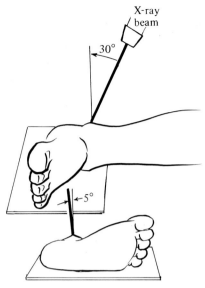

Fig. 4.10. Superoinferior oblique lateral projection (Merrill).

X-ray
beam

30°

5°

A

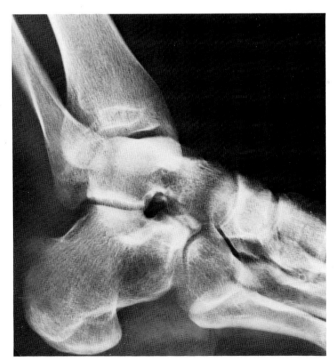

B

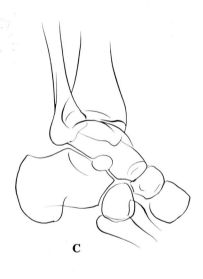

C

Fig. 4.11. Oblique dorsiplantar view (lateromedial oblique projection; Feist-Mankin position).

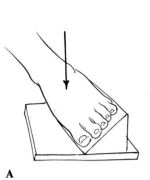

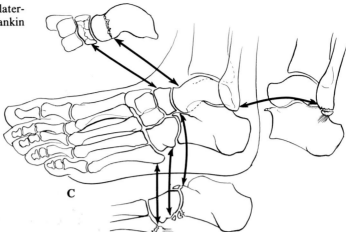

A

C

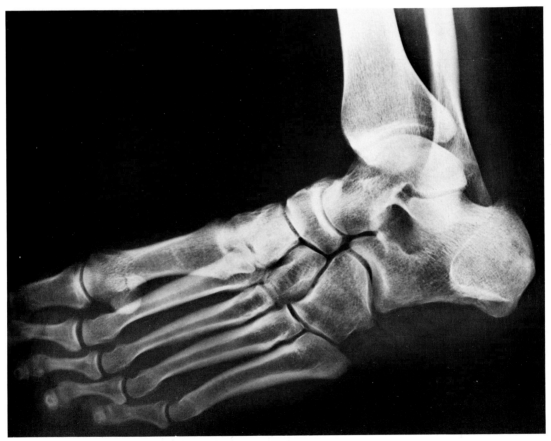

B

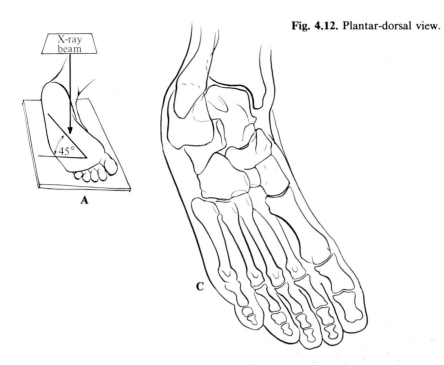

Fig. 4.12. Plantar-dorsal view.

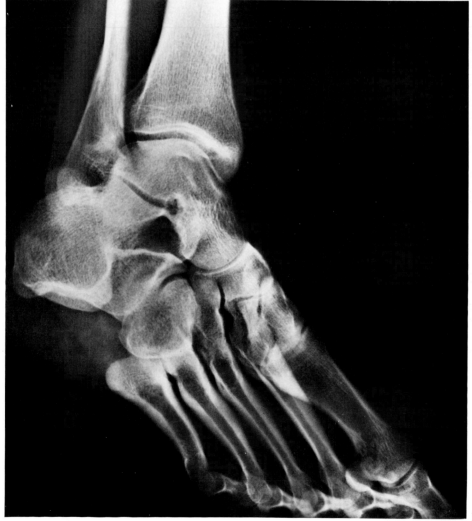

This view allows visualization of the supinator line [25]. It reveals the neck of the talus, the posterior subtalar joint, the medial, intermediate, and lateral cuneiforms, and the beak of the apophyses of the calcaneus, as well as the metatarsal and the tarsal bones in true lateral projection.

The Plantar-Dorsal View

If further projections are necessary, a plantar-dorsal position can be obtained to project the tarsometatarsal joints and the tarsal bones (Fig. 4.12) [109].

Discussion

To recapitulate, frontal views include the standard AP as well as the mortise projections. The latter view is obtained with the limb in sufficient internal rotation (10–30°) to place the intermalleolar line in the frontal plane, parallel with the X-ray cassette or table. The central ray is applied perpendicular to the ankle and parallel to the articular surfaces of the tibia and talus. With this projection, the joint spaces between these parts should be uniform, most distinct, and clearly defined [85]. Oblique projections, most usually obtained at 45° of internal and external rotation, with variations for special circumstances, have been described. A lateral view may be taken, either from medial to lateral, or lateral to medial, as preferred and permitted by patient circumstances.

Ankle studies should include an oblique dorsiplantar projection of the foot so as to identify supinator line injuries. Moreover, the entire leg, from the ankle to the knee, must be surveyed in the AP and lateral views if one suspects either an indirect supramalleolar injury of the fibula (Figs. 4.13, 11.9, and 11.10) or a fracture-dislocation of the ankle due to posterior dislocation of the fibula (Figs. 4.14 and 6.15).

In the aforementioned Bosworth lesion [11], the pathognomonic finding on X-ray examination is that of an apparent anatomic inconsistency: an anteroposterior view of the knee joint concurrent with a lateral view of the talus and foot. The fibula is seen to cross the tibia from the lateral to the medial side, and it is clearly trapped

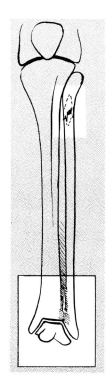

Fig. 4.13. Maisonneuve combination—injury to the ankle and supramalleolar portion of the fibula.

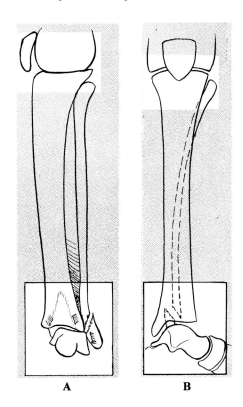

A   B

Fig. 4.14. Bosworth injury illustrated in lateral (**A**) and anteroposterior (**B**) projections.

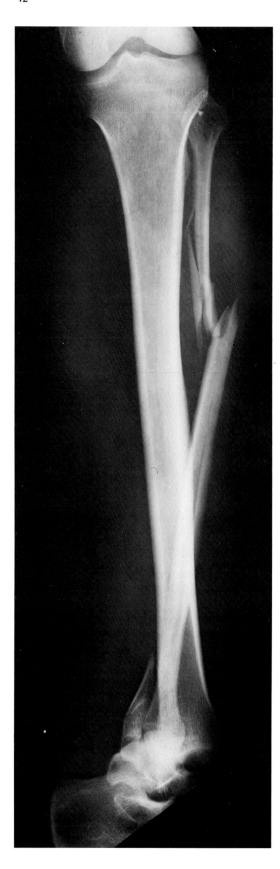

in this abnormal position (Fig. 4.15) [130]. In the full-length lateral view, the fibula is seen to be posterior to the tibia throughout its entire length. If the distal fibula is fractured, the lateral malleolus will project even further posterior to the shaft of the fibula in the lateral projections of the lower limb. The lateral malleolus is always the most posteriorly projected structure in the lateral position under these circumstances. One should especially look for these strange and rare entrapments of the fibula with a fixed and ostensibly irreducible dislocation of the ankle joint [42,95,98,107,165].

Paramount in any assessment of the ankle is soft tissue integrity. This can only be accurately determined by history and physical examination—and frequently, stress testing and arthrography. The "isolated" nondisplaced fibular fracture is a major problem for the uninitiated. This is usually associated with failure of the anterior inferior tibiofibular ligament, but often cannot be demonstrated radiographically. It is important in this situation to exclude an associated deltoid ligament lesion, whose existence renders this lesion potentially unstable. In doubtful cases, stress films performed in external rotation and/or abduction may be required (Fig. 10.17).

So-called "stove-in" deformities, occurring medially in adduction (Fig. 8.17A,B) and laterally in abduction injuries, reveal themselves at the angle between the trochlea of the talus and its corresponding malleolus. These should be carefully scrutinized in the AP, mortise, and oblique views.

The subtle osteochondral flake fractures of the talus are usually missed unless they are sought [20,76,114,145]. These more hidden talar dome fractures may require neutral, plantar-, and dorsiflexion views in the AP, mortise, and oblique projections, in addition to inversion and eversion stress films. Magnification and high resolution radiography may help to discern these minute fragments [59], which conspire to evade detection in plain film views. Tomograms, computed to-

◁

Fig. 4.15. Bosworth injury—posterior dislocation of the talus and distal fibula. In this instance, there was an associated posterior tibial lip fracture but no distal fibular fracture.

mography (CT) scanning, and arthrography may prove necessary. If the flakes are purely cartilaginous, and do not opacify, it is necessary to proceed with gas-enhanced arthrography. Recently, high resolution computed tomography has been successfully employed to detect both the osteochondral and purely cartilaginous lesions as to site and extent, and affecting either the distal tibia or talus [132].

Stress Projections

A caveat must be placed upon any undue reliance on findings in most stress films. There are simply far too many false-negative and false-positive results. These projections are valuable only if interpreted in a proper clinical context; they are complementary and adjunctive to clinical examination and are not mutually exclusive. In order to be reliable, such testing must be performed under effective local, regional, or general anesthesia. The jig-related or manual forces must be applied by someone knowledgeable in the mechanisms productive of the lesions under consideration.

The Eversion (Abduction) Stress View

Most authorities do not consider isolated eversion stress testing (Fig. 4.16) either informative or particularly reliable in assessment of medial ligamentous attenuations. In normal ankles, however, there should be little tilting or valgus deformity of the talus when subjected to stress in this plane. More than 10° of tilting of the talus into abduction is considered pathologic, as are an increase of more than 2 to 3 mm of the medial clear space and movement of the talus laterally at its contact points along the tibial plafond.

Since isolated rupture of the deltoid ligament is rare, testing must consider the entire restraining complex, including the anterior tibiofibular ligament, the tibiofibular joint and its entire syndesmosis, plus the fibula [82]. Rotatory stress testing is therefore considered more appropriate in this regard.

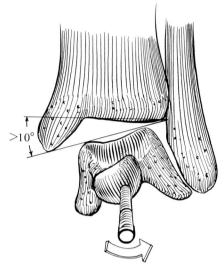

Fig. 4.16. Abduction stress testing: more than 10° of talar tilt is considered pathologic.

The External Rotatory Stress View

External stress applied to an abnormally lax deltoid complex should reveal more than 3 mm widening of the medial clear space, as compared to the width of the clear space at the lateral aspect of the tibiotalar joint—the usual displacement expected whenever the deep portion of the deltoid ligament is attenuated or ruptured (Figs. 4.17, 10.16, 10.17, and 11.11). It is the exception for such to exist in isolation, however, and involvement of the tibiofibular ligaments and/or fracture of the fibular malleolus usually coexist. These associated injuries may not be readily demonstrable even on stress films, since they often take the form of rotational rather than translational instability. Their presence must be inferred on the basis of such a degree of medial instability.

The Inversion (Adduction) Stress View

An approach to the diagnosis of lateral ligamentous insufficiency of the ankle has involved stressing the talus in inversion (or more properly, adduction) to demonstrate tilting of the talus within the tibiofibular mortise (Figs. 4.18 and 8.15) [26].

The stress tests are variable and the reports in the literature provide conflicting results. Chapman [26] has summarized his impressions on the

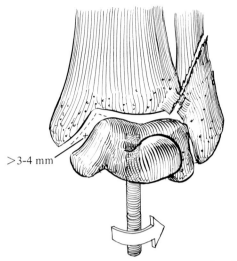

Fig. 4.17. External rotatory stress testing: widening of the medial clear space more than 3–4 mm indicates insufficiency of the deep deltoid ligament.

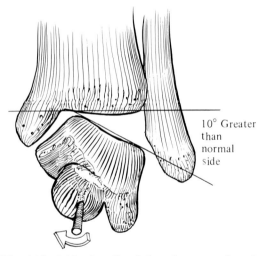

Fig. 4.18. Adduction tilt of the talus more than 8–10° in excess of the normal side suggests significant lateral ligamentous injury.

reliability and applicability of the applied ankle inversion (adduction and supination of the heel and subtalar joints) stress tests; his article provides a prudent and circumspect analysis. Inversion testing is most often only marginally reliable and verifiable, and then only in an ideal setting.

Whenever adduction tilt of the lateral aspect of the talus occurs, it must be compared to the opposite ankle. For the test to be considered positive, the adduction tilt of the suspected ankle

should always exceed that of the uninjured ankle by at least 6°. Stewart, as cited by Canale [19], states that 8–10° of tilt in excess of the normal ankle is indicative of a significant lateral ligament complex injury. Even so, a disparity of 10° can be seen in 3% of normal persons—hence, the need to interpret this test in the appropriate clinical context. A talar tilt in excess of 25–30°, however, must in the vast majority of cases be considered indicative of a complete tear of the lateral collateral ligaments. Old and hitherto undisclosed injuries, eccentric hypermobility, and congenitally lax ligaments combine to misrepresent the comparative findings.

These tests should be imaged in a neutral position of dorsiflexion, and then in some 20 or more degrees of plantarflexion and internal rotation in order to be reliable [32]. Plantarflexion and internal rotation removes the blocking action of the lateral malleolus, which acts as a bony buttress when the ankle is dorsiflexed to neutral. Whatever the position of plantarflexion referable to the foot and ankle relative to the tibia, and whatever the degree of internal rotation of the leg relative to the central ray, they should be exactly the same for both ankles.

The patient should be properly anesthetized to relieve the generalized protective muscular hypertonia, to minimize focal peroneal spasm, and to relieve attendant pain. Slowly and gradually applied stress, utilizing manual forces or special technical jigs, however, is believed to circumvent the need for local or general anesthesia. Colton [32] describes and illustrates the use of a simple wrench to accomplish the appropriate strain.

The Sagittal Anterior Transpositional Stress View

The anterior stress radiograph is considered useful in discriminating anterior talofibular ligament tears in isolation, and is performed in the lateral projection as one attempts to manually displace the talus anteriorly out of the ankle mortise (Fig. 4.19A,B) [25,50]. The amount of metric measurement indicating pathologic displacement is unsettled: minimum estimates range from 3 to 8 mm. The manner of measurement varies and is dependent upon relative points of reference between talus and tibia. Comparison with the assumed normal ankle may be necessary in questionable cases.

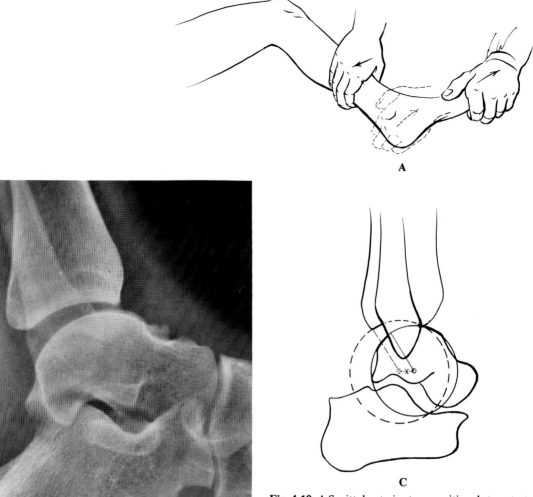

A

B

Fig. 4.19. A Sagittal anterior transpositional stress test. **B** Radiograph obtained in this position. **C** Schematic indicating degree of displacement of reference points.

The examiner can usually see and palpate a sulcus, thus observing the peculiar and characteristic sucking-in actions of the soft tissues, which occur anteriorly and medially over the ankle joint as the heel and foot are drawn forward, while the tibia is thrust backward. The foregoing is an important visual and palpable impression of subluxation when accomplished manually, without resorting to special equipment or imaging, although several jigs and static loading methods have been described. This forward sliding study may be practically painless for the patient as compared with other stress testing.

With combined medial (deltoid) and lateral ligamentous insufficiency, anterior drawer testing

will produce straight anterior translation of the talus with respect to the distal tibia and fibula. With isolated lateral ligament injury, only the lateral aspect of the trochlea tali can be translated anteriorly, resulting in internal rotation of the talus about a medial tether provided by the intact deltoid ligament, the so-called anterolateral rotatory instability (Fig. 4.20) [24,128]. These two phenomena can usually be distinguished clinically but are frequently confused radiographically. Since the anterior drawer test is generally obtained with the foot maintained in contact with the X-ray table or cassette, anterolateral rotatory instability is usually manifested radiographically as excessive external rotation of the proximal

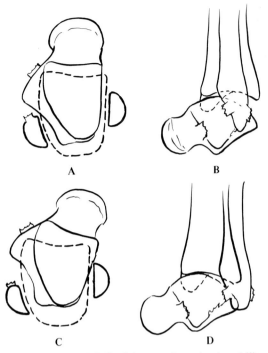

A   B

C   D

Fig. 4.20. **A** and **B** Straight anterior talar instability. **C** and **D** Anterolateral rotatory instability of the talus. Since radiographs are usually obtained with the foot in contact with the X-ray table or cassette, internal rotation of the talus will be manifest radiographically as external rotation of the tibiofibular mortise.

limb with respect to the talus. It should, therefore, be suspected whenever the sagittal anterior transpositional stress view demonstrates anterior translation of the talus in association with posterior migration of the fibula—indicating external rotation of the limb and tibiofibular mortise.

The Subtalar Stress View

The tests to discover subtalar ligament attenuations are described by Kleiger [82], and these are projected in the AP and lateral views. Subtalar inversion instability is usually seen in complex supinator line injuries, and frequently occurs in conjunction with lateral ligament tears of the ankle. Severe injuries to the calcaneofibular ligament frequently involve subcrural dissociation, allowing the normal relationship of the talus and calcaneus to be disturbed when inversion stress is applied. Both ankle and subtalar instability

can occur as isolated phenomena, but are more often associated. These particular problems are to be sought more often in old recurrent instability.

Discussion

Given the morass of conflicting reports regarding variants and degrees and millimeters of tilt accepted within the parameters of normal, many experienced observers are cautious in reference to stress-testing procedures, especially if utilized in isolation. The tilt motions employed are complex and movements are seldom elicited in purely one plane [128]. These tests are to be considered as complementary [72]. Consideration of rotational instability must be incorporated in any properly exhaustive analysis seeking strain-related talar translation.

Glasgow, et al. [50] have analyzed instability of the ankle after recent and old injuries to the lateral ligaments of the ankle; they recommend anterior stress testing measurement. Anterior subluxation of the talus can be measured in sagittal stress films [50]. When the anterior fibulotalar ligament is torn, this test is more reliable than that of Inversion Stress. If the lateral ligaments and capsular soft tissues are defective, any forward drift of the talus, with its tendency to subluxate, is bound to be magnified. In the final analysis, the anterior stress test is most valuable in subtle discrimination of isolated tears of the anterior talofibular ligament complex.

Specific techniques for accomplishing eversion, inversion, rotatory, and anterior stress and strain, with radiographic imaging, are well described in the current literature [19,25,26,32,36,50,56,65, 72,79,82,92,111,128,140].

Arthrography

The use of arthrography in a properly exhaustive search for acute ligamentous injuries is a well-accepted and commonly employed procedure. In acute traumatic soft tissue and joint attenuations of the syndesmosis and mortise, where discrimination between the conjoined lateral ligaments is desired, valuable information can often be obtained [160,161]. Arthrography is especially helpful when radiographic plain film techniques and stress testing are unrewarding or remain equivocal. Although arthrography cannot take the place of common sense and careful clinical inspection, it plays an important part in the step-by-step discrimination of acute ankle lesions. For a variety of interconnecting mortise and tenon injuries, it is occasionally indispensable.

Arthrography is considered to be more than reasonably reliable in discernment of acute deltoid and anterior talofibular ligament tears, but only when accomplished soon after trauma. The test is best employed within the first 24 to 48 h, and never later than 1 week following an acute injury. A sealing of rents by clot and fibrin, especially in partial, yet significant, deltoid ligament tears, has been observed as early as 48 h postinjury.

Reliability exists only when techniques are carefully and properly accomplished. The arthrographic procedure demands a mastery of detail in technique and proper and accurate interpretation requires experience and skill. Although arthrography is a statistically safe and essentially harmless method, it is neither altogether simple nor innocuous as an approach. It is decidedly invasive and must be used judiciously.

Indications

Arthrographic examination of the ankle is generally indicated in the presence of the following:

1. Old supportive tissue laxity, chronic ligamentous lesions, and especially chronic recurrent syndromes of instability suggesting a need for ligamentous reconstructive procedures.
2. Intraarticular craters and osteocartilaginous loose bodies.
3. Signs and symptoms of joint catching and locking indicative of minute flakes of joint cartilage.

Technique

The joint must be positioned in advance for imaging of the needle and in anticipation of the routine projections, which include AP, oblique, and lateral views, in addition to any difficult and special projections that become necessary. The ankle should be cleansed, prepared, and draped as in any surgical procedure.

The local anesthetic employed, the detailed and precise regional introduction of a proper-caliber needle, its positioning and placement well away from the site of suspected injury, and the amount, force, and speed of instillation of opacifying materials require a meticulous methodology.

A large needle (18 to 22 gauge and 1.5 in.) is preferred for acute injuries to facilitate joint aspiration and lavage. The insertion of the needle should be remote from any major lesion under suspicion. When inserted anteromedially, the needle should be placed between the anterior tibial and extensor hallucis longus tendons, opposite the most prominent portion of the medial malleolus. The dorsalis pedis artery should be identified and avoided. Image amplification and television screening are preferable to plain film imaging for determination of needle placement.

The joint is first aspirated to remove any effusion. Lavage is necessary for removal of blood and clots that may interfere with the instillation and dispersion of contrast material.

Contrast material is then introduced; the materials preferred, and their volumes, are somewhat variable. Currently, 60% methylglucamine diatrizoate (Renographin) in volumes of between 6 and 12 ml, or 50% diatrizoate (Hypaque) diluted to 25% with sterile water in volumes usually not exceeding 10 ml, have been recommended. Some prefer a combination of contrast material and local anesthetic, with an instilled volume ranging from 6 to 12 ml (8 ml of contrast material and 4 ml of 1% xylocaine). The single positive and single negative contrast arthrogram is utilized for discernment of loose bodies—the positive contrast for acute and chronic ligamentous injuries. The double contrast technique is usually reserved for study of the articular contour and detection of surface defects, and it is advised that the materials combine 6 to 8 ml of air with a very small amount of positive contrast material.

During insertion of the material, a respect for resistance and ease of instillation may invite smaller or larger volumes of material. On occasion, as little as 4 ml or as much as 20 ml are utilized. When a felt resistance is met to the slow, gradual, and steady introduction of material, it usually signifies proper filling and distention of the joint cavity. Rapid egress of injected material through a major rent may result in failure to reveal all of the associated defects. Too forceful or too rapid instillation may rupture frangible, old, and weakened tissues, and excessive pressure may rupture normal tissues—inviting extravasations that will confuse interpretation. Extracapsular introduction of contrast material must be avoided, and careful monitoring of the first few drops of material by fluoroscopic technique is advised to be certain of intraarticular instillation.

After the material is introduced, the surface area is carefully wiped clean and a sterile compression dressing is applied and maintained while the ankle is passively and actively exercised through a repeated range of motion. This will facilitate complete dispersion of the material within the interstices of the joint space.

A detailed discussion of the special surgical techniques of local instillation of anesthesia, needle insertions, and the type and dilutions of opaque materials for peroneal tendon sheath injections is included in the recent edition of *Campbell's Operative Orthopaedics* [19].

Interpretation

In the presence of anterior tibiofibular ligament rupture, there will be filling of the syndesmotic recess beyond its usual 4-mm width and height of 1–2.5 cm. This is best visualized in the mortise and internal oblique views. The extravasation of contrast material reveals upward egress. The lateral view reveals this as a proximal and posterior tracking; projections of the dye can also frequently be noted anteriorly in its forward extension through the syndesmotic recess and up into the interosseous region. The proximal extravasations can be noted in all views. These findings lend strong presumptive support for some degree of tibiofibular diastasis (Fig. 13.7).

Whenever the intraarticularly instilled dye comes to final rest immediately anterior to and against the tibia, directly opposed to and in front of the syndesmosis, it is considered to be proof of a rupture of the anterior tibiofibular ligament of the syndesmosis.

Extreme caution must be taken against misinterpreting any other anterior tibial dye migrations. Some may be coming from the far lateral positions, and are indicative of lateral ligamentous rupture. These are due to extravasations from rents and tears of the lateral collateral ligaments, and not syndesmotic lesions. Whenever dye egresses from lateral tears, it not only rests inferior and superficial to the lateral malleolus, but can track forward across the front of the joint to appear as a collection of dye anterior to the distal tibia at the syndesmosis. In this situation, however, the dye is never contiguous and directly applied to the syndesmosis; rather, it is separated by a distinct clear space. There is no anterior clear space when the dye extravasates from the syndesmotic recess.

Deltoid ligament injuries, which rarely occur as isolated and complete lesions, are demonstrated at arthrography by extravasation of contrast medium below and medial to the distal tibia, and are best discerned in the AP projection.

Discussion

It is suggested that arthrographic results are occasionally inconsistent and unreliable in ankle injuries, since false-negative and false-positive results are not uncommon. Proper interpretation requires a full understanding of variants and natural egress along tendon sheaths and into adjacent subtalar joints, as discussed by Bröstrom [13–15] and others (Fig. 4.21) [1,4,8,18,44,51, 52,54,74,90,133].

Special Studies

Xeroradiography

Clarification of the borders and edges between superimposed bony elements—e.g., the flattened plane border of the fibular incisura and syndesmotic projections comprising the anterior and posterior tubercles of the tibia—can be best detailed by the technique of xeroradiography. This procedure utilizes a physicoelectric process as opposed to the photochemical process employed in the X-ray film technique.

Xeroradiography allows for edge enhancements when a reusable selenium plate is exposed. It serves as a valuable extension of standard radiographic techniques, allowing a much larger exposure range, with detailed delineation of the

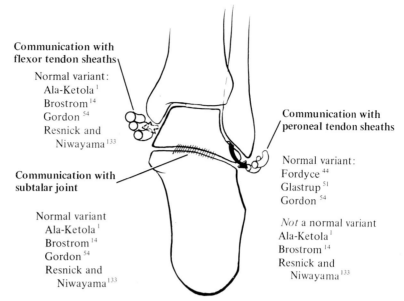

Communication with
flexor tendon sheaths

Normal variant:
Ala-Ketola[1]
Brostrom[14]
Gordon[54]
Resnick and
Niwayama[133]

Communication with
subtalar joint

Normal variant
Ala-Ketola[1]
Brostrom[14]
Gordon[54]
Resnick and
Niwayama[133]

Communication with
peroneal tendon sheaths

Normal variant:
Fordyce[44]
Glastrup[51]
Gordon[54]

Not a normal variant
Ala-Ketola[1]
Brostrom[14]
Resnick and
Niwayama[133]

Fig. 4.21. Arthrography of the Ankle: Communications between the ankle joint and subtalar joint or flexor tendon sheaths are generally accepted as normal variants. There is no consensus, however, as to whether communications with the peroneal tendon sheaths are normal variants or traumatic in origin.

soft tissue elements about the ankle. In particular, the tendo Achilles and its juxtaposed bursae are easily discerned. Changes in density within the tendon and its integrity are clearly revealed as compared to routine radiography.

The major advantage of xeroradiography is its representation of osseous contours: contours are intensified so that the boundary lines between areas of different thickness or density (e.g., bones against soft tissues) are especially pronounced [139]. Fine calcifications are especially clearly defined, as are small foreign bodies and metallic markers. When small and poorly defined changes about the ankle and tarsal bones are being sought, especially in a postreduction film of the plaster-encased extremity, it can allow fine visualization of bony alignment that is not possible otherwise. This technique is particularly valuable in discernment of intraosseous cysts and tumors, and allows observation of extensions beyond the confines of the bone.

The xeroradiography image can be visualized with top illumination, and can be produced in both a positive and negative mode. Faulty exposure in xeroradiography is unusual. It is, however, a more expensive technique than standard radiography, and the X-ray exposure is certainly greater.

Tomography

This technique is especially valuable in the imaging of pain-mediating nidi buried or sequestered within the bone about the ankle, peculiar to osteoid osteoma of the talus and abscesses about the distal tibia. It also is effective in delineating osteochondral defects on the surface of the talar dome and at the trochlear edges (Fig. 4.22). Post-traumatic syndesmotic bony coalescences, non-unions, sinus tarsi fractures, and subtalar osseous defects, plus tarsal coalitions, may sometimes only be revealed in this particular fashion.

By the simultaneous movement of X-ray tube and X-ray film in opposite directions, a clear image in one plane will occur, with blurring of other planes and their images. This differs from the simple plain film in that it represents a specific slice at a particular depth from among the usually superimposed images.

Nuclear Scanning

Inflammatory reactions within bone and soft tissue can be discerned earliest by utilizing gallium and technetium-99m pyrophosphate scanning.

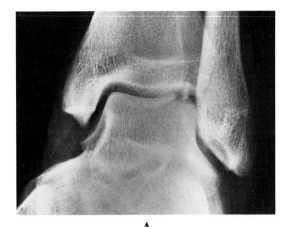

A

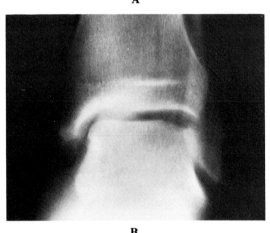

B

Fig. 4.22. Osteochondral fracture of the talus, suggested on plain films (**A**) and confirmed on anteroposterior tomograms (**B**).

Technetium scans are particularly valuable in detection of occult fractures. This is especially so during the evolution of stress fractures, where detection can be accomplished long before their appearance on plain films [6].

Although highly sensitive, these skeletal scans lack specificity: it is often impossible to differentiate between the reactive and inflammatory elements of osteoarthroses, fracture, tumor, or infection. Increased activity is discerned in reflex sympathetic dystrophy and avascular necrosis, but increased activity about joints due to nonspecific and traumatic hyperemia and synovitis may be misleading. Moreover, the use of scanning in detecting delayed union of fractures is debated, and some recent studies suggest it is not helpful in this respect [71].

The use of gallium scintigraphy is especially valuable in detection of soft tissue infection about the ankle, but it too is not infallible, even in acute osteomyelitis; therefore, a negative scan may be erroneous [47].

Pain in the environs of the foot and ankle may be related to an occult osteoid osteoma situated in the talus, and scanning elsewhere in the leg may be required in addition [93,99].

Magnification Roentgenography

Magnification roentgenography and its enlargement of images can help to detect subtle changes, such as those found in small avulsion fractures [59].

Computed Axial Tomography

Views of the ankle and foot utilizing high resolution cross-sectional scanning are employed for detection of a variety of obscure and deeply hidden lesions, and can provide information that would otherwise be unobtainable (Fig. 13.2) [49]. It allows detection of osteochondritis dissecans of the talus. Moreover, syndesmotic lesions can be detected by horizontal slices [132]. The subtalar joint can also be specially viewed with this procedure [49].

Conclusion

It is important to stress that radiographic findings constitute an aid to diagnosis, not a mechanism for establishing a conclusive diagnosis [35]. Those of us dealing with these problems must adhere to the dictum that "however important it may be, the radiograph must nevertheless still be looked upon as one of several aids to diagnosis and management" [78].

References

1. Ala-Ketola L, Puranen J, Koivisto E: Arthrography in the diagnosis of ligament injuries and classification of ankle injuries. Radiology 125:63, 1977.
2. American Roentgen Ray Society. Syllabus for the Categorical Course on the Skeletal System. Annual Meeting, Washington, D.C., 1976, pp. 387.
3. Arimoto HK, Forrester DM: Classification of ankle fractures; an algorithm. Am J Roentgenol

135:1057, 1980.

4. Arndt R-D, Horns JW, Gold RH: Clinical Arthrography. Baltimore, Williams & Wilkins, 1981, pp. 141.

5. Ashhurst APC, Bromer RC: Classification and mechanism of fractures of the leg bones involving the ankle. Arch Surg 4:51, 1922.

6. Batillas J, Vasilas A, Pizzi WF, Gokcebay T: Bone scanning in the detection of occult fractures. J Trauma 21:564, 1981.

7. Bauer M, Bergstrom B, Hemborg A: Arthrosis of the ankle evaluated on films in weight-bearing position. Acta Radiol Diagn 20:88, 1979.

8. Berridge FR, Bonnin JG: The radiographic examination of the ankle joint including arthrography. Surg Gynecol Obstet 79:383, 1944.

9. Bohler L: The Treatment of Fractures, Vol. 3. Translated by A. Wallner and O. Russe. New York, Grune & Stratton, 1958.

10. Bolin H: The fibula and its relationship to the tibia and talus in injuries of the ankle due to forced external rotation. Acta Radiol Scand 29:439, 1961.

11. Bosworth DM: Fracture-dislocation of the ankle with fixed displacement of the fibula behind the tibia. J Bone Joint Surg 29:130, 1947.

12. Brand RL, Collins MDF, Templeton T: Surgical repair of ruptured lateral ankle ligaments. Am J Sports Med 9:40, 1981.

13. Bröstrom L: Sprained ankles. Acta Chir Scand 128:483, 1964.

14. Bröstrom L: Sprained ankles. Acta Chir Scand 130:560, 1965.

15. Bröstrom L, Liljedahl S-O, Lindvall N: Sprained ankles. Acta Chir Scand 129:485, 1965.

16. Buckingham WW: Subtalar dislocation of the foot. J Trauma, 13:753, 1973.

17. Burwell HN, Charnley AD: The treatment of displaced fractures at the ankle by rigid internal fixation and early joint movement. J Bone Joint Surg 47B:634, 1965.

18. Callaghan JE, Percy EC, Hill RO: The ankle arthrogram. J Assoc Canad Radiol 21:74, 1970.

19. Canale ST: Miscellaneous affections of bones and joints. In Edmonson AS, Chrenshaw AH (eds): Campbell's Operative Orthopaedics, Vol. 1, 6th ed. St. Louis, Mosby, 1980, p. 1163.

20. Canale ST, Belding RH: Osteochondral lesions of the talus. Jefferson Orthop J 8:26, 1979.

21. Canale ST, Kelly F: Fractures of the neck of the talus. J Bone Joint Surg 60A:143, 1978.

22. Cave EF, Burke JF, Boyd RJ: Trauma Management. Chicago, Year Book Medical, 1974.

23. Cedell C-A: Ankle lesions. Acta Orthop Scand 46:425, 1975.

24. Cedell C-A: Supination—outward rotation injuries of the ankle. Acta Orthop Scand (Suppl) 110:1, 1967.

25. Chapchal G (ed): Injuries of the Ligaments and Their Repair. Littleton, PSG, 1977.

26. Chapman MW: Sprains of the ankle. II. In: Instructional Course Lectures. Am Acad Orthop Surg 24:294, 1975.

27. Charnley J: The Closed Treatment of Common Fractures, 3rd ed. Baltimore, Williams & Wilkins, 1970.

28. Church CC: Radiographic diagnosis of acute peroneal tendon dislocation. Am J Roentgenol 129:1065, 1977.

29. Cimmino CV: Fracture of the lateral process of the talus. Am J Roentgenol Radium Ther Nucl Med 90:1277, 1963.

30. Close RJ: Some applications of the functional anatomy of the ankle joint. J Bone Joint Surg 38A:761, 1956.

31. Cobb N: Oblique radiography in diagnosis of ankle injuries. Proc Roy Soc Med 58:334, 1965.

32. Colton CL: Injuries of the ankle. In Wilson JN (ed): Watson-Jones Fractures and Joint Injuries, Vol. 2, 5th ed. Edinburgh, Churchill Livingstone, 1976, p. 1091.

33. Colton CL: The treatment of Dupuytren's fracture–dislocation of the ankle. J Bone Joint Surg 53B:63, 1971.

34. Conrad JJ, Tannin AH: Trauma to the ankle. In Jahss MH (ed): Disorders of the Foot, Vol. 2. Philadelphia, Saunders, 1982, p. 1543.

35. Coulam CM, Erickson JJ, Rollo FD, James AE: The Physical Basis of Medical Imaging. New York, Appleton, 1981.

36. Cox JS, Hewes TF: "Normal" talar tilt angle. Clin Orthop Rel Res 140:37, 1979.

37. Daffner RH: Pseudofracture of the dens: Mach bands. Am J Roentgenol 128:607, 1977.

38. Dalinka MA: Ankle fractures. In Feldman F (ed): Radiology, Pathology, and Immunology of Bones and Joints: A Review of Current Concepts. New York, Appleton, 1978, p. 229.

39. Danielsson LG: Avulsion fracture of the lateral malleolus in children. Br J Accident Surg 12:165, 1980.

40. Dunn AR, Jacobs B, Campbell RD: Fractures of the talus. J Trauma 6:443, 1966.

41. Eisenberg RL, Amberg JR (ed): Critical Diagnostic Pathways in Radiology: An Algorithmic Approach. Philadelphia, Lippincott, 1981.

42. Fahey JJ, Schlenker LT, Stauffer RC: Fracture dislocation of the ankle with fixed displacement of the fibula behind the tibia. Am J Roentgenol Radium Ther Nucl Med 76:1102, 1956.

43. Ferreira AP, De Wet IS, Dommisse GF: Fractures and dislocations of the ankle joint. South Afr Med J 54:1095, 1978.

44. Fordyce AJW, Horn CV: Arthrography in recent injuries of the ligaments of the ankle. J Bone Joint Surg 54B:116, 1971.

45. Freiberger RH: Principles of radiology. In Owen R, Goodfellow J, Bullough P (eds): Scientific Foundations of Orthopaedics and Traumatology. Philadelphia, Saunders, 1980, p. 329.

46. Frisby JP: Seeing Illusion, Brain and Mind. Oxford, Oxford University Press, 1980.

47. Garnett ES, Cockshott WP, Jacob J: Classical acute osteomyelitis with a negative bone scan. Br J Radiol 50:757, 1977.

48. Gaston SR, MacLaughlin HL: Complex fractures of the lateral malleolus. Trauma 1:68, 1961.

49. Genant HK, Wilson JS, Bovill EG, Brunelle FO, Murray WR, Rodrigo JJ: Computed tomography of the musculoskeletal system. J Bone Joint Surg 60A:1088, 1980.

50. Glasgow M, Jackson A, Jamieson AM: Instability of the ankle after injury to the lateral ligament. J Bone Joint Surg, 62B:196, 1980.

51. Glastrup H: Arthrographies in acute ankle joint injuries. Acta Orthop Scand 36:281, 1965.

52. Goergen TG, Danzig LA, Resnick D, Owen CA: Roentgenographic Evaluation of the Tibiotalar Joint. J Bone Joint Surg 59A:874, 1977.

53. Goldman AB, Katz MC, Freiberger RH: Posttraumatic adhesive capsulitis of the ankle: arthrographic diagnosis. Am J Roentgenol 127:585, 1976.

54. Gordon RB: Arthrography of the ankle joint. Experience in 107 studies. J Bone Joint Surg 52A:1623, 1970.

55. Gould N: Articular osteoid osteoma of the talus: A case report. Foot Ankle 1:284, 1981.

56. Gould N, Seligson D, Gassman J: Early and late repair of lateral ligament of the ankle. Foot Ankle 1:84, 1980.

57. Grath GB: Widening of the ankle mortise. Acta Chir Scand (Suppl) 263:1, 1960.

58. Grech P: Casualty Radiology: A Practical Guide for Radiological Diagnosis. London, Chapman and Hall, 1981.

59. Griffiths HJ, DeHaven KE: Magnification and high-resolution radiography in sports-related injuries. Am J Sports Med 9:394, 1981.

60. Harrington ED: Degenerative arthritis of the ankle secondary to longstanding lateral ligament instability. J Bone Joint Surg 61A:354, 1979.

61. Harris JH, Harris WH: The Radiology of Emergency Medicine, 2nd ed. Baltimore, Williams & Wilkins, 1975, p. 593.

62. Hendelberg T: The roentgenographic examination of the ankle joint in malleolar fractures. Acta Radiol 27:23, 1946.

63. Heppenstall RB: Fracture Treatment and Healing. Philadelphia, Saunders, 1980.

64. Heppenstall RB, Farahvar H, Balderston R, Lotke P: Evaluation and management of subtalar dislocations. J Trauma 20:494, 1980.

65. Horstman JK, Kantor GS, Samuelson KM: Investigation of lateral ankle ligament reconstruction. Foot Ankle 1:338, 1981.

66. Hug G, Dixon AStJ: Ankle joint synoviography in rheumatoid arthritis. Ann Rheumatic Dis 36:532, 1977.

67. Hughes J: The medial malleolus in ankle fractures. Orthop Clin North Am 11:649, 1980.

68. Hughes JL, Weber H, Willenegger H, Kuner EH: Evaluation of ankle fractures: Nonoperative and operative treatment. Clin Orthop Rela Res 138:111, 1979.

69. Husfeldt E: Significance of roentgenography of ankle joint in oblique projection in malleolar fractures. Hospitalstid 80:788, 1937.

70. Ihle CL, Cochran RM: Fracture of the fused os trigonum. Am J Sports Med 10:47, 1982.

71. Jacobs RR, Jackson RP, Preston DF, Williamson JA, Gallagher J: Dynamic Bone Scanning in Fractures. Br J Accident Surg 12:455, 1980.

72. Johannsen A: Radiological diagnosis of lateral ligament lesions of the ankle. Acta Orthop Scand 49:295, 1978.

73. Joy G, Patzakis MJ, Harvey JP: Precise evaluation of the reduction of severe ankle fractures. J Bone Joint Surg 56A:979, 1974.

74. Kaye JJ, Bohne WHO: A radiographic study of the ligamentous anatomy of the ankle. Radiology 125:659, 1977.

75. Keats TE: An Atlas of Normal Roentgen Variants that May Simulate Disease. Chicago, Year Book Medical, 1973.

76. Kenny CH: Inverted osteochondral fracture of the talus diagnosed by tomography. J Bone Joint Surg 63A:1020, 1981.

77. Kenzora JE, Abrams RC: Problems encountered in the diagnosis and treatment of osteoid osteoma of the talus. Foot and Ankle 2:172, 1981.

78. Kessel L: Clinical and radiographic diagnosis. In Wilson JN (ed): Watson-Jones Fractures and Joint Injuries, Vol. 1, 5th ed. Edinburgh, Churchill Livingstone, 1976, p. 249.

79. Kleiger B: The ankle. In Jahss MH (ed): Disorders of the Foot, Vol. 1. Philadelphia, Saunders, 1982, p. 776.

80. Kleiger B: Injuries of the talus and its joints. Clin Orthop Rel Res 121:243, 1976.

81. Kleiger B: Mechanisms of ankle injury. Orthop Clin North Am 5:127, 1974.

82. Kleiger B, Greenspan A, Norman A: Roentgenographic examination of the normal foot and ankle. In Jahss MH (ed): Disorders of the Foot, Vol. 1. Philadelphia, Saunders, 1982, p. 116.

83. Kohler A, Zimmer EA: Borderlands of the Normal and Early Pathologic in Skeletal Roentgenology. New York, Grune & Stratton, 1968.

84. Lauge-Hansen N: Fractures of the ankle. II. Combined experimental-surgical and experimental-roentgenologic investigations. Arch Surg 60:957, 1950.

85. Lauge-Hansen N: Fractures of the ankle. III. Genetic roentgenologic diagnosis of fractures of the ankle. Am J Roentgenol Radium Ther Nucl Med 71:456, 1954.

86. Lauge-Hansen N: Ligamentous ankle fracture: diagnosis and treatment. Acta Chir Scand 97:544, 1949.

87. Lee CK, Hansen HT, Weiss AB: Supramalleolar fracture of the ankle (Malgaigne's fracture). Am Surg 43:589, 1977.

88. Letts RM, Gibeault D: Fractures of the neck of the talus in children. Foot Ankle, 1:74, 1980.

89. Lewis R: The Joints of the Extremities, A Radiographic Study. Springfield, Ill., Thomas, 1955.

90. Lindholmer E, Foged N, Jensen JT: Arthrogra-

phy of the ankle. Acta Radiol Diagn 19:585, 1978.

91. Lindsjo U, Hemmingsson A, Sahlstedt B, Danckwardt-Lilliestrom G: Computed tomography of the ankle. Acta Orthop Scand 50:797, 1979.

92. Lindstrand A: New aspects in the diagnosis of lateral ankle sprains. Orthop Clin North Am 7:247, 1976.

93. Lisbona R, Rosenthall L: Role of radionuclide imaging in osteoid osteoma. Am J Roentgenol 132:77, 1979.

94. London PS: A Practical Guide to the Care of the Injured. Edinburgh, Livingston, 1967.

95. Lovell ES: An unusual rotatory injury of the ankle. J Bone Joint Surg 50A:163, 1968.

96. Lucht U, Sigurd P, Termansen V: Lateral ligament reconstruction of the ankle with a modified Watson-Jones operation. Acta Orthop Scand 52:363, 1981.

97. Mandell J: Isolated fractures of the posterior tibial lip at the ankle as demonstrated by an additional projection, the "poor" lateral view. Diagn Radiol 101:319, 1971.

98. Mayer PJ, Evarts M: Fracture-dislocation of the ankle with posterior entrapment of the fibula behind the tibia. J Bone Joint Surg 60A:320, 1978.

99. McCauley RGK, Goldberg MJ, Schwartz AM: Referred pain in the lower leg, A cause of delayed diagnosis. Skeletal Radiol 6:39, 1981.

100. McDade W: Treatment of ankle fractures. I. In: Instructional Course Lectures. Am Acad Orthop Surg 24:251, 1975.

101. McDaniel WJ, Wilson FC: Trimalleolar fractures of the ankle. Clin Orthop Rel Res 122:37, 1977.

102. McReynolds IS: Trauma to the os calcis and heel cord. In Jahss MH (ed): Disorders of the Foot, Vol. 2. Philadelphia, Saunders, 1982, p. 1497.

103. Menelaus MB: Injuries of the anterior inferior tibiofibular ligament. Aust NZ J Surg 30:279, 1961.

104. Merrick MV, Smith MA: Radioisotopes in orthopaedic surgery. In Owen R, Goodfellow J, Bullough P (eds): Scientific Foundations of Orthopaedics and Traumatology. Philadelphia, Saunders, 1980, p. 342.

105. Merrill V: Atlas of Roentgenographic Positions and Standard Radiologic Procedures, Vol. 1, 4th ed. St. Louis, Mosby, 1975.

106. Meyer JM, Lagier R: Posttraumatic sinus tarsi syndrome. Acta Orthop Scand 48:121, 1977.

107. Meyers MH: Fracture about the ankle joint with fixed displacement of the proximal fragment of the fibula behind the tibia. J Bone Joint Surg 39A:441, 1957.

108. Mitchell WG, Shaftan GW, Sclafani SJA: Mandatory open reduction: Its role in displaced ankle fractures. J Trauma 19:602, 1979.

109. Montagne J, Chevrot A, Galmiche J-M: In Chafetz N (ed): Atlas of Foot Radiology. New York, Mason, 1981.

110. Moppes FI, van den Hoogenband CR, Betts-Brown A: Filling of lymphatic vessels in ankle arthrography. Diagn Imaging 49:171, 1980.

111. Mortensson AL: Anterior instability in the ankle joint following acute lateral sprain. Acta Radiol Diagn 18:529, 1977.

112. Murray RO, Jacobson HG: The Radiology of Skeletal Disorders, Vol. 2, 2nd ed. Edinburgh, Churchill Livingstone, 1977.

113. Murray RO, Jacobson HG: The Radiology of Skeletal Disorders, Vol. 3, 2nd ed. Edinburgh, Churchill Livingstone, 1977.

114. Newberg AH: Osteochondral Fractures of the Dome of the Talus. Br J Radiol 52:105, 1979.

115. Nicholas JA: Ankle injuries in athletes. Orthop Clin North Am 5:153, 1974.

116. Niedermann B, Andersen A, Andersen SB, Funder V, Jørgensen JP, Lindholmer E: Rupture of the lateral ligaments of the ankle: operation or plaster cast? Acta Orthop Scand 52:579, 1981.

117. Nofray JF, Rogers LF, Adamo GP, Groves HC, Heiser WJ: Common calcaneal avulsion fracture. Am J Roentgenol 134:119, 1980.

118. Olding-Smee W, Crockard A (eds): Trauma Care. London, Academic Press, 1981.

119. Olson RW: Arthrography of the ankle. Its use in the evaluation of ankle sprains. Radiology 92:1439, 1969.

120. Ozonoff MB: Pediatric Orthopedic Radiology, Vol. 15. Philadelphia, Saunders, 1979.

121. Pankovich AM: Acute indirect ankle injuries in the adult. In Kane WJ (ed): Current Orthopaedic Management. Edinburgh, Churchill Livingstone, 1981, p. 266.

122. Pankovich AM: Adult ankle fractures. J Continuing Educ Orthop 7:17, 1979.

123. Pankovich AM: Fractures of the fibula proximal to the distal tibiofibular syndesmosis. J Bone Joint Surg 60A:221, 1978.

124. Parkes JC, Hamilton WG, Patterson AH, Rawles JG: The anterior impingement syndrome of the ankle. J Trauma 10:895, 1980.

125. Pennal GF: Fractures of the talus. Clin Orthop Rel Res 30:53, 1963.

126. Penny JN, Davis LA: Fractures and fracture-dislocations of the neck of the talus. J Trauma 10:1029, 1980.

127. Peterson L, Goldie IF, Irstam L: Fracture of the neck of the talus. Acta Orthop Scand 48:696, 1977.

128. Rasmussen O, Tovborg-Jensen I: Anterolateral rotational instability in the ankle joint. Acta Orthop Scand 52:99, 1981.

129. Rechfeld H: Ruptures of ligaments in the ankle and foot. In Chapchal G (ed): Reconstruction Surgery and Traumatology, Vol. 15. Basel, Karger, 1976, p. 70.

130. Reckling FW, McNamara GR, DeSmet AA: Problems in the diagnosis and treatment of ankle injuries. J Trauma 21:943, 1981.

131. Redler I, Brown GG, Williams JT: Operative

treatment of the acutely ruptured lateral ligament of the ankle. South Med J 70:1168, 1977.

132. Reis ND, Zinman C, Besser MIB, Shifrin LZ, Folman Y, Torem S, Froindlich D, Zaklad H: High-resolution computerised tomography in clinical orthopaedics. J Bone Joint Surg 64B:20, 1982.

133. Resnick D, Niwayama G: Diagnosis of Bone and Joint Disorders, Vol. 1. Philadelphia, Saunders, 1981, p. 44, 254–312, 510–613.

134. Rogers LF, Campbell RE: Fractures and dislocations of the foot. Sem Roentgenol 13:157, 1978.

135. Rüedi TP, Allgöwer M: The operative treatment of intra-articular fractures of the lower end of the tibia. Clin Orthop Rel Res 138:105, 1979.

136. Samuelson KM, Harrison R, Freeman MAR: A roentgenographic technique to evaluate and document hindfoot position. Foot Ankle 1:286, 1981.

137. Sanders HWA: Ankle arthrography and ankle distortion. Radiol Clin Biol 46:1, 1977.

138. Schatzker J, McBroom R, Dzioba R: Irreducible fracture dislocation of the ankle due to posterior dislocation of the fibula. J Trauma 17:397, 1977.

139. Schertel L, Puppe D, Schnepper E, Witt H, zum Winkel K: Atlas of Xeroradiography. Philadelphia, Saunders, 1976.

140. Sedlin ED: A device for stress inversion or eversion roentgenograms of the ankle. J Bone Joint Surg 42A:1184, 1960.

141. Shelton ML, Anderson RL: Complications of fractures and dislocations of the ankle. In: Complications in Orthopaedic Surgery, Ed by Charles H. Epps Jr Vol. 1. Philadelphia, Lippincott, 1978, p. 535.

142. Shelton ML, Pedowitz WJ: Injuries to the talus and midfoot. In Jahss MH (ed): Disorders of the Foot, Vol. 2. Philadelphia, Saunders, 1982, p. 1463.

143. Singh Mac S, Kleiger B: The early complications of subtalar dislocation. Foot Ankle, 1:270, 1981.

144. Skinner EH: The mathematical calculation of prognosis in fractures of the ankle and wrist. Surg Gynecol Obstet 18:238, 1914.

145. Smith GR, Winquist RA, Allan TNK, Northrop CH: Subtle transchondral fractures of the talar dome. A radiological perspective. Diagn Radiol 124:667, 1977.

146. Sneppen O, Christenson SB, Krogsoe O, Lorentzen J: Fracture of the body of the talus. Acta Orthop Scand 48:317, 1977.

147. Spiegel PK, Staples OS: Arthrography of the ankle joint. Problems in diagnosis of acute lateral ligament injuries. Radiology 114:587, 1975.

148. Squire LF: Fundamentals of Roentgenology. Cambridge, Harvard University Press, 1964.

149. Staples OS: Injuries to the medial ligaments of the ankle. J Bone Joint Surg 42A:1287, 1960.

150. Staples OS: Ruptures of the fibular collateral ligaments of the ankle. J Bone Joint Surg 57A:101, 1975.

151. Steel MW, Johnson KA, DeWitz MA, Ilstrup DM: Radiographic measurements of the normal adult foot. Foot Ankle 1:151, 1980.

152. Stepanuk M: Arthrography of the ankle joint in diagnosis of acute ankle sprains. Am Orthop Assoc 76:530/82–536/88, 1977.

153. Stover CN: Recognition and management of soft tissue injuries of the ankle in the athlete. Primary Care 7:183, 1980.

154. Sumner-Smith G (ed): Bone in Clinical Orthopaedics. Philadelphia, Saunders, 1982.

155. Surgical Staff, The Hospital For Sick Children, Toronto: Care for the Injured Child. Baltimore, Williams & Wilkins, 1975.

156. Tansey WJ: Low-intensity x-ray-imaging scope (Lixiscope). Am J Sports Med 9:360, 1981.

157. Tinnemans JGM, Severijnen RSVM: The triple fracture of the distal tibial epiphysis in children. Br J Accident Surg 12:393, 1980.

158. Towbin R, Dunbar JS, Towbin J, Clark R: Teardrop sign. Plain film recognition of ankle effusion. Am J Roengenol 134:985, 1980.

159. Vainionpää S, Kirves P, Laike E: Lateral instability of the ankle and results when treated by the Evans procedure. Am J Sports Med 8:437, 1980.

160. Vuust M: Arthrographic diagnosis of ruptured calcaneofibular ligament. I. A new projection tested on experimental injury postmortem. Acta Radiol Diagn 21:123, 1980.

161. Vuust M, Niedermann B: Arthrographic diagnosis of ruptured calcaneofibular ligament. II. Clinical evaluation of a new method. Acta Radiol Diagn 21:231, 1980.

162. Weseley MS, Koval R, Kleiger B: Roentgen measurement of ankle flexion-extension motion. Clin Orthop Rel Res 65:167, 1969.

163. Wheelhouse WW, Rosenthal RE: Unstable ankle fractures. Comparison of closed versus open treatment. South Med J 73:45, 1980.

164. Williams JGP: Color Atlas of Injury in Sport. Chicago, Year Book Medical, 1981, p. 441.

165. Woods RS: Irreducible dislocation of the ankle-joint. Br J Surg 29:359, 1942.

166. Yablon IG, Heller FG, Shouse L: The key role of the lateral malleolus in displaced fractures of the ankle. J Bone Joint Surg 59A:169, 1977.

167. Yablon IG, Wasilewski S: Isolated fracture of the lateral malleolus. Orthopedics 4:301, 1981.

168. Yde J: The Lauge-Hansen classification of malleolar fractures. Acta Orthop Scand 51:181, 1980.

169. Yde J, Kristensen KD: Inferior tibio-fibular diastasis treated by staple fixation. J Trauma 21:483, 1981.

170. Zatkin H: Trauma to the foot. Semin Roentgenol, 5:419, 1970.

Chapter 5 Overuse Syndromes

Eric L. Hume

The term "overuse" is misleading in that it implies the existence of a standardized definition of normal use; this obviously is not so. Normal use varies considerably from culture to culture, person to person, and even from time to time during the life span of an individual. "Overuse" in the context of this chapter will refer to injury resulting from excessive repetition of a common activity or performance of an activity to which an individual is not accustomed.

Most overuse syndromes involve an anatomic or physiologic weak link that is compromised as a result of repetitive minor insults. Training stresses the body sufficiently to produce gains in strength and stamina, while minimizing the small physical insults that might compromise a weak link. The ability of individuals to tolerate and repair these insults varies considerably. Since few individuals can consistently control their activity level, and even fewer are aware of their tolerance limits, overuse syndromes are commonly encountered in clinical practice but most have no lasting significance. Mechanical trauma is a common precipitating event, although the etiology of these conditions involves anatomic, metabolic, and vascular factors. This text is concerned with traumatic disorders of the ankle, but the discussion that follows will necessarily include nontraumatic factors in an attempt to place the pathophysiology of these bone and soft tissue "injuries" into proper perspective [4]. In order to understand the contribution of these other factors, it is necessary to review the histology, physiology, and mechanical properties of the tissues involved.

Musculotendinous Unit

The musculotendinous unit is best considered in terms of five different areas: tendon, muscle belly, musculotendinous junction, origin, and insertion (Fig. 5.1).

Tendon

Tendon is a relatively simple material. Grossly, it consists of a cord of dense pliable tissue with high tensile strength. Tensile strength is a function of the tendon's cross-sectional area and is estimated to be 15,000 pounds per square inch [26]. Because tendon is noncontractile, it does

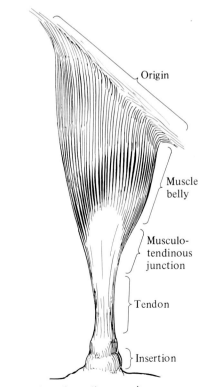

Fig. 5.1. Musculotendinous unit.

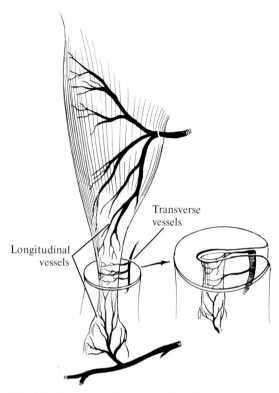

Transverse
vessels

Longitudinal
vessels

Fig. 5.2. Musculotendinous unit blood supply.

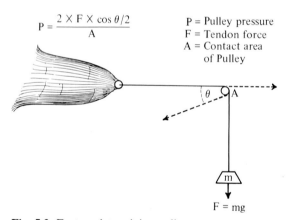

$$P = \frac{2 \times F \times \cos\theta/2}{A}$$

P = Pulley pressure
F = Tendon force
A = Contact area
of Pulley

$$F = mg$$

Fig. 5.3. Factors determining pulley pressure.

no work; therefore, it does not require energy to transfer force and its vascular requirement is minimal.

Histologically, tendon is composed of axially organized bundles of collagen with scattered cells and a sparse capillary network. The tendon's meager vascular supply is proportionate to its minimal basal metabolic requirements. It consists of longitudinal arterioles that course the length

of the tendon as well as arterioles which traverse the mesotenon from surrounding tissues (Fig. 5.2). These mesotenon vessels are especially important at the midportion of long tendons where the longitudinal vessels are far removed from their source.

The meager blood supply of tendon is adequate under normal conditions. With the increased metabolic demand of repair, however, the blood supply of tendon can easily become inadequate, resulting in relative ischemia with delayed or poor healing. The ingrowth of new vessels from the paratenon enhances blood supply, but the process can interfere with normal tendon motion. The opposite is true also; tendon motion may interfere with the ingrowth of required vessels from the paratenon. The long supply line of the longitudinal vessels prohibits significant neovascularization from this source.

The predominance of either of these two modes of neovascularization dictates the type of tendon repair possible, i.e., intratenon or paratenon. Intratenon repair permits good sliding function, but owing to the limited vascular supply available, healing is slow. Paratenon healing occurs by ingrowth of vessels from surrounding tissues and therefore is faster and stronger; tendon excursion, however, may necessarily be restricted by associated paratenon scarring. An increase in either tendon strength or function, therefore, occurs at the other's expense.

Localized pressure can abrade tendon substance as well as impair the local blood supply. This phenomenon occurs commonly where a tendon angles around a bone or retinacular pulley [37]. Decreasing the pulley surface area, increasing the angulation of the tendon, and/or increasing the muscle force all serve to exaggerate local pressure at the tendon-pulley interface (Fig. 5.3). The net result is local inflammation, gradual progressive weakening, or both; the problem becomes clinically evident as either tendonitis or tendon rupture.

Muscle and Musculotendinous Junction

Histologically, muscle is composed of parallel contractile fibers with a fibrous skeleton for attachment at both ends of the structure. Muscle is highly vascularized, commensurate with its rapid metabolic rate during and after contraction.

Hence, vascular supply for healing is abundant (Fig. 5.2).

Muscle force is estimated to be 42 pounds per square inch [14] or roughly 0.3% that of tendon. Muscle cross-sectional area, however, is many times larger than the tendon associated with it. This large cross-sectional area enables more muscle fibers to function in parallel, so that muscle is able to generate a force nearer to the tensile strength of tendon.

Unlike tendon, muscle force is a function of length. At normal resting length, the muscle force occurs predominantly as a result of contractility. Near maximum length, however, the fibrous connective tissue around individual fibers and bundles of fibers contributes a greater percentage of the generated force. Because the resulting force-length relationship is a double-peaked curve, the muscle's ability to resist applied force is a function of the muscle length at the time of injury [14]. The relative content of muscle fiber and fibrous tissue varies from muscle to muscle as well as from point to point along a given muscle belly. In unipenate muscles with long tendon excursions, the muscle fibers terminate rather abruptly on a small area of the tendon. This arrangement predisposes the musculotendinous junction of unipenate muscles to a higher incidence of failure than that of bipenate muscles. These factors determine the location of the weakest area within the muscle belly and musculotendinous junction.

Origin and Insertion

Muscle origin and insertion are considered together because both are transitional areas and therefore possess characteristics of two overlapping tissue types.

The **origin** consists of Sharpey's fibers, which blend intimately with osseous and muscular tissue. The muscle blood supply is excellent and the cross-sectional area is often large. Therefore, this region is strong and heals predictably if injured.

The **insertion** is also composed of Sharpey's fibers. They create a strong transition from tendon to bone, but usually over a smaller area than at the muscle origin. Because of this, the musculotendinous unit is more likely to fail at insertion than at origin. Healing may be prolonged because of the relatively poor vascular supply of tendon and of bone.

Pathophysiology of Failure

McMaster [25] arrived at the following conclusions from experimental studies: (1) muscle can be disrupted by direct/indirect and acute/chronic trauma; (2) overuse phenomena are likely to result in tendon rupture; and (3) acute severe trauma most likely causes musculotendinous junction disruption or avulsion fracture at origin/insertion (Fig. 5.4).

McMaster isolated rabbit femur-gastrocnemius-os calcis preparations and applied tensile force until failure. He found that failure occurred at all sites except within tendon (Fig. 5.4C). This test system however was not physiologic because it eliminated the contractile ability of muscle to resist elongation. Since intentional and reflex muscle activities were eliminated, McMaster overestimated the relative frequency of muscle belly and musculotendinous junction disruption. The important observation he made was that normal tendon did not fail.

McMaster also tested specimens after an area of Achilles tendon had been rendered ischemic

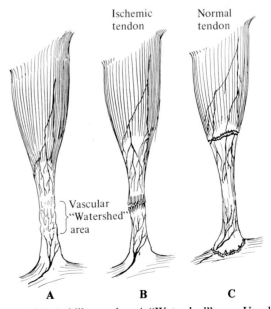

Fig. 5.4. Achilles tendon. A "Watershed" area. Usual sites of rupture of ischemic (**B**) and normal (**C**) tendon.

by circumferential ligatures applied in vivo several weeks before testing. These specimens failed between the ligatures, suggesting that ischemia had weakened tendon tissue (Fig. 5.4B). This observation emphasized the relative importance of vascular supply and, when combined with later microvascular injection studies that demonstrated impoverished or "watershed" areas within certain human tendons, helped to explain many common clinical conditions (Figs. 5.4A and 5.5).

In healthy individuals with normal bone and tendon, the weak link may be muscle belly, origin, insertion, or musculotendinous junction. Avulsion from origin or insertion occurs if the local bony architecture predisposes or if bone is weakened as a result of a disease process. Repeated low-level injury, collagen vascular disease, inflammatory arthritides, and local anatomic conditions that promote ischemia and/or exaggerate local pressure will decrease tendon strength and predispose to tendon rupture.

Biomechanical Considerations

The musculotendinous units about the ankle add dynamic stability to the static stability created by the osseous configuration and collateral ligaments. The musculotendinous unit has the intermittent requirement of locomotion superimposed upon its continuous reflex activity for balance. Depending on the lever arm and the specific function of the musculotendinous unit, forces equivalent to several times body weight may be generated within a particular unit.

Musculotendinous units can be considered in two groups when discussing dynamic ankle stability. The gastrocnemius-soleus complex and the tibialis anterior muscle control ankle motion in the sagittal plane. The tibialis anterior and posterior muscles on the medial side and the peroneal muscles on the lateral side contribute to frontal plane stability of the ankle and hindfoot [37].

During locomotion, the gastrocnemius-soleus has the largest power requirement of all the musculotendinous units about the ankle. The ratio of the lever arm over which gravity acts to the lever arm over which the gastrocnemius-soleus group functions is approximately 2.5:1 (Fig. 5.6A). Therefore, a simple toe raise requires the development of tension within the Achilles ten-

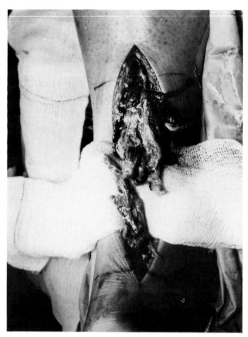

Fig. 5.5. Achilles tendon rupture in the "watershed" area. Patient was a 42-year-old male with a 6-month history of Achilles tendon pain on activity.

don equivalent to 2.5 times body weight. This is multiplied several times in a sprinter accelerating out of the blocks or in a dancer jumping several feet.

The tibialis anterior, however, simply supports the forefoot during swing phase and decelerates the body at heel strike, with a mechanical advantage of 1:1 (Fig. 5.6B). This function is obviously less demanding than that imposed on the gastrocnemius-soleus group. The peronei (Fig. 5.6C) and both tibialis muscles (Fig. 5.6D) in the frontal plane generate small forces to control inversion-eversion, with mechanical advantage also of approximately 1:1 at the subtalar joint. Therefore, on the basis of mechanical advantage and locomotion requirements, the gastrocnemius-soleus complex must generate the greatest force.

Clinical Syndromes and Their Treatment

Gastrocnemius-Soleus/Tendo Achilles

The soleus muscle originates from the proximal one-third of the fibula and tibia as a dense apo-

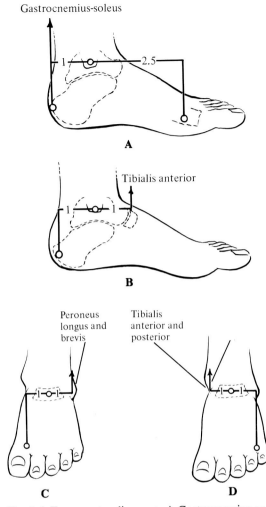

Gastrocnemius-soleus

A

Tibialis anterior

B

Peroneus longus and brevis

Tibialis anterior and posterior

C   **D**

Fig. 5.6. Force vector diagrams. **A** Gastrocnemius-soleus, **B** Tibialis anterior. **C** Peroneus longus and brevis. **D** Tibialis anterior and posterior.

neurosis. The gastrocnemius muscle arises from a medial and a lateral head on the femoral condyles. The two muscles share a common tendon, the tendo Achilles, which has a broad insertion onto the posterior aspect of the calcaneus. The anatomy permits two large muscles to act where large forces are required. The broad area of origin and insertion makes failure at these sites very uncommon.

Brewer [4] noted that the musculotendinous units most commonly injured have three characteristics: (1) the musculotendinous unit in question crosses two joints; (2) other musculotendinous units function at the same joints; and (3) several other musculotendinous units contribute

to provide a full range of joint motion. Of the musculotendinous units functioning about the ankle, these characteristics are true only for the gastrocnemius-soleus unit.

A vascular "watershed" area is present in the tendo Achilles approximately 4.5 cm proximal to the calcaneus [36]. The poor local vascularity would be expected to render this area susceptible to chronic inflammation (Fig. 5.4A) [13] and ultimately rupture (Figs. 5.4B and 5.5) [6,7]. This expectation agrees with clinical experience. Rupture of the tendo Achilles in a healthy individual without prior symptoms is extremely rare. However, rupture at this site in older patients or after a significant period of prodromal pain is not uncommon [4,11].

Achilles tendonitis presents as pain exacerbated by activity. The pain is often in the heel or just proximal to it, with local tenderness 3–5 cm above the calcaneus. Included in the differential diagnosis is retrocalcaneal bursitis; this tenderness, however, is usually localized anterior to the tendo Achilles [6]. Although steroid injection is helpful for bursitis, many authors now believe that local steroids have no place in the treatment of Achilles tendonitis [7,13]. Rather, a trial of rest, oral antiinflammatory agents, and stretching is preferred. Improvement may be seen up to 8 weeks later. If nodular or fusiform swelling develops, this suggests the occurrence of a partial tear and a period of prolonged rest or early surgical exploration is recommended [6]. Although equinus casting is adequate treatment for most individuals with partial rupture [11], surgical exploration is frequently advisable for competitive athletes and dancers [7,37]. In a recent study, it was noted that no dancer returned to the profession once actual rupture had occurred [28]. At surgery, the inflamed peritendineum and nodules should be removed, and partial tears should be repaired by suture. The removal of peritendineum is important to facilitate good vascular ingrowth and strong healing.

Tendo Achilles rupture is frequently overlooked initially. The patient, often a middle-aged male, frequently hears a "pop" but has relatively little pain and walks after the rupture. The examiner can usually palpate a gap in the tendo Achilles and can usually demonstrate decreased plantarflexion actively or passively with calf squeeze (Thompson test) [40]. This test is especially useful in differentiating plantaris tendon rupture from tendo Achilles rupture. Both conditions can present with a similar history, but with plantaris rupture the Thompson test evokes a normal plantarflexion response. Distinction between these two entities is important since tendo Achilles rupture will require specific treatment, but plantaris tendon rupture only requires symptomatic treatment until the acute symptoms subside. Neither long-term symptoms nor disability have been described following plantaris rupture.

Achilles tendon rupture should be treated with casting in equinus with or without surgical repair, depending on the age, general medical condition, and expected functional capacity of the patient. Closed treatment by immobilization in equinus position may leave the patient with impaired strength and endurance and is associated with a significant incidence of rerupture [17,32]. Operative treatment incurs the risk of delayed skin healing and wound breakdown [32]. A technique of percutaneous repair has been described also [24].

Generally, sedentary individuals can be satisfactorily treated by immobilization alone, whereas healthy active individuals are best treated by operative repair [17,18,32,33]. Conflicting results are described in the literature, and some series suggest no difference in functional results or major complication rates between closed vs. open treatment methods [20,21,29]. Percutaneous repair is allegedly applicable to all age groups if the technique can be satisfactorily mastered. It apparently avoids the major complications of both open and closed techniques [12,24].

Closed Treatment

Lea and Smith [20,21] treated all ruptures of the Achilles tendon with a below-knee cast and reported good functional results. Rerupture occurred in seven of 65 patients; four of these patients, however, had only been immobilized for 6 weeks [20].

In **closed treatment**, the patient sits on the edge of the examining table with his foot in a relaxed equinus position. Flexing the knee to 90° relaxes the gastrocnemius muscle. A short leg cast with walking heel is applied. Full weight-bearing ambulation is permitted as soon as the plaster is dry. Lea and Smith [20,21] emphasized the importance of 8 weeks of cast immobilization,

because in their experience the rerupture rate was higher when immobilization was limited to 6 weeks. After cast removal, a 1-in. heel lift is prescribed and active gastrocnemius exercises are performed for 4 more weeks. Full activity is allowed at 24 weeks.

Open Repair

The patient is placed in a prone position with a pneumatic tourniquet about the proximal thigh [33]. A 15-cm incision is made along the medial edge of the Achilles tendon; distally, the incision is curved slightly anterior to avoid placing the scar directly over the prominence of the os calcis. Full thickness skin and subcutaneous flaps are created. The tendo Achilles sheath is split longitudinally. The plantaris tendon is identified and divided as far proximally as possible. Using a Gallie needle, the plantaris tendon is woven first medial to lateral in the proximal portion of the Achilles tendon, then lateral to medial in the distal portion; this is repeated as many times as the length of tendon will permit. The anastomosis site is then reinforced with nonabsorbable sutures, as are the areas of plantaris-Achilles tendon contact (Fig. 5.7A). If the plantaris tendon

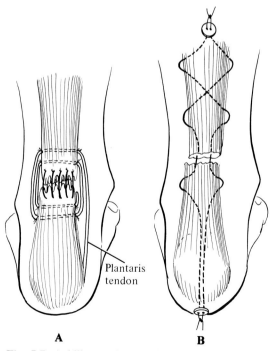

Plantaris tendon

A   **B**

Fig. 5.7. Achilles tendon repair (after Quigley [33]). **A** With plantaris tendon. **B** With Bunnell suture.

is not available (20% congenital absence), a wire Bunnell pull-out suture can be used instead (Fig. 5.7B). The sheath of the Achilles tendon should be closed if possible. Postoperatively, the patient is immobilized in an above-knee cast with the ankle in equinus and the knee in 30° of flexion. At 4 weeks, this is changed to a short leg cast with the ankle in equinus. Immobilization is discontinued at 6 weeks and heel lifts of decreasing height are prescribed: 19 mm the first week; 13 mm the second week; and 6 mm the third week. At 3 months following surgery, backward stair walking and toe circles are initiated.

Lindholm [23] has described methods of reinforcing the acute repair with gastrocnemius fascia. He initially utilized a central flap but discovered a repair to be necrotic when he explored it for rerupture. He subsequently recommended that small medial and lateral flaps be rotated down over the repair.

Bosworth [3] used gastrocnemius fascia and Bugg and Boyd [5] used fascia lata and a modified Bunnell suture to bridge a gap when chronic unrecognized rupture was associated with gastrocnemius-soleus muscle contracture. The approach and aftercare are similar to those described for acute ruptures.

Percutaneous Repair

The procedure is performed in the prone position (Fig. 5.8) [24]. Local, regional, or general anesthesia can be used. A tourniquet is not usually employed. Two stab incisions, one medial and one lateral, are placed 2.5 cm proximal to the site of rupture. A heavy, nonabsorbable suture on a Keith needle is then passed transversely through the lateral stab incision to penetrate the center of the tendon and emerge in the medial stab incision (Fig. 5.8A). A second Keith needle is then applied to the free end of the suture and the proximal stump is traversed at 45° angles from both medial and lateral sides (Fig. 5.8B). At the sites of needle penetration, additional medial and lateral stab incisions are made. A curved needle is used to advance the lateral suture to the level of the calcaneal tendon stump where a fifth stab incision is made (Fig. 5.8C). The curved needle is then replaced with a Keith needle to traverse the distal stump from lateral to medial at a level 1.2 cm distal to the rupture

gap. The sixth stab incision is placed at this site (Fig. 5.8D). A curved needle is then used to advance the same end of the suture proximally to the middle of the medial stab incisions (Fig. 5.8E), where the suture is tightened and tied (Fig. 5.8F). At each of the six stab wounds, care is taken to blindly dissect the subcutaneous tissue free from the sheath without cutting the sheath or tendon. This prevents soft tissue entrapment when passing and tightening the suture. The stab wounds are not approximated. A non-weight-bearing short leg cast is applied with the ankle in equinus position. At 4 weeks, a heel-bearing below-knee cast is applied and maintained for 4 additional weeks.

Peroneal Muscles

The peroneus brevis originates from the distal two-thirds of the fibula and inserts on the base of the fifth metatarsal. The peroneus longus originates from the lateral tibial condyle and proximal two-thirds of the fibula and inserts on the plantar aspect of the first metatarsal base and adjacent cuneiform. Both tendons run through a pulley mechanism behind the distal fibula where they undergo an acute change in direction (Fig. 1.14). The walls of the pulley tunnel are (1) the lateral malleolus, anteriorly and superiorly; (2) the superior and inferior peroneal retinacula, laterally; and (3) the fibulocalcaneal ligament, medially.

Theoretically, the peroneal tendons should be susceptible to tendinitis and rupture within this pulley mechanism. Although tendinitis does occur at this level, it is uncommon. Rupture at this site also is rare, probably because these tendons are characterized by relatively low force transmission; or perhaps single tendon rupture occurs but is overlooked because the remaining peroneal musculotendinous unit can perform the eversion function.

Peroneal rupture through tendon or muscle belly is a rare occurrence [1,9,37]. The weak link of the peroneal system seems to be the osseous architecture at the insertion of the peroneus brevis, such that the usual mode of failure is avulsion fracture at this site. Another failure mode is pulley disruption, which allows peroneal tendon subluxation or dislocation. This is a relatively rare occurrence to be considered in the differential diagnosis of lateral ankle sprain.

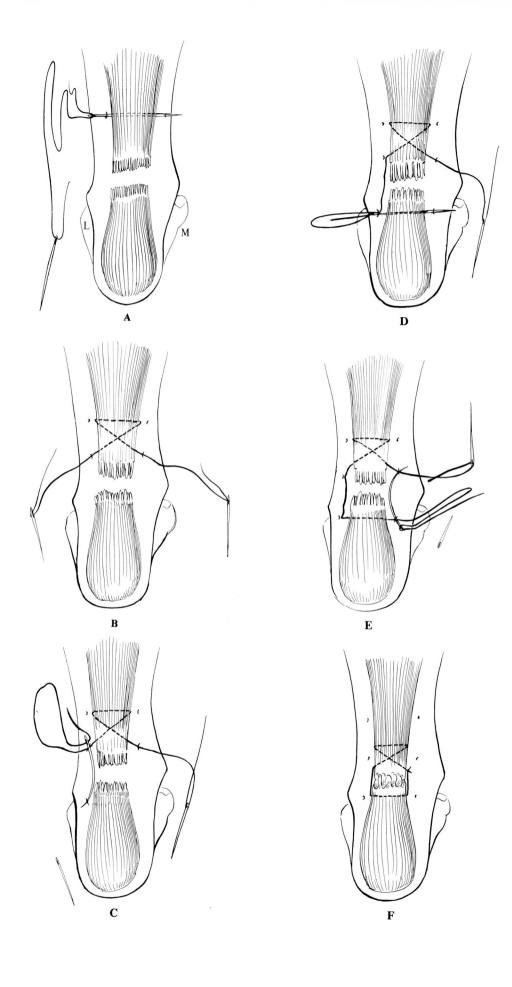

A

B

C

D

E

F

L   M

Tibialis Anterior

The tibialis anterior muscle originates from the proximal two-thirds of the tibia, the lateral tibial condyle, and the interosseous membrane. It pursues an essentially straight course under the superior extensor retinaculum to the medial side of the foot where it inserts on the navicular, first metatarsal base, and first cuneiform. Its straight course and minimal mechanical demands are consistent with its rare involvement by inflammation or rupture. When it does occur, rupture generally involves older patients and symptoms frequently mimic radiculopathy with foot drop [10,27]. Avulsion fracture at its insertion can occur. Most of these injuries, however, can be adequately treated by immobilization. If the avulsed fragment is displaced more than 5 mm, surgical reduction and fixation are recommended [37].

Toe Extensors

The extensor digitorum longus originates from the lateral tibial condyle and from the proximal fibula and interosseous membrane in continuity with the extensor hallucis longus. Together, these tendons pass distally under the extensor retinaculum. The little force they generate and the minimal physical disability associated with rupture probably explain why rupture is not a significant clinical problem. Tendinitis mimicking compartment syndrome has been described but is unusual. "Lace bite" or pain from local pressure of foot wear is more common. This entity comprises extensor synovitis, anterior tibial neuritis, or a combination of both. Pain may be severe enough to mimic an anterior compartment syndrome [22]. This is an excellent example of a functionally reduced pulley area caused by shoelaces that localize pressure onto the dorsum of the foot and ankle (Fig. 5.9B) rather than distributing it over the gradual curve normally created by the retinaculum (Fig. 5.9A). Treatment consists primarily of mechanical measures to better distribute the pressure in this area, although

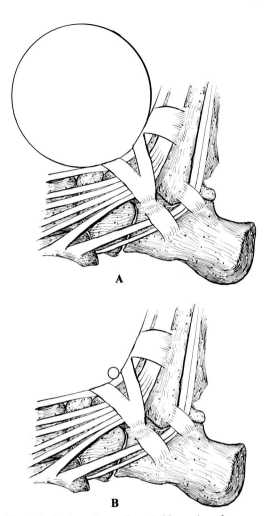

Fig. 5.9. Retinacular pulley. **A** Normal surface area. **B** Pulley surface area reduced by tight shoelaces.

a period of rest and antiinflammatory agents may be indicated acutely. Retinaculum disruption has been described [2] but is uncommon.

Toe Flexors

The flexor hallucis longus originates from the distal two-thirds of the fibula and interosseous septum. It joins the flexor digitorum longus to pass through the tarsal tunnel. The pulley mechanism at this site puts the flexor hallucis longus at risk if high physical demands are imposed.

In classical ballet, which requires women to dance "on pointe," a high force is generated within the flexor hallucis longus to accomplish

---

◁

Fig. 5.8. Percutaneous repair (after Ma and Griffith [24]).

and maintain toe raise. As one might expect, flexor hallucis tendonitis is a significant problem in this group of patients. It presents as pain behind the medial malleolus, with radiation into the plantar aspect of the foot and toes; it may radiate proximally into the leg as well [15]. Triggering of the hallux is a frequent early complaint [34]. Disability from tendinitis, triggering, and potential rupture demands early surgical exploration in professional dancers. Early surgery has allowed some patients to return to dancing. Release of the laciniate ligament usually demonstrates fusiform swelling suggestive of disruption of the central fibers of the flexor hallucis longus [35]. Release of the ligament seems to be adequate treatment. Several bilateral cases have been described. A traumatic case of rupture has been reported [19].

Tibialis Posterior

This musculotendinous unit arises from the interosseous membrane, tibia, and fibula and travels posterior to the medial malleolus to insert on the navicular, cuneiform, and bases of the second, third, and fourth metatarsals. Especially in planovalgus feet is a significant pulley pressure generated. The associated tenosynovitis is most common in patients 40 to 60 years of age. Treatment includes antiinflammatory agents and medial plantar wedges [37] to reduce the tendon forces generated. Local steroids should be used with caution since rupture of this tendon has been described under these circumstances. Systemic disease must also be considered [30].

Bone

According to Wolff's law, bone responds by remodeling to best resist applied stress. Overuse syndromes result when the stress occurs in excess of the bone's remodeling ability.

Anterior ankle joint osteophytes are probably a response to repeated forced ankle plantar- and dorsiflexion [15,28,31,38]. Bone overgrowth (Fig. 5.10) at the site of impingement creates osteophytes. These osteophytes predispose to further impingement and painful inflammation ensues. An alternative explanation is that these osteophytes are caused by capsular traction and subperiosteal disruption, secondary to forced plantar- or dorsiflexion of the ankle. Excision of osteophytes that cause recurrent symptoms and restrict motion offers significant relief in this entity [38].

Stress fractures are more obviously an overuse phenomenon [38]. Repeated microfractures can be created at a rate that exceeds repair. The initial symptom is pain, but if overuse continues the ultimate outcome is fracture. This is analogous to the tendinitis and rupture sequence encountered in the musculotendinous unit. Theoretically, any bone can be involved. The most common sites about the ankle are the tibia, metatarsals (especially the second), and less commonly the fibula (Fig. 5.11) and neck of the talus. Stress fractures present as discomfort associated with activity. There is usually local tenderness. Radiographs will not be positive for 2 to 3 weeks, although a bone scan will frequently be positive within 2 to 5 days of onset of symptoms. Treat-

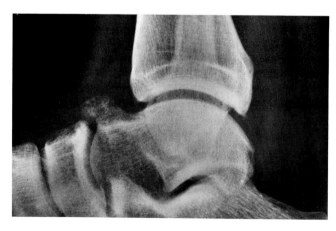

Fig. 5.10. Anterior ankle joint osteophyte associated with impingement syndrome.

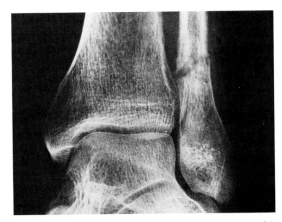

Fig. 5.11. Stress fracture of the distal fibula in an elderly patient, who had been placed on a graduated walking program by his cardiologist.

ment is symptomatic and should include at least temporary cessation of the offending activity [8,39].

References

1. Abraham E, Stirnaman JG: Neglected rupture of the peroneal tendons causing recurrent sprains of the ankle. J Bone Joint Surg 61A:1247, 1979.
2. Akhtar M, Levine J: Dislocation of extensor digitorum longus tendons after spontaneous rupture of the inferior retinaculum of the ankle. J Bone Joint Surg 62A:1210, 1980.
3. Bosworth DM: Repair of defects in the tendo Achilles. J Bone Joint Surg 38A:111, 1956.
4. Brewer BJ: Mechanism of injury to the musculotendinous unit. Instructional Course Lectures. Am Acad Orthop Surg 17:354, 1960.
5. Bugg EI Jr, Boyd BM: Repair of neglected rupture or laceration of the Achilles tendon. Clin Orthop Rel Res 56:173, 1968.
6. Clancy WG: Runners' injuries. II. Am J Sports Med 8:287, 1980.
7. Clancy WG, Neidhart D, Brand RL: Achilles tendonitis in runners. A report of 5 cases. Am J Sports Med 4:46, 1976.
8. Daffner RH, Martinez S, Gehweiler JA: Stress fractures in runners. JAMA 247:1039, 1982.
9. Davies JAK: Peroneal compartment syndrome secondary to rupture of the peroneus longus. J Bone Joint Surg 61A:783, 1979.
10. Dooley BJ, Kudelka P, Menelaus MB: Subcutaneous rupture of the tendon of the tibialis anterior. J Bone Joint Surg 62B:471, 1980.
11. Fox JM, Blayina ME, Jobe FW, Kerlan RK, Carter VS, Shields CL, Carlson GJ: Degeneration and rupture of the Achilles tendon. Clin Ortho Rel Res 107:221, 1975.
12. Good R, Brumback R: Personal communication, 1982.
13. Gould N, Korson R: Stenosing tenosynovitis of the pseudosheath of the tendo Achilles. Foot Ankle 1:179, 1980.
14. Guyton AC: Textbook of Medical Physiology. Philadelphia, Saunders, 1971, pp. 85, 89.
15. Hamilton WG: Tendonitis about the ankle joint in classical ballet dancers. Am J Sports Med 5:84, 1977.
16. Hovelius L, Palmgren H: Laceration of tibial tendons and vessels in ice hockey players. Am J Sports Med 7:297, 1979.
17. Inglis AE, Scott WN, Sculco TP, Patterson AH: Ruptures of tendo Achilles. J Bone Joint Surg 58A:990, 1976.
18. Jacobs D, Martens M, VanAudekercke R, Mulier JC: Comparison of conservative and operative treatment of Achilles tendon rupture. Am J Sports Med 6:107, 1978.
19. Krackow KA: Acute traumatic rupture of flexor hallucis longus tendon. Clin Orthop Rel Res 150:261, 1980.
20. Lea RB, Smith L: Nonsurgical treatment of tendo Achilles rupture. J Bone Joint Surg 54A:1398, 1972.
21. Lea RB, Smith L: Rupture of the Achilles tendon—nonsurgical treatment. Clin Orthop Rel Res 60:115, 1968.
22. Lindenbaum BL: Ski boot compression syndrome. Clin Orthop Rel Res 140:109, 1979.
23. Lindholm Å: A new method of operation in subcutaneous rupture of the Achilles tendon. Acta Chir Scand 117:261, 1959.
24. Ma GWC, Griffith TG: Percutaneous repair of acute closed ruptured tendo calcaneus. Clin Orthop Rel Res 128:247, 1977.
25. McMaster PE: Tendon and muscle ruptures. J Bone Joint Surg 15:705, 1933.
26. Mears DC: Materials in Orthopaedic Surgery. Baltimore, Williams & Wilkins, 1979.
27. Meyn MA: Closed rupture of the anterior tibial tendon. Clin Orthop Rel Res 113:154, 1975.
28. Miller EH, Schneider HJ, Bronson JL, McLain D: A new consideration in athletic injuries: The classical ballet dancer. Clin Orthop Rel Res 111:181, 1975.
29. Nistor L: Surgical and nonsurgical treatment of Achilles tendon rupture. J Bone Joint Surg 63A:394, 1981.
30. Norris SH, Mankin HJ: Chronic tenosynovitis of the posterior tibial tendon with new bone formation. J Bone Joint Surg 60B:523, 1978.
31. Parkes JC, Hamilton WG, Patterson AH, Rawles JG Jr: The anterior impingement syndrome of the ankle. J Trauma 20:895, 1980.
32. Percy EC, Conochu LB: The surgical treatment of ruptured tendo Achilles. Am J Sports Med 6:132, 1978.
33. Quigley TB, Scheller AD: Surgical repair of the ruptured Achilles tendon. Am J Sports Med 8:244, 1980.

34. Quirk RP: Patterns of injury in ballet dancers. J Bone Joint Surg 58B:259, 1976.

35. Sammareo GJ, Miller EH: Partial rupture of flexor hallucis longus tendon in classical ballet dancers. J Bone Joint Surg 61A:149, 1979.

36. Schatzker J, Branemark P: Intravital observations on the microvascular anatomy and microcirculation of the tendon. Acta Orthop Scand (Suppl) 126:1, 1969.

37. Scheller AD, Kasser JR, Quigley TB: Tendon injuries about the ankle. Orthop Clin North Am 11:801, 1980.

38. Slocum DB: Overuse syndromes of the lower leg and foot in athletes. Instructional Course. Am Acad Orthop Surg 17:359, 1960.

39. Stanitski CL, McMaster JH, Scranton PE: On the nature of stress fractures. Am J Sports Med 6:391, 1978.

40. Thompson TC: A test for rupture of the tendo Achilles. Acta Orthop Scand 32:460, 1962.

Chapter 6   Malleolar Fractures and Dislocations of the Ankle

William C. Hamilton

Ankle injuries are usually the result of indirect or torsional violence [5,31,32,41] which distorts the normal relationship between the talus and the tibiofibular mortise. Most commonly, the foot is fixed and the injury is sustained as a result of the tibiofibular mortise moving against the talus [77,83]. Most authors, however, have found it more convenient to speak in terms of motion of the talus with respect to the tibiofibular mortise [44]; this custom shall be observed in this text.

The talus is the key to understanding ankle fractures. Every fractured malleolus is either pushed off or pulled off by the talus undergoing pathologic motion (Fig. 6.1) [66,101]. Pathologic talar motion can be comprised of entirely unphysiologic motion, an excessive degree of motion in a physiologic plane, or a combination of both. The ankle can tolerate large loads in compression [34], but the forces required to produce injuries by rotation are small [34,55]. This explains how severe ankle injuries may sometimes result from apparently trivial violence [58,90,97,98,103].

Prior to the 18th century, serious ankle injuries were regarded as dislocations without mention of associated fractures [6]. Petit, in 1723, 172 years before the advent of radiography, postulated that luxations could only arise if one or both malleoli were fractured [49,59,80,91]. We now know that, due to the efficiency of the mortise, subluxation or dislocation of the ankle without fracture is quite rare [22,40,41,92]. In fact, the present tendency is to concentrate on the fractures, sometimes at the exclusion of the associated soft tissue disruption [6]. This represents a serious error, however. By virtue of its design, the ankle has minimal inherent stability and relies heavily on ligaments to bind the bony structures in a stable relationship. Also, the complicated patterns of ankle injury can only be properly understood if they are analyzed in light of associated ligament injuries [8]. Ligament injuries, therefore, are just as important as fractures and deserve the same degree of careful attention for diagnosis and treatment [44,79,83,90].

Most indirect ankle fractures have associated ligament injury of some degree [15], but ligament injury commonly exists without fracture [44]. Although fractures are easily demonstrated on radiographs, ligament injuries are more subtle [44], and their existence must often be inferred by less precise means, such as mechanism of injury and/or physical findings [6]. Neer [71] pointed out that the ankle was a closed circle analogous to the pelvis (Fig. 6.2), such that disruption at one site frequently produces pathology

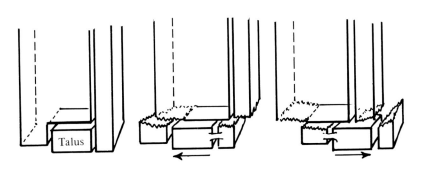

Fig. 6.1. All (indirect) malleolar fractures are produced by the talus.

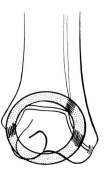

Fig. 6.2. The tibia, fibula, talus, and connecting ligaments form a closed circle—interruption at one site is usually associated with remote injury [71].

Table 6.1. Classification of Ankle Fractures.

Anatomic
Unimalleolar
Bimalleolar
Trimalleolar

Ashhurst and Brömer
External rotation
Abduction
Adduction
Compression

Lauge-Hansen
Supination-Eversion (external rotation)
Pronation-Eversion (external rotation)
Supination-Adduction
Pronation-Abduction
Pronation-Dorsiflexion

at a distance. As a general rule, one can assume that the amount of ligament damage is always greater than routine radiographs suggest [34,55]. An apparently "minor fracture" that represents the origin or insertion of a critical ligament can significantly jeopardize the effect of that ligament on ankle function [44,53,95].

In the treatment of ankle injuries, the commonest errors are the result of nondiagnosis or faulty assessment of ligament lesions [90]. If it were not for ligament injury, treatment of malleolar fractures would be greatly simplified [89]. Ankle fractures, therefore, cannot be studied or treated out of context, but rather must be viewed as part of an injury complex [78,90,99] whose degree of severity may range from mild, transient subluxation to frank, complete, and fixed dislocation of the tibiotalar, tibiofibular, and/or talofibular joints. The resultant injury will be a function of the starting position of the foot, the direction and degree of applied forces, and the relative resistance of the joint structures [44].

Classification of Ankle Fractures

To facilitate patient care, as well as comparison and communication among clinicians, it is essential that some form of classification system be available (Table 6.1). Attempts at classification based on morbid radiographic anatomy—unimalleolar, bimalleolar, and trimalleolar [20, 31,41,72,80,91,94,97]—are notoriously inaccurate because they fail to consider the degree of displacement or associated ligament damage [28,62,95].

Classification of fractures according to mechanism provides much more helpful information. Along these lines, the first comprehensive classification of ankle injuries was proposed by Ashhurst and Bromer in 1922 [3]. Their effort marked the first significant American contribution to the study of traumatic ankle pathology [26]. In an extensive treatise, based on experimental cadaver and radiographic studies, Ashhurst and Bromer concluded that ankle fractures could be caused by four different mechanisms: external rotation, abduction, adduction, and compression. They also attempted to grade injuries according to severity, depending on the number of malleoli involved. Unfortunately Ashhurst and Bromer did not place significant emphasis on associated soft tissue damage [26,28,41].

Lauge-Hansen, in a series of articles initiated in 1948 [49–53], presented a more complete classification system that placed appropriate emphasis on concomitant ligamentous injuries. The principles were similar to those employed by Ashhurst and Bromer [3], but the terminology was different and, unfortunately, confusing at times. Like Ashhurst and Bromer, Lauge-Hansen's conclusions were also based on experimental production of fractures in cadaver limbs [50,53]. He classified ankle fractures into five categories, using a *dual designation* where the first word of the designation referred to the *position of the foot at the moment of injury* and the second word detailed the *specific direction of talar motion*

[50]. Differentiation was based primarily on the appearance and location of the fibular fracture [51]. Lauge-Hansen's scheme distinguished between external rotation fractures that occurred when the foot was supinated and those that occurred when the foot was pronated. It included the pronation and supination fractures of Ashhurst and Bromer, and added a fifth type, pronation-dorsiflexion, to explain fractures resulting primarily from axial compression forces.

Unfortunately, Lauge-Hansen used the term "eversion" inappropriately to signify external rotation of the talus with respect to the tibia [11,62]. Although his true intention was later clarified by Kristensen [46,47], this misnomer continues to represent a source of confusion to many clinicians, who cannot understand how an ankle can be supinated and everted simultaneously.

Lauge-Hansen identified the specific sequence of bone and ligament injury and different stages of severity for each mechanism. With this information, it became possible to analyze radiographs of an injured ankle and infer what ligament injuries had occurred earlier in the sequence [2, 11,23,62,83,95]. As demonstrated by Grath [30], the collateral ligaments as well as those of the syndesmosis have a definite but variable "successive protective function"; each ligament assumes its protective task before its predecessor has failed completely, so that there is frequently some anatomic overlap between one stage of injury and another. In terms of functionally significant disruption, however, the identification of different stages has proved valid.

Lauge-Hansen believed that an exact "genetic" roentgenographic diagnosis permitted more accurate reduction by retracing the path of the original injury [51,53]. Others have also found this to be true [4,23,46,62].

The Lauge-Hansen classification is the most comprehensive and accurate scheme available today [11,14,23,62,79,90,95,103,104]. It permits one to categorize well over 95% of all indirect ankle injuries [4,11,21,51,56,63,95,103], and to utilize radiographic fracture patterns to recognize occult ligament injuries [83]. It is also helpful as an investigative tool to group fractures and facilitate comparison between various forms of treatment [103]. This system, with certain exceptions and variations to be noted, will be utilized throughout this text.

The Danis-Weber classification system, based on the appearance and location of the fibular fracture (Fig. 6.3), is a helpful teaching model

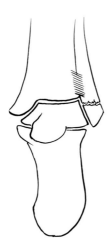 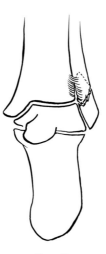 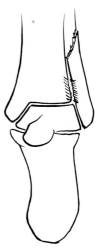

Type A	Type B	Type C
Transverse, avulsion fracture of lateral malleolus at or below the level of the ankle joint (corresponds to the supination-adduction mechanism of Lauge-Hansen).	Spiral fracture of the lateral malleolus at the level of the tibial plafond (corresponds to the supination-external rotation and pronation-abduction mechanisms of Lauge-Hansen.	Fracture of the fibula above the syndesmosis associated with rupture of the tibiofibular ligaments (corresponds to the pronation-external rotation mechanism of Lauge-Hansen).

Fig. 6.3. Danis-Weber classification [70,100].

[35,36,70,100]. It simplifies classification by fibular fracture type [56], but unlike the Lauge-Hansen scheme, it does not permit categorization of injuries according to severity. Although it provides a statistical incidence of syndesmosis injury for each fracture type, this scheme does not permit one to predict the degree of such injury in any given situation.

Instability

Fracture stability, in general, is a function of soft tissue integrity [43]. An ankle fracture can be considered stable if it is not significantly displaced and, with minimal or no protection, is not likely to displace during the period of observation. The prognosis for complete pain relief and functional recovery should be excellent. At the other extreme, a displaced ankle fracture with extensive soft tissue disruption that is difficult to reduce or maintain is obviously unstable [91].

It is with the intermediate degrees of instability that assessment and treatment become difficult [91]. It cannot be overemphasized that radiographs of a traumatized ankle demonstrate the injury at only one point in time. The apparent degree of displacement should be regarded as the minimum deformity possible, with the understanding that the ankle at the moment of injury may have been characterized by much more (but never less) displacement [14,40,45]. With this in mind, even minimally displaced fractures will be approached with considerable caution.

In general, fracture of a single malleolus, without soft tissue tenderness or swelling of the opposite malleolar region, can tentatively be considered stable [18,33,41,45,66,71], and treatment is simplified. If, however, there are symptoms or findings related to two different malleolar regions, the injury must be considered at least potentially unstable and treated more aggressively [45]. Stress radiographs performed with adequate anesthesia will often be revealing in this latter situation (Fig. 6.4) [60,71,78].

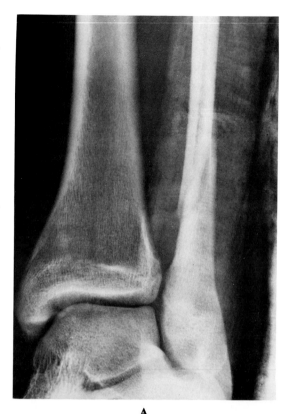

A

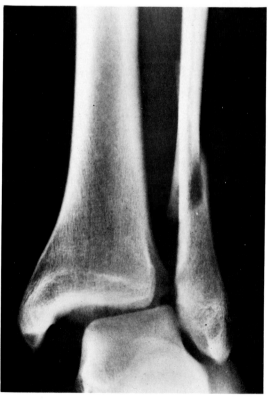

B

▷

Fig. 6.4. A Spiral supramalleolar fracture of fibula associated with medial ankle tenderness. **B** Radiograph obtained during application of external rotation stress, demonstrating obvious deltoid ligament insufficiency.

The Lauge-Hansen classification system [50,53], to be described in subsequent chapters, provides a means to predict associated ligament damage and facilitates estimation of relative fracture stability.

Diastasis

Varying degrees of injury to the tibiofibular ligaments may occur in association with malleolar fractures or collateral ligament injuries. This pathologic condition has engendered the use of numerous descriptive terms, including the following:

Diastasis (total, ligamentous, partial, anterior, intraosseous)
Widening of the syndesmosis
Widening of the mortise (or malleolar fork)
Rupture of the syndesmosis
Lateral instability of the ankle
Sprung mortise

These terms are frequently confusing and have unfortunately been utilized in the literature for many years without standardized definitions.

Tibiofibular Diastasis

Tibiofibular diastasis has been regarded by some (but not all) authors to indicate lateral translation of the fibula with respect to the tibia that can be demonstrated on radiographs [10,29,41, 44,95]. By strict definition, however, distal tibiofibular diastasis only implies separation of the distal tibia and fibula. It does not describe the degree of separation or, for that matter, the direction that the tibia and fibula pursue with respect to one another. Technically, it does not even apply to complete rupture of all the tibiofibular ligaments, if the tibia and fibula, by any chance, happen to resume their normal relationship after injury. For our purposes, we shall accept the definition of Bonnin that diastasis involves "any degree of separation of the tibia from the fibula at the lower tibiofibular joint beyond the normal elasticity of the ligaments" [7].

Total diastasis (ligamentous diastasis, classical diastasis) will be reserved for that condition characterized by *complete* distal tibiofibular ligamentous violation with *displacement* or the *potential for displacement* of the entire distal fibula with respect to the fibular incisura of the tibia (Fig. 6.5A). This implies complete rupture of the anterior inferior tibiofibular ligament, posterior inferior tibiofibular ligament, inferior transverse tibiofibular ligament, and interosseous ligament [17,38,69,98] (in association with medial ankle instability) (Fig. 6.5B) [16,30,92]. It represents a serious and relatively uncommon degree of injury. Total diastasis, in this context, corresponds to "diastasis of the third degree" as defined by Bonnin.

Lesser degrees of syndesmosis injury may permit excessive external rotation of the fibula with respect to the tibia without vertical or horizontal translation. This occurs as a result of disruption of the anterior inferior tibiofibular ligament [80]. Since the remaining tibiofibular ligaments are situated posterior to the axis of fibular rotation, they are not very effective in limiting external rotation of this bone. This situation, whereby the anterior borders of the distal tibia and fibula separate or have the potential to separate, has been appropriately referred to as **anterior diastasis** or **widening of the anterior syndesmosis** (Fig. 6.7) [29,69]. The term "partial diastasis" has little value since it does not imply direction or degree. It is frequently used to refer to anterior inferior tibiofibular ligament insufficiency, but for this condition, "anterior diastasis" is a more descriptive and appropriate designation.

Widening of the syndesmosis implies "ligamentous tibiofibular diastasis," and unfortunately these two terms are sometimes used interchangeably. "Widening of the syndesmosis," however, inadvertently suggests that the tibiofibular distortion is limited to lateral displacement of the fibula with respect to the tibia—ignoring the possibility of displacement in other planes. "Widening of the syndesmosis" is also easily confused with "widening of the malleolar fork (or mortise)." To appreciate the subtle distinction between these two terms, it is necessary to realize that the tibiofibular syndesmosis and the ankle mortise are not one and the same. (Fig. 6.8). The tibiofibular syndesmosis is but one component of the ankle mortise; the mortise may fail (widen) at the syndesmosis or at another site.

Complete ligamentous diastasis with widening of the syndesmosis will permit widening of the mortise (Fig. 6.5). Widening of the mortise, how-

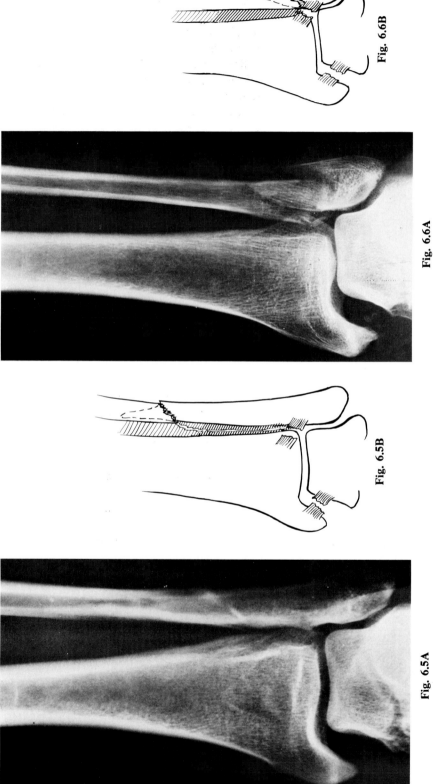

Fig. 6.6B

Fig. 6.6A

Intraosseous diastasis

Supination-external rotation injury, stage IV. Anterior and posterior inferior tibiofibular ligaments are ruptured; interosseous ligament, however, remains intact.

Fig. 6.5B

Fig. 6.5A

Ligamentous diastasis

Pronation-external rotation injury, stage IV. All tibiofibular soft tissues are ruptured proximally to the level of the fibular fracture.

Fig. 6.5 and 6.6. Widening of the malleolar mortise (lateral ankle instability)

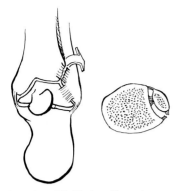

Fig. 6.7. Anterior tibiofibular diastasis.

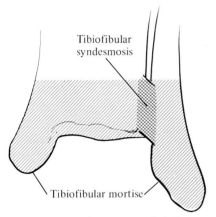

Fig. 6.8. The tibiofibular syndesmosis is but one part of the tibiofibular mortise.

ever, can occur in the absence of complete ligamentous diastasis or widening of the syndesmosis, if a lateral malleolar fracture occurs below the level of the syndesmosis (Fig. 6.6) [44]. Hence, the terms "ligamentous diastasis" (with implied widening of the syndesmosis) and "widening of the ankle mortise (or malleolar fork)" are not truly synonymous. Although ligamentous diastasis implies widening of the mortise, the converse is not true, since widening of the mortise may occur as a result of either ligamentous diastasis or distal fibular fracture. Widening of the mortise in the absence of a distal fibular fracture, however, implies that all the syndesmotic ligaments have ruptured [1,10,22,66]. In this event, the fibula usually fractures at a proximal level (Fig. 6.5) or the proximal tibiofibular joint is disrupted [11,16,17,69].

Iselin and de Vellis [39] used the term **diastasis intraperonier** to refer to the widening of the malleolar fork in association with distal fibular fracture (Fig. 6.6). Burwell and Charnley [11] have translated this term to mean **intraosseous diastasis.** This indicates that the distal tibiofibular separation (diastasis) occurs through the fibular fracture site, rather than through ligamentous tissue. Even with a distal fibular fracture characterized by severe displacement of the talus and lateral malleolus, when both the anterior and posterior tibiofibular ligaments have been violated, the proximal fibular fragment maintains its normal connections to the distal tibia via the interosseous ligament and membrane (Fig. 6.6B). Therefore a total ligamentous diastasis has not occurred.

Kleiger [42–44] has coined the term **lateral ankle instability** to represent lateral shift of the talus, permitted by either complete ligamentous diastasis (widening of the syndesmosis) (Fig. 6.5) or fracture of the lateral malleolus (Fig. 6.6), in association with medial ankle injury. Although this concept is valid, the term "lateral ankle instability" may lead to confusion with the condition of lateral collateral ligament insufficiency.

At the other extreme, it is quite possible to sustain a severe, unstable subluxation or dislocation of the talus with fractures of both malleoli, and yet not have ligamentous diastasis or widening of the malleolar mortise. The distal tibiofibular relationship is preserved, and the relationship of the malleoli with respect to the talus and each other is maintained, despite the severity of the injury (Fig. 6.9) [29].

Obviously none of these terms will be particularly helpful in a diagnostic or therapeutic sense until there is general agreement concerning their significance and implications. In the meantime, the specific pathologic components of ankle injuries should be described so as to avert confusion.

Eponyms

The history of ankle injuries is graced by the names of many famous clinicians. A complete historical review is beyond the scope of this text and, for this purpose, the reader is referred to several excellent monographs [3,7,26,37,45,49]. Since the use of eponyms is not entirely avoidable, however, some of the more commonly employed designations will be summarized here.

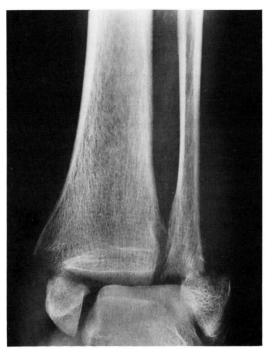

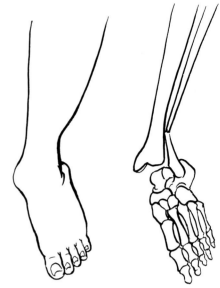

Fig. 6.10. Pott's fracture.

Fig. 6.9. Unstable fracture—dislocation of the ankle. The distal tibiofibular relationship is maintained as is the relationship between the talus and both malleoli.

Pott's Fracture

In 1756, Percival Pott, while recovering from an open fracture of the tibia and fibula (probably diaphyseal), wrote several monographs [28,84]. One of these, entitled *Some Few General Remarks on Fractures and Dislocations* [81], described a serious ankle injury characterized by a nearly transverse fibular fracture occurring 2–3 in. above the malleolar tip with rupture of "those strong tendinous attachments which connect the lower end of the tibia with the astragalus and os calcis" (deltoid ligament), and resultant outward dislocation of the talus with respect to the tibiofibular mortise. Pott believed that the mechanism was forced abduction of the foot. Although he made no mention of the condition of the tibiofibular ligaments [28,75], his illustration, which has become classic, suggests that they remained intact and acted as a hinge about which the distal fibular fragment rotated (Fig. 6.10) [54].

Ashhurst and Bromer [3] later concluded that Pott had described a fracture which really did not exist. To date, there is no agreement as to

exactly what injury most closely resembles the lesion originally described by Pott [20,32,80, 86,93], and therefore the term probably should not be used except in the most general sense [28,48]. Bonnin [7] stated that the designation "Pott's fracture" is "no more an accurate diagnosis than the term jaundice."

Without the benefit of radiographs, it is easy to understand how Pott's interpretation of the injury developed. It is difficult to understand how the term Pott's fracture came to be used to describe fractures of the medial and lateral malleoli [80,88]. Nowhere in Pott's treatise is there any mention of a medial malleolar fracture, and there is nothing to suggest that he even considered this possibility.

Pott's most significant contribution to the treatment of ankle injuries was to advocate reduction and splinting with the limb in a flexed attitude to reduce spasm, as opposed to the then-popular Hippocratic method characterized by limb extension [26,37].

Dupuytren's Fracture

Baron Dupuytren was the first to emphasize the distinction between relatively benign *direct* fractures of the fibula and those caused by violent actions "through the medium of the foot" (*indi-*

rect or malleolar fractures) [25]. In this latter group of more severe and potentially disabling injuries, Dupuytren postulated that injury could be caused by "violent motions of the foot inward or outward" (adduction-abduction). Whether he appreciated the significance of external rotation in the production of these injuries is uncertain [21,26,73].

Dupuytren commended Pott for the accurate description of what he also thought was the typical (abduction) fracture of the distal fibula [28]. The injury originally described by Pott came to be known in France as Dupuytren's fracture [80]. Some subsequent authors referred to this injury as Pott-Dupuytren fracture, recognizing the contributions of both men [20,32,80]. In fact, however, the injury as illustrated did not really exist or at least does not correspond to any fracture pattern that we recognize today.

Dupuytren, like Pott, apparently overlooked injury to the tibiofibular ligaments in the typical fracture [26,75]. Among the nearly 200 injuries that he reported, however, there was one instance of proximal and lateral talar dislocation, where Dupuytren observed that the tibiofibular ligaments were torn [24]. For this reason, he has sometimes been credited with discovery of ligamentous diastasis of the distal tibiofibular syndesmosis [26,75]:

Eighth complication. Dislocation of the foot outwards and upwards.

This form of displacement is so rare that I have only seen it once in nearly 200 cases of fractured fibula which have fallen under my observation in the last 15 years. It involves not only fracture of the fibula, but also laceration of the strong tibio-peroneal ligaments, which generally resist the force to which the osseous tissue itself yields. [24]

Dupuytren's name, therefore, has been associated with two different ankle injuries: one that really "does not exist" (Pott's fracture) and the other (tibiofibular diastasis) whose discovery is usually credited to Maisonneuve. Although Dupuytren's contributions to the study of ankle injuries were many, the term Dupuytren's fracture is misleading.

Maisonneuve Fracture

J.G. Maisonneuve [61] was a pupil of Dupuytren. He is credited with being the first person to recog-

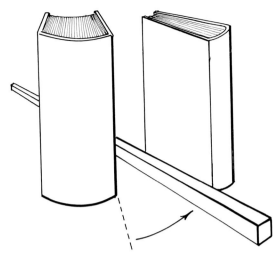

Fig. 6.11. Maisonneuve's explanation of external rotation ("divulsion") injury.

nize the role of external rotation ("divulsion") as a cause of ankle injury [7,13,23,28,69,80]. His experiment, using two books and a ruler, has become a familiar illustration (Fig. 6.11) [28].

Maisonneuve postulated that external rotation caused the typical oblique fracture of the distal fibula (probably the fracture referred to by Pott and Dupuytren) [32,80] if the distal tibiofibular ligaments remained intact [26,82]; but under other circumstances, external rotation could cause a proximal fibular fracture associated with tibiofibular ligamentous disruption—"fracture par diastase" [59,61]. It is ironic that, although the former injury is more common and clinically significant, it is the latter injury which bears Maisonneuve's name. His contributions to the study of ankle injuries were extensive and far reaching.

Wagstaffe (LeFort) Fracture

Wagstaffe (1875) [96] reported on two patients with vertical fractures of the distal fibula. One patient healed with a painful anterior prominence. The other patient died and, at postmortem examination, was found to have a transverse fracture of the distal fibula associated with a vertical fracture of the distal fibular fragment. Neither lesion was illustrated and Wagstaffe made no attempt to explain the mechanism of this fracture.

LeFort (1886) described three instances of isolated fracture of the anterior margin of the lateral malleolus [49]. The fracture fragment included the attachments of both the anterior talofibular and anterior tibiofibular ligaments; LeFort concluded that the fracture was caused by avulsion forces transmitted through the anterior talofibular ligament as a result of forced supination-adduction of the foot. Bonnin [7], however, did not think that the strength of the anterior talofibular ligament would permit an avulsion fracture of this size.

Pankovich [76] has described three different types of Wagstaffe lesion (Fig. 6.12):

Type I   Avulsion fracture: fragment maintains attachment to both the anterior talofibular and anterior inferior tibiofibular ligaments.

Type II   Associated with oblique fracture of the fibula originating distal to the anterior inferior tibiofibular ligament insertion ("mixed oblique fracture"): Wagstaffe fragment postulated to be produced by impingement of the dislocating talus on the spike of the proximal fibular fragment. This is probably analogous to the original injury dissected by Wagstaffe. After the spike is fractured off the proximal fibular fragment, the fibular fracture sometimes appears relatively transverse in nature.

Type III Associated with fracture of the anterior tibial tubercle: this probably occurs as a result of avulsion fracture of the anterior tibial tubercle, followed by oblique fracture of the distal fibula with superimposed type II Wagstaffe fracture.

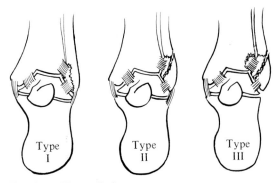

Fig. 6.12. Wagstaffe fractures.

Volkmann-Tillaux Fracture

R. von Volkmann (1875) was apparently the first to describe a fracture of the anterolateral tibia [49]. His illustrations suggest that he believed the fragment could be small or quite large (Fig. 6.13). Somehow, however, the designation "Volkmann's fragment" evolved in such a way that it is frequently used to refer to fracture of the posterior lip of the tibia [36,70,85].

Later, Tillaux (1890), while trying to refute Maisonneuve's findings, produced avulsion fractures of the lateral tibia with abduction stress. He did not comment specifically on their origin, but diagrams published posthumously demonstrated avulsions from both the anterior and posterior tubercles of the distal tibia [49]. He is commonly credited, however, with describing avulsion fracture of the anterior tibial tubercle.

Cotton's Fracture

In 1915, Frederic J. Cotton [19] called attention to what he considered "a new type of ankle fracture," characterized by fracture of the posterior lip of the tibia, as well as both medial and lateral malleoli, with resultant posterior dislocation of the foot (Fig. 6.14). Henderson, in 1932 [32], coined the term "trimalleolar fracture" to describe this entity. In point of fact, this injury had been previously described by Sir Astley Cooper in 1822 [18,65]. Nevertheless, Cotton deserves credit for emphasizing the nature of this injury and distinguishing it, both diagnostically and therapeutically, from the so-called Pott's fracture.

Bosworth Fracture

In 1947, Bosworth [9] described five patients with injuries consisting of lateral malleolar fracture and dislocation of the ankle that were irreducible by closed means, because the proximal fibular fragment had become entrapped behind the posterior tubercle of the tibia (Fig. 6.15). Three of these patients required open reduction; the other two patients were diagnosed late and required arthrodesis. At surgery, Bosworth observed that the proximal fibular fragment was held firmly in the dislocated position by the intact interosse-

Fig. 6.13. von Volkmann's illustrations. *Left* An actual case presenting fractures of the fibula, and anterolateral tibia. *Right* von Volkmann's theoretical explanation for fractures of the anterolateral tibia and medial malleolus. From Lauge-Hansen N: Fractures of the ankle. Arch Surg 56:277, 1948. Copyright 1948, American Medical Association. Reprinted with permission.

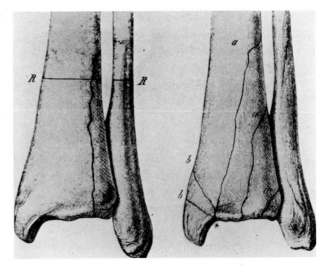

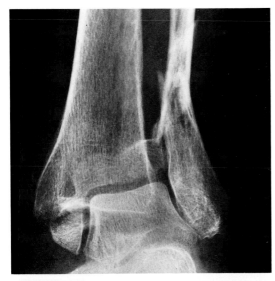

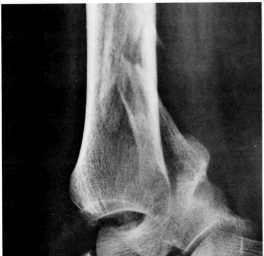

Fig. 6.14. Cotton's fracture (trimalleolar).

ous membrane; considerable force was required to pry it back into place. Closed reduction had not been possible because the fibular fracture had severed all connection between the proximal fibular fragment and the foot. Bosworth postulated that this injury was caused by external rotation and believed that the fibular dislocation occurred prior to the distal fibular fracture. This fracture is best explained as an atypical supination-external rotation injury (Chapter 10).

To date, approximately 30 cases of this injury have been reported in the literature [12,27,57, 64,67,68,74,87,102]. Three of these patients demonstrated posterior dislocation and entrapment of the fibula without fibular fracture [64,74,102], suggesting that the sequence postulated by Bosworth is correct. Although most patients with this injury have required open reduction, Mayer and Evarts [64] were able to effect reduction by

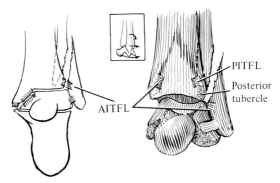

Fig. 6.15. Bosworth fracture.

closed means in three of the four patients they encountered. They attributed their success to early diagnosis and the application of direct anterolateral pressure to the back of the fibular shaft concomitant with attempts to reduce the talus. The radiographic criteria which should suggest the existence of this lesion have been well publicized and are detailed in Chapter 4.

References

1. Alldredge RH: Diastasis of the distal tibiofibular joint and associated lesions. JAMA 115:2136, 1940.
2. Arimoto HK, Forrester DM: Classification of ankle fractures: an algorithm. Am J Roentgenol 135:1057, 1980.
3. Ashhurst APC, Bromer RS: Classification and mechanism of fractures of the leg bones involving the ankle. AMA Arch Surg 4:51, 1922.
4. Bistrom O: Conservative treatment of severe ankle fractures. A clinical and follow-up study. Acta Chir Scand (Suppl) 168:1, 1952.
5. Bohler L: The Treatment of Fractures, 5th ed. New York, Grune & Stratton, 1956.
6. Bolin H: The fibula and its relationship to the tibia and talus in injuries of the ankle due to forced external rotation. Acta Radiol 56:439, 1961.
7. Bonnin JG: Injuries to the Ankle. New York, Grune & Stratton, 1950.
8. Bonnin JG: Injury to the ligaments of the ankle. J. Bone Joint Surg 47B:609, 1965.
9. Bosworth DM: Fracture-dislocation of the ankle with fixed displacement of the fibula behind the tibia. J Bone Joint Surg 29:130, 1947.
10. Burns BH: Diastasis of the inferior tibio-fibular joint. Proc Roy Soc Med 36:330, 1943.
11. Burwell HN, Charnley D: Treatment of displaced fractures at the ankle by rigid internal fixation and early joint movement. J Bone Joint Surg 47B:634, 1965.
12. Cabrera C, Simonovich S: Major fractures of the ankle and their sequelae. Ed: J. Delchef, R de Marneffe, E Vander Elst. Proceedings of the 12th Congress of the International Society of Orthopaedic Surgery and Traumatology, Tel-Aviv, Oct 9–12 1972. Excerpta Medica, Amsterdam, 1973.
13. Cave F (Ed): Ankle Injuries. Fractures and Other Injuries. Chicago, Year Book Medical, 1958.
14. Cedell CA: Supination-outward rotation injuries of the ankle. Acta Orthop Scand (Suppl) 110:1, 1967.
15. Cedell CA: Ankle lesions. Acta Orthop Scand 46:425, 1975.
16. Close R: Some applications of the functional anatomy of the ankle joint. J Bone Joint Surg 38A:761, 1956.
17. Colton CL: Fracture-diastasis of the inferior tibio-fibular joint. J Bone Joint Surg 50B:830, 1968.
18. Cooper AP: On dislocations of the ankle joint. Clin Orthop 42:3, 1965.
19. Cotton FJ: A new type of ankle fracture. JAMA 64:318, 1915.
20. Cox FJ, Laxson WW: Fractures about the ankle joint. Am J Surg 83:674, 1952.
21. Dabezies E, D'Ambrosia R, Shoji H: Classification and treatment of ankle fractures. Orthopedics 1:365, 1978.
22. D'Anca AF: Lateral rotatory dislocation of the ankle without fracture. A case report. J Bone Joint Surg 52A:1643, 1970.
23. DeSouza Dias L, Foerster TP: Traumatic lesions of the ankle joint. The supination-external rotation mechanism. Clin Orthop Rel Res 100:219, 1974.
24. Dupuytren G: On the Injuries and Diseases of Bones. Translated by F. LeGros Clark. London, The Syndenham Society, 1847.
25. Dupuytren G: Of Fractures of the Lower Extremity of Fibula and Luxations of the Foot. Med Classics 4:151, 1939.
26. Ellison AE: A brief review of the literature on the ankle joint. Am J Sports Med 5:226, 1977.
27. Fahey JJ, Schlenker LT, Stauffer RC: Fracture dislocation of the ankle with fixed displacement of the fibula behind the tibia. Am J Roetgenol Radium Ther Nucl Med 76:1102, 1956.
28. Ferreira AP, DeWet IS, Dommisse GF: Fractures and dislocations of the ankle joint. S Afr Med J 54:1095, 1978.
29. Golterman AFL: Diagnosis and treatment of tibiofibular diastasis. Arch Chir Neerl 16:185, 1964.
30. Grath G: Widening of the ankle mortise. A clinical and experimental study. Acta Chir Scand (Suppl) 263:1, 1960.
31. Harvey JP Jr: Fractures of the ankle. A clinical survey of 181 cases. Clin Orthop 42:57, 1965.
32. Henderson MS: Fractures of the ankle. Wisc Med J 31:684, 1932.
33. Henderson MS, Stuck WG: Fractures of the ankle. Recent and old. J Bone Joint Surg 15:882, 1933.
34. Hirsch C, Lewis J: Experimental ankle-joint fractures. Acta Orthop Scand 36:408, 1965.
35. Hughes J: The medial malleolus in ankle fractures. Orthop Clin North Am, 11:649, 1980.
36. Hughes JL, Weber H, Willenegger H, Kuner EH: Evaluation of ankle fractures. Non-operative and operative treatment. Clin Orthop Rel Res 138:111, 1979.
37. Hughes SPF: An historical review of fractures involving the ankle joint. Mayo Clin Proc 50:611, 1975.
38. Hughes SPF: External rotational injury of the ankle joint with displacement of the talus. Ann

Roy Coll Surg 59:61, 1977.

39. Iselin M, deVellis H: La primauté du péroné dans les fractures' du cou-de-pied. Mém Acad Chir 87:399, 1961.

40. Jergesen F: Open reduction of fractures and dislocations of the ankle. Am J Surg 98:136, 1959.

41. Key JA, Conwell HE: Injuries in the Region of the Ankle. The Management of Fractures, Dislocations and Sprains, 6th ed. St. Louis, Mosby, 1956.

42. Kleiger B: The diagnosis and treatment of traumatic lateral ankle instability. NY State J Med 54:2573, 1954.

43. Kleiger B: Treatment of oblique fractures of the fibula. J Bone Joint Surg 43:969, 1961.

44. Kleiger B: Mechanisms of ankle injury. Orthop Clin North Am 5:127, 1974.

45. Klossner O: Late results of operative and nonoperative treatment of severe ankle fractures. Acta Chir Scand (Suppl) 293:1, 1962.

46. Kristensen T: Treatment of malleolar fractures according to Lauge-Hansen's method. Preliminary results. Acta Chir Scand 97:362, 1949.

47. Kristensen T: Fractures of the ankle. VI. Follow-up studies. AMA Arch Surg 73:112, 1956.

48. Lane WA: The operative treatment of simple fractures. Surg Gynecol Obstet 8:344, 1909.

49. Lauge-Hansen N: Fractures of the ankle. Arch Surg 56:259, 1948.

50. Lauge-Hansen N: Fractures of the ankle. II. Combined experimental-surgical and experimental-roentgenologic investigations. Arch Surg 60:957, 1950.

51. Lauge-Hansen N: Fractures of the ankle. IV. Clinical use of the genetic roentgen diagnosis and genetic reduction. Arch Surg 64:488, 1952.

52. Lauge-Hansen N: Fractures of the ankle. V. Pronation-dorsiflexion fracture. Arch Surg 67:813, 1953.

53. Lauge-Hansen N: Fractures of the ankle. III. Genetic roentgenologic diagnosis of fractures of the ankle. Am J Roentgenol 71:456, 1954.

54. Lewin P: Fractures of the Bones of the Foot and Ankle. Philadelphia, Lea & Febiger, 1959.

55. Lewis JL: The effect of ankle-injury forces. J Bone Joint Surg 46A:1380, 1964.

56. Lindsjo U: Operative treatment of ankle fractures. Acta Orthop Scand (Suppl) 189:1, 1981.

57. Lovell ES: An unusual rotatory injury of the ankle. J Bone Joint Surg 50A:163, 1968.

58. MacKinnon AP: Fracture of the lower articular surface of the tibia in fracture dislocation of the ankle. J Bone Joint Surg 10:352, 1928.

59. Magnusson R: On the late results in non-operated cases of malleolar fractures. I. Fractures by external rotation. Acta Chir Scand (Suppl) 84:1, 1944.

60. Magnusson R: Ligament injuries of the ankle joint. Acta Orthop Scand 36:317, 1965.

61. Maisonneuve MJG: Fractures du péroné. Arch Gen Med 1:165, 1840.

62. Malka JS, Taillard W: Results of non-operative and operative treatment of fractures of the ankle. Clin Orthop Rel Res 67:159, 1969.

63. Mast JW, Teipner A: A reproducible approach to the internal fixation of adult ankle fractures. Rationale, technique, and early results. Orthop Clin North Am 11:661, 1980.

64. Mayer PJ, Evarts CMcC: Fracture-dislocation of ankle with posterior entrapment of the fibula behind the tibia. Recognition and management. J Bone Joint Surg 60A:320, 1978.

65. McDaniel WJ, Wilson FC: Trimalleolar fractures of the ankle. An end result study. Clin Orthop Rel Res 122:37, 1977.

66. McLaughlin HL: Trauma. Philadelphia, Saunders, 1960.

67. Meyers MH: Fracture about the ankle joint with fixed displacement of the proximal fragment of the fibula behind the tibia. J Bone Joint Surg 39A:441, 1957.

68. Meyers MH: Fracture about the ankle joint with fixed displacement of the proximal fragment of the fibula behind the tibia. Clin Orthop Rel Res 42:67, 1965.

69. Monk CJE: Injuries of the tibiofibular ligaments. J Bone Joint Surg 51:330, 1969.

70. Müller ME, Allgöwer M, Schneider R, Willenegger H: Manual of Internal Fixation. New York, Springer-Verlag, 1979.

71. Neer CS II: Injuries of the ankle joint. Evaluation. Conn State Med J 17:580, 1953.

72. Neufeld AJ: Ankle joint fractures and their treatment. Clin Orthop 42:91, 1965.

73. Nyström G: A contribution to the treatment of fractures of the posterior border of the tibia by malleolar fractures. Acta Radiol 25:672, 1944.

74. Olerud S: Subluxation of the ankle without fracture of the fibula. A case report. J Bone Joint Surg 53A:594, 1971.

75. Pankovich AM: Fractures of the fibula proximal to the distal tibiofibular syndesmosis. J Bone Joint Surg 60A:221, 1978.

76. Pankovich AM: Fractures of the fibula at the distal tibiofibular syndesmosis. Clin Orthop Rel Res 143:138, 1979.

77. Pankovich AM: Adult ankle fractures. JCE Orthop 7:17, 1979.

78. Phillips RS, Balmer GA, Monk CJE: The external rotation fracture of the fibular malleolus. Br J Surg 56:55, 1969.

79. Phillips WA, Spiegel PG: Evaluation of ankle fractures, non-operative vs. operative. Clin Orthop Rel Res 138:17, 1979.

80. Platt H: Introduction to a discussion on fractures in the neighborhood of the ankle-joint. Lancet 1:33, 1926.

81. Pott P: Some Few General Remarks on Fractures and Dislocations. London, Hawes, Clarke and Collins, 1768. Reprinted in Med Classics 1:329, 1936.

82. Purvis GD: The unstable oblique distal fibular fracture. Clin Orthop Rel Res 92:330, 1973.

83. Quigley TB: Analysis and treatment of ankle injuries produced by rotatory, abduction and adduction forces. Instructional Course Lectures Am Acad Orthop Surg 19:172, 1970.

84. Rang M: Anthology of Orthopaedics. Edinburgh, Churchill Livingstone, 1966.

85. Rütt A: Surgery of the Lower Leg and Foot. Translated by G. Stiasny. Philadelphia, Saunders, 1980.

86. Sarkisian JS, Cody GW: Closed treatment of ankle fractures. A new criterion for evaluation—a review of 250 cases. J Trauma 16:323, 1976.

87. Schatzker J, McBroom R, Dzioba R: Irreducible fracture dislocation of the ankle due to posterior dislocation of the fibula. J Trauma 17:397, 1977.

88. Sisk TD: In Edmonson AP, Crenshaw AH (eds): Campbell's Operative Orthopaedics, 6th ed. St. Louis, Mosby, 1980.

89. Solonen KA, Lauttamus L: Treatment of malleolar fractures. Acta Orthop Scand 36:321, 1965.

90. Solonen KA, Lauttamus L: Operative treatment of ankle fractures. Acta Orthop Scand 39:223, 1968.

91. Staples OS: Injuries to the medial ligaments of the ankle. J Bone Joint Surg 42A:1287, 1960.

92. Staples OS: Ligamentous injuries of the ankle joint. Clin Orthop 42:21, 1965.

93. Stimson LA: Pott's fracture at the ankle. NY Med J 55:701, 1892.

94. Tanton J: Fractures du Membre Inferieur. Librairie J.-B. Bailliere et Fils Paris, 1916.

95. Vasli S: Operative treatment of ankle fractures. Acta Chir Scand (Suppl) 226:1, 1957.

96. Wagstaffe WW: An unusual form of fracture of the fibula. St Thomas Hosp Rep 6:43, 1875.

97. Walheim T: Intra-articular malleolar fractures. A survey. Acta Chir Scand 79:166, 1937.

98. Walsh WM, Hughston JC: Unstable ankle fractures in athletes. Am J Sports Med 4:173, 1976.

99. Watson-Jones R: Fractures and Other Joint Injuries, 4th ed. Baltimore, Williams & Wilkins, 1955.

100. Weber BG: Die Verletzungen des oberen Sprunggelenkes. In: Aktuelle Probleme in der Chirurgie. Bern, Verlag Hans Huber, 1966.

101. Wilson FC Jr, Skilbred LA: Long-term results in the treatment of displaced bimalleolar fractures. J Bone Joint Surg 48A:1065, 1966.

102. Woods RS: Irreducible dislocation of the anklejoint. Br J Surg 29:359, 1942.

103. Yde J: The Lauge-Hansen classification of malleolar fractures. Acta Orthop Scand 51:181, 1980.

104. Yde J, Kristensen KD: Ankle fractures. Supination-eversion fractures stage II. Primary and late results of operative and non-operative treatment. Acta Orthop Scand 51:695, 1980.

Chapter 7 Malleolar Fractures and Dislocations of the Ankle: Treatment

WILLIAM C. HAMILTON

Initial Evaluation and Care

Historical information concerning the mechanism of ankle injury is notoriously inaccurate for treatment or investigative purposes, since the patient is rarely able to describe either the direction or degree of ankle distortion that occurred at the moment of injury [13,64,95].

Physical examination is of prime importance. It should include careful inspection of the entire lower limb for deformity, instability, soft tissue swelling, and tenderness [6]. Knowledge of ligamentous anatomy permits accurate localization of pathology by the site of tenderness and soft tissue swelling [13,50]. This is best accomplished within the first few hours after injury. Beyond this time, tenderness becomes diffuse and soft tissue swelling confluent, so that precise localization is difficult or impossible. Similarly, clinical testing for stability can frequently be accomplished without anesthesia immediately after the injury, before discomfort and muscle spasm have developed to such a degree that testing becomes painful and unreliable [106,119]. Specific testing techniques and their significance will be covered in subsequent chapters.

Fractures of the tibial or fibular shaft, especially those with spiral configuration, should prompt a careful clinical and radiologic examination of the ankle region. Hedström and Sundgren [48] observed that ankle injury complicated 14% of all tibial and fibular shaft fractures. Lucas [77] distinguished between "obliquely transverse" fractures of the tibia, which were rarely (0.6%) accompanied by ankle injury, and spiral fractures of the tibia, which were commonly associated with ankle fracture (33%); occasionally, ankle involvement was secondary to intra-articular extension of the primary tibial fracture, but in most instances the ankle injury represented a remote lesion. Similarly, spiral fractures of the fibular shaft must necessarily be associated with fracture of the tibial shaft or injury to the tibiofibular syndesmosis; the latter can be easily overlooked during a cursory examination.

Examination of an injured ankle is not complete without observing the condition of the distal circulation. Pulsations in the posterior tibial and dorsalis pedis vessels, as well as the color, temperature, and capillary refill of the toes should be noted. Peripheral nerve injuries are relatively uncommon except with the more severe ankle injuries, but should be carefully sought by noting any disturbance of distal motor or sensory function.

Radiographs should be taken promptly in at least two planes. If at all possible, four views should be obtained: anteroposterior, lateral, mortise, and external oblique [4,124]. In certain cases, specialized studies, such as arthrography [4,61, 106,124],stress films, or axial tomography [4, 13,61,66,106,119,124,128], will be required to determine the full extent of injury (Chapter 4).

If definitive treatment of a displaced ankle fracture is to be delayed for any reason, especially if the skin is under tension or the distal circulation is impaired, an early attempt at provisional reduction is mandatory [6,11,66,89]. The extremity should then be carefully splinted in the reduced position. This is best accomplished by using a circumferential compression dressing with a posterior or stirrup splint (Fig. 7.1); this provides firm, well-distributed pressure and thereby minimizes swelling and the likelihood of bleb formation.

Definitive treatment should be accomplished as soon as possible depending on the patient's general health, associated injuries, and other practical considerations.

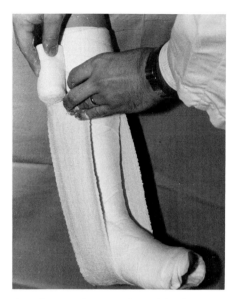

Fig. 7.1. Compression dressing with plaster stirrup splint.

Objectives of Treatment

The object of treatment is the restoration of complete function with the least risk to the patient, and the least anxiety to the surgeon.

Robert Jones, 1913 [59]

In order to accomplish this goal in the treatment of ankle fractures, satisfactory fracture position and ligament apposition need to be obtained and maintained during the period of healing and convalescence. Exactly what constitutes satisfactory position and which methods are best suited to obtain and maintain this position with minimal risk and inconvenience to the patient continue to be sources of some controversy. Fortunately, most ankle fractures are not characterized by significant displacement and, therefore, closed treatment will usually suffice [67]. Displaced ankle fractures, however, are another matter.

Over the years, numerous attempts have been made to compare the results of open and closed treatment of displaced ankle injuries [17,34, 49,56,67,81,116,121,124,134,137,138]. Unfortunately, the studies available to date have been too small, the observation period too short, or the evaluation criteria too varied to permit meaningful comparisons [17,18,56,67,81,100,116, 124,138]. Two other factors have complicated

attempts to compare operative and closed treatment. First, open reduction and internal fixation, in many series, has only been employed to treat the more difficult fractures not amenable to treatment by closed means; these more severe injuries are necessarily associated with a less desirable prognosis irrespective of treatment [9,60,67, 81,124,129]. Second, many earlier studies compared results by closed reduction with results obtained by open reduction and internal fixation, using reduction criteria and fixation techniques which presently would be considered inadequate [76]; these reports may have presented an unduly pessimistic assessment of the results achievable with operative means.

It is generally accepted that anatomic reduction of the mortise is a prerequisite to restoration of normal ankle function [9,11–13,18,76,81, 83,100,121,124,128]. At one time, the major emphasis was on restoring normal relationship of the talus to the distal tibia and medial malleolus [12,27,47,67]; the fibular fracture was treated by closed means, and frequently incomplete reduction was accepted [67,76,116,124].

Lane [72], as early as 1912, emphasized the importance of restoring fibular length and "form." Fairbank [35], in 1926, stated that "the slightest tilt of the lower fragment of the fibula spoils the fit of the bones forming the ankle joint, and any instability in the joint means grave risk of arthritis and disability." The scientific basis for these observations was not provided until much later. Lambert [69] demonstrated that the fibula carries 16% of the static load during weight bearing. Riede et al. [108] demonstrated experimentally that as little as 2 mm displacement of the lateral malleolus will result in lateral talar displacement of 1–2 mm, as well as talar external rotation of 1–2°, with a resultant 51% reduction of the tibiotalar contact surface. Similarly, Ramsey and Hamilton [107] showed that the first 1 mm of lateral talar displacement reduces the tibiotalar contact surface by 46%, with further reduction occurring in smaller increments with additional talar displacement (Fig. 7.2).

As a result of these observations, more attention has been paid recently to correction of fibular shortening, rotation, and displacement to restore tibiofibular and talofibular anatomy, as a desirable end in itself as well as a means of ensuring satisfactory restoration of the ankle mortise

Fig. 7.2. Reduction of contact surface o. the tibiotalar joint occurring as a result of lateral talar displacement. **A** Specimen immediately prior to testing. **B** Graph summarizing average reduction with each millimeter of talar displacement.

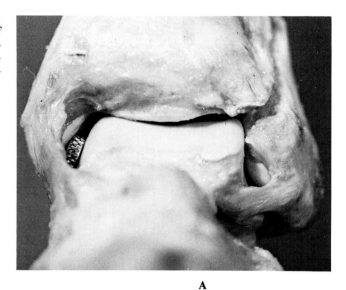

A

[18,30,88,91,103,114,130,131,132,135]. Fibular restoration, however, is difficult to accomplish by closed measures [17,31,76,90,91,95,121,131] since the distal fibular fragment can only be controlled indirectly by its ligamentous attachments to the talus [101,135]. Therefore, the current trend is toward more liberal utilization of operative treatment [34,82,111,115,120,131,133,135]. To date, however, clinical evidence for the superiority of the operative approach remains lacking [100]. Provided satisfactory reduction can be achieved and maintained, results with open and closed treatment seem quite comparable [37, 60,67,68,81,133,137]. For many injuries, however, truly satisfactory reduction can only be accomplished by operative means [28,67,92, 100,116,124].

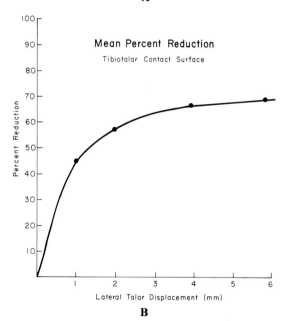

B

Selection of Treatment

As is true of any medical or surgical condition, the selection of treatment for ankle injury must be individualized. No text can begin to include all of the variables that need to be considered before a recommendation is made to the individual patient. The decision must necessarily be based upon the nature and degree of the injury, the circumstances and needs of the patient, and the capabilities of the surgeon and his environment.

As a result of improved surgical techniques, more reliable implants, and increased awareness of biomechanical requirements, a trend has developed toward expanded utilization of operative treatment for fractures in general, and especially for those that involve joints. Internal fixation of ankle fractures has become the "industry standard" in some centers. With this in mind, the advantages and disadvantages of open reduction, as compared to closed treatment, will be discussed.

The **advantages** of operative treatment can be summarized as follows:

1. Allows precise reduction.
2. Reduces the extent and/or duration of immobilization.
3. Maintains reduction and eliminates need for repeat manipulations and plaster changes.
4. Eliminates the need to immobilize the ankle in an unphysiologic position.
5. Permits removal of interposed soft tissue from joint and fracture site(s).
6. Allows inspection of the joint surface and replacement or removal of bone/cartilage fragments.

(1) Allows Precise Reduction [31,70,82,83]

"The shape and dimensions of the bones of a limb correspond exactly and in detail to those which optimally fulfill the functional requirements. The ability of the organism to adapt to certain types of skeletal deformity is remarkable. Nevertheless there is no doubt that integral restoration is necessary for complete recovery of the extent, force, and precision of normal movement. . . . Even radiography too often gives an excessively optimistic picture."

Danis, 1949 [31]

Lane [71–73] and Lambotte [70] are generally credited with being the first to emphasize the value of internal fixation to the restoration of normal anatomy. Later authors, regardless of their preference for operative or closed treatment, have almost universally shared the belief that the clinical results following ankle injuries are generally proportional to the adequacy of reduction [8,67,113,120]. Distortion of bone and ligament relationships will alter ankle weight bearing and motion. Normal motions may be limited and abnormal motions permitted. The mechanical disturbance itself may cause pain and dysfunction, and with time, changes in the weight-bearing surface due to malalignment, incongruity, and instability will frequently lead to eccentric loading of articular cartilage and resultant degenerative arthritis.

Generally, given a good anatomic result, the functional result is satisfactory [101]. Unfortunately, however, there is no general agreement as to what represents a satisfactory reduction. Various radiographic criteria have been proposed by Magnusson [80], Kristensen [68], Vasli [124], Klossner [67], Burwell and Charnley [13], Solonen and Lauttamus [115], Weber [131], Cedell [17], Joy et al. [60], and Sarkisian and Cody [112].

However, with the exception of certain fracture components (e.g., large posterior lip fragments), the fine distinction between acceptable and unacceptable reduction remains unclear. Also, conventional radiographic study provides a relatively crude two-dimensional analysis and is not likely to demonstrate subtle anatomic distortions, especially those involving rotation. Successful operative treatment obviates both of these concerns as it will usually permit true "millimetric" reduction of fracture fragments and torn ligaments under direct vision.

If, however, as a result of surgical intervention, anything less than anatomic reduction is realized, then neither of the above concerns is eliminated and the operation may be considered as meddlesome [15]. As emphasized by Charnley, the only justification for operative treatment (Pott's injury) is "absolutely perfect hairline reposition of the fragments" [21].

Occasionally, a patient with an apparently satisfactory reduction develops painful joint degeneration [27,63,67,90,115,134]. This may occur because the radiograph has provided too optimistic an assessment [7] or because of occult injury to the articular cartilage or its nutritional mechanism [27]. Therefore, even perfect reduction cannot guarantee an excellent result [58,67].

At other times, a patient with a markedly deformed ankle may demonstrate a considerable degree of painless, useful function [51,70,80]. This, however, attests more to the remarkable "ability of the organism to adapt to . . . skeletal deformity," rather than to the efficacy of treatment. It is fortunate when nature is kind under these circumstances, but nature is unpredictable and cannot be relied upon by the surgeon.

(2) Reduces the Extent and/or Duration of Immobilization [28,72,83,88,124,128]

With adequate internal fixation, external immobilization can frequently be reduced in extent or duration. Ideally, when the patient is reliable and the fixation is rigid, external immobilization can be avoided entirely, and early exercises can be initiated [11,13,18,31,70,96,116]. This approach appears to shorten convalescence by eliminating the so-called "fracture disease" characterized by joint stiffness, contracture, and atrophy [55,96,124]. Whether immediate immobilization improves the long-term results is unknown at present.

Although this concept is appealing, no attempt has been made to separate the benefits derived from rigid internal fixation in anatomic position from the benefits accruing as a result of the immediate mobilization. It may be that the risk of plaster has been exaggerated [17,18] and that anatomic reduction is the more important ingredient in the apparent success of the aggressive operative approach.

By reducing the extent and/or duration of external immobilization, adequate internal fixation will also facilitate care of local soft tissue injuries as well as associated musculoskeletal and visceral trauma. Reducing or eliminating external immobilization, however, assumes that satisfactory fixation has been achieved [124]. If for any reason this is not the case, fracture position should not be jeopardized by institution of premature exercises [84].

(3) Maintains Reduction and Eliminates the Need for Repeat Manipulation and Plaster Changes

Reliable internal fixation should eliminate the need for frequent cast changes and repeat manipulations necessitated by fracture displacement. When anatomic reduction is sought by closed means, repeat manipulation is required with considerable frequency [7,9,14,39,124]. Repeat manipulation, besides exposing the patient to another anesthetic, imposes additional trauma to articular cartilage and periarticular soft tissues [14,34].

(4) Eliminates Need to Immobilize the Ankle and/or Limb in an Unphysiologic Position [12,28,58,135]

When external immobilization is employed, following open reduction and internal fixation of ankle fractures, it usually takes the form of a protective cast or splint, applied with the ankle in/or near neutral position. To maintain fracture position following closed reduction, however, the ankle and limb frequently need to be immobilized in an exaggerated attitude; this may damage articular cartilage, stretch important soft tissue structures, and/or encourage joint contracture in an undesirable position.

(5) Permits Removal of Interposed Soft Tissue from Joint and/or Fracture Site(s) [58,128]

Open reduction eliminates possible interposition of soft tissue within the joint and/or fracture site(s) that might otherwise jeopardize reduction or prevent prompt bone healing [129].

Prevention of talar reduction by interposition of ruptured deltoid ligament has been observed quite commonly [24,37,47,83,94]. Rarely, the posterior tibial tendon or other medial structure becomes interposed between the medial malleolus and the talus, preventing satisfactory reduction and necessitating open treatment [37,38,65, 94,128].

When medial injury is characterized by fracture rather than deltoid ligament rupture, periosteum frequently becomes invaginated into the fracture site [6,11,17,83,87,93,116,124,128,134]. Burwell and Charnley [13] demonstrated periosteal interposition in more than 50% of the medial malleolar fractures they treated surgically.

Also, operative treatment permits approximation of ligament ends, ensuring that they are not retracted or separated by interposed tissue that might prevent secure healing.

(6) Allows inspection of Joint Surface and Replacement or Removal of Bone and/or Cartilage Fragments [11,82,83,128,129]

With operative treatment, the joint surface can be inspected directly and articular damage visualized. This will permit replacement of large osteochondral fragments or removal of small ones, which if neglected could become joint mice and further irritate the synovium and/or articular cartilage. Hughes [55] observed significant intraarticular bone fragments in eight of 25 patients with medial malleolar fractures caused by abduction or external rotation violence. Also, inspection of the joint surface will sometimes correct an otherwise favorable but misleading prognosis.

The disadvantages of open reduction can be summarized as follows:

1. Requires operation with its attendant risks.
2. Introduces a quantity, sometimes considerable, of metallic hardware that might require subsequent removal.

(1) Requires Operation with Its Attendant Risks

Since adequate closed reduction usually requires an anesthetic, the additional risks incurred by open reduction–internal fixation are limited to those directly attributed to the procedure: technical failure to achieve anatomic reduction/secure fixation; infection; and incisional skin necrosis.

Technical Failure

Failure to achieve anatomic reduction for technical reasons should be a rare occurrence if the physician is experienced and exercises good judgment in selecting patients and planning the procedure. Certain comminuted fractures are not amenable to internal fixation, except by surgeons very experienced in the technique; some fractures are not amenable to fixation by even the most experienced surgeons [81]. The primary objective of treatment is to provide optimal fracture reduction. If, for any reason (nature/severity of the injury, expertise of the treating physician with closed manipulation, or lack of expertise with open techniques), a superior reduction cannot be achieved by open reduction, then there is little to recommend this form of treatment [15,81].

Infection

Deep infection complicating open reduction of ankle fractures is a serious problem that usually compromises the result and may culminate in arthrodesis or amputation. In this event, the result is usually less desirable than the anticipated outcome with closed treatment.

Superficial infection (which is frequently confused with incisional skin necrosis) occurs with a frequency as high as 5.9% [11,13,17,67] but usually responds to local treatment. Deep infection, fortunately, is much less common, with a reported incidence of 0.3–2.2% [11,13,17,67, 90,124]. The incidence of infection can be reduced to a minimum by careful timing, meticulous skin preparation, and expeditious surgery [58]. The use of prophylactic antibiotics should be considered at least in those situations where host resistance is thought to be compromised.

Incisional Skin Necrosis

Significant skin necrosis can generally be avoided by appropriately placed incisions, careful handling of skin edges, and closure without excessive or concentrated tension [18,58,115]. Minor degrees of skin necrosis usually respond to local measures without affecting the final result [124]. Occasionally, skin loss is caused by intrinsic, irreversible damage incurred at the moment of injury and, under these circumstances, is unavoidable to some degree with either operative or closed treatment. With proper precautions, this potential problem should not significantly affect the decision to employ open reduction–internal fixation but might alter the timing of proposed surgery, so as to optimize skin condition.

(2) Introduces Metallic Hardware

The development of efficient, inert metallic appliances has minimized the short-term problems of device failure and local tissue reaction, provided that the devices are employed properly and adequately covered by soft tissue.

For the long-term application, however, there are many unanswered questions concerning the mechanical effects of these implants on bone and the possible biologic effects on contiguous soft tissue and remote viscera [1,5,86,124]. Until these questions are answered, removal of implants, after they have served their purpose, should be seriously considered. Implant removal requires a second operative procedure and another period of protection to permit bone healing and remodeling. This, however, may be a small price to pay if maximal functional recovery, permitted by anatomic reduction, cannot be obtained by other means.

General Principles of Closed Reduction

Although closed reduction techniques vary [14,21,25,89], several principles are generally agreed upon in the available literature to date:

1. For closed reduction to be successful, it must be attempted as early as possible after injury, preferably within the first few hours [14, 50,63,67,101,115,129]. Satisfactory assistance and complete anesthesia with muscular relaxation are required [50,65,68,101,129]. Attempted closed reduction in an emergency room without assistance or anesthesia is, at best, a nominal attempt.

2. Generally, fractured malleoli remain attached to the talus by ligament structures. Intact malleoli are separated from the talus by ligament rupture. Malleoli cannot be replaced directly by closed means but can only be reduced indirectly by repositioning the talus [21,63]. Great force should not be required to obtain reduction [14]. If so, the possibility of soft tissue interposition within the joint or fracture surfaces must be suspected [21,38,47].

3. Plaster technique is critical [115]. The cast should be snug and well molded, and must satisfactorily prevent recurrence of the pathologic talar motion that was initially responsible for the injury [50,68,129]. For external rotation injuries, this usually means extending the plaster above the flexed knee [65,106,136].

4. Satisfactory reduction should be documented by radiographic examination before termination of the anesthetic [51].

5. Since these are intra-articular fractures, weight bearing should be avoided, at least early in the course of treatment [21,50, 63,84,103,104,106].

6. Careful follow-up with serial radiographic examination is mandatory for all but the most stable injuries [21,47,63]. The physician must be able and willing to change the plasters [8,11], remanipulate the ankle [11, 14,63,115], or resort to operative treatment [101,133] if satisfactory reduction cannot be secured and maintained during the period of healing [58].

7. When closed reduction has been successful, the period of immobilization, although variable, should be kept to a minimum so as to prevent unnecessary joint stiffness [50,96].

General Principles of Open Reduction–Internal Fixation

Since the overall results with closed treatment of ankle fractures are generally satisfactory [21,34,50,101,120,134], open reduction should only be undertaken if conditions are optimal and surgery is likely to improve upon these results. This presumes that the surgeon is adequately trained [21,58], works in a satisfactory facility with knowledgeable assistants, and has available all of the equipment and devices for which a need might arise during the course of the operative procedure [15,82,83]. One must think not only in terms of the final radiograph but also how efficiently and safely the internal fixation or repair has been accomplished. The goal should be "hairline" reduction and stable fixation of as many components of the injury as possible (Fig. 7.3) [21,31,124].

The ideal timing of surgery is not generally agreed upon [11,13,34,50,67,81–83,88]. In general, the procedure should be performed as soon as circumstances permit [12,84], depending upon the patient's general condition and associated injuries [15,82], but not before the prerequisites specified above have been fulfilled. In some situations, these requirements can be fulfilled immediately; in others, it is more prudent to delay surgery until these conditions can be met. Provided talar displacement is corrected and the limb is well immobilized, little is usually lost by a delay of 1 or 2 days [13,116]. If, however, talar displacement cannot be reduced to a minimum, then the skin and other soft tissues remain under tension and operative intervention becomes urgent [8].

Ideally, skin and soft tissue should be in optimal condition, free of contusion, abrasions, blebs, and inordinate swelling before surgery is performed [15,58,124,128,129]. In certain situations, however, this requirement cannot be observed. Whether to proceed with operative intervention when skin conditions are less than ideal is a matter of clinical judgment that must be individualized. The surgeon must carefully weigh the potential risks and difficulties likely to be incurred by deferring internal fixation [50,82,84] until skin integrity has been restored (occasionally up to several weeks) [58,124] versus the risk of proceeding with open reduction in the presence of

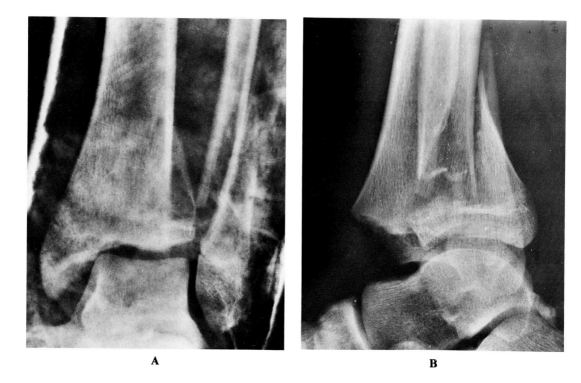

A   B

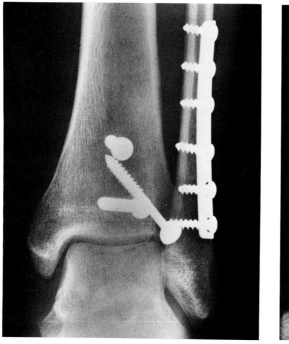

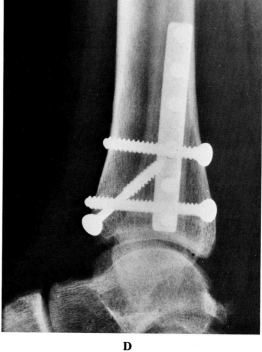

C   D

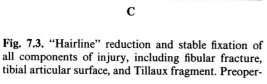

Fig. 7.3. "Hairline" reduction and stable fixation of all components of injury, including fibular fracture, tibial articular surface, and Tillaux fragment. Preoper- ative anteroposterior (**A**) and lateral (**B**) views, postop- erative anteroposterior (**C**) and lateral (**D**) views.

compromised soft tissues [8]. This will depend, to a large degree, on the nature of the soft tissue damage and whether other forms of treatment are likely to produce an acceptable end result.

Prior to the procedure, the surgeon should carefully review the available radiographs and obtain any other views or studies that are necessary to appreciate the full extent of injury [55]. In this manner, a tentative approach can be formulated preoperatively [82].

Satisfactory general [11,81] or regional [16] anesthesia with muscular relaxation is a prerequisite for formal open reduction. A pneumatic tourniquet is generally employed unless there is a specific contraindication such as vascular insufficiency [12,13,15,81,116,124]. The tourniquet should be placed above the knee [11]. Ischemia time should be minimized; generally, all but the most severe and complex ankle injuries can be satisfactorily repaired with 60 min or less of tourniquet ischemia.

Radiographic capability in the operating room, though not absolutely necessary, is obviously highly desirable [12,89,128]. The surgeon's impression of the reduction was more optimistic than the radiograph in 22% of the cases reviewed by Lindsjo [76].

For most procedures, the patient should be positioned supine. A small pack or sandbag under the ipsilateral buttock will greatly facilitate exposure of the distal fibula, lateral malleolus, and syndesmosis, usually without jeopardizing access to the medial side of the ankle [11,128]. If necessary, however, the pack can be removed during the procedure by an unsterile assistant or circulating nurse. Rarely is it necessary to place a pack under the contralateral hip to gain access to the medial malleolus, since the lower extremity naturally falls into external rotation. For exploration of the posterior tibial margin via the posterolateral approach, a sandbag under the ipsilateral buttock is essential or the operation should be performed with the patient in the prone or lateral decubitus position [82].

The entire limb should be prepared and draped free using stockingette [84,128]. If there is any possibility that bone graft will be required (e.g., pilon fracture), then the selected donor site (proximal tibia, distal femur, greater trochanter, or iliac crest) should be prepared and readily accessible.

It matters little which component of the injury is explored initially; however, the order of repair is sometimes critical. In general, it is better to fix fractures before ligaments are repaired, since bone stabilization will have a protective effect on the sutured ligament [58]. If fracture fixation will jeopardize visualization of the torn ligament, sutures can be inserted in the ligament initially but not tied until after the fracture has been fixed.

During the course of surgery, meticulous sterile technique needs to be observed and both soft tissues and bone must be handled with extreme care [82]. Excessive dissection and retraction is traumatic and undesirable [15]; bone fragments should be gently manipulated, lest they become devitalized or comminuted [70,82,128].

Exploration of the joint cavity for fragments and evidence of cartilage damage is an integral part of the procedure and should not be omitted [128]. The ankle has many recesses that can conceal loose bodies and these can be easily overlooked if a diligent search is not made [55].

Operative treatment of ankle injuries presumes perfect reduction and firm fixation of all fractures, as well as meticulous repair of ruptured ligaments. Implants should be strong and manufactured precisely from high grade surgical metals [31,72,84]. These devices should be carefully sized to their specific function and placed so that soft tissue coverage will be adequate. Employing too little or too much metal is undesirable [58].

After repair has been completed, hemostasis should be obtained prior to closure. Closed suction for 1 to 2 days is frequently desirable [116]. The wound should be approximated gently with care to minimize resultant skin tension. If closure will place excessive tension on already traumatized skin, it is frequently better to leave the wound open and plan on delayed primary closure or skin grafting at a later date [15].

The decision to employ a long leg cast, short leg cast, or no cast at all must be made by the operating surgeon, based on the degree of fixation provided at the time of surgery. Even when internal fixation is deemed to be self-sufficient, however, the limb should be carefully dressed and immobilized after surgery to provide compression and at least temporary support and protection [55,81,82,84,91]. It is a rare patient who is willing and able to exercise his ankle effectively within the first few hours after surgery.

Weight Bearing

It is generally accepted that weight bearing should be avoided initially in fractures that involve the articular surface of the talus or distal tibia, as well as in instances where temporary tibiofibular screw fixation has been employed [76,82,89]. Stable "unimalleolar" injuries, that do not require reduction, can probably be safely allowed to bear weight if they are adequately immobilized.

However, for displaced fractures, that require closed or open reduction, opinions vary widely. For fractures treated by internal fixation, recommendations range from almost immediate weight bearing in a short leg cast [76]; to weight bearing in plaster, as soon as satisfactory motion has been regained (2–3 weeks) [13,124]; to avoidance of weight bearing for most of the time spent in plaster (6–8 weeks) [17,58,67,138]. Where plaster immobilization is avoided entirely, weight bearing should be prohibited, or at least limited, until some healing has occurred [11,88,90].

Factors to be considered in deciding when weight bearing should be instituted include the original degree of fracture instability or displacement; the degree of stability restored by internal fixation; the adequacy of external immobilization (depending on soft tissue swelling and limb size); the weight and activity level of the patient; as well as the risk, inconvenience, and social disruption likely to be incurred by avoidance of weight bearing. This latter consideration is especially important for older patients, since prohibition of weight bearing makes ambulation difficult, may predispose to reinjury, and frequently prevents the patient, at least temporarily, from returning home and functioning in a familiar environment.

Other Treatment Modalities

Occasionally, the nature of the injury or the circumstances of the patient are such that neither closed manipulation nor open reduction represents the preferred treatment. Instead, one of the following specialized techniques may be required.

Quigley Suspension

Quigley has described a technique which simultaneously provides limb elevation as well as reduction of certain fracture-dislocations caused by abduction and/or external rotation (Fig. 7.4) [105,106].

The entire lower limb is encased in stockingette which is suspended from the distal end. The knee is kept semiflexed by a sling under the distal thigh. Since the lower extremity at rest falls into external rotation, the distal extremity will necessarily rotate internally, placing the foot and ankle in supination (plantarflexion, internal rotation, adduction)—tending to correct external rotation and lateral displacement of the talus. While in this suspension, radiographs are obtained at 12 and 24 h; if satisfactory position has been achieved and swelling reduced to an acceptable degree, plaster is applied without moving the patient.

This technique is contraindicated for supination-adduction injuries as well as for external rotation injuries characterized by basal fracture of the medial malleolus, since there is no bony buttress to prevent overreduction of the talus (Fig. 7.5). This technique cannot be expected to correct the fibular shortening observed in some displaced external rotation injuries. Quigley suspension places the ankle in equinus and immobilization in this position is frequently undesirable. Use of this suspension for an extended period of time may cause discomfort or skin breakdown over the posterolateral heel or lateral malleolus.

Skeletal Traction (Os Calcis)

Except for comminuted fractures of the tibial plafond, skeletal traction through the os calcis has limited usefulness in the treatment of fracture-dislocations of the ankle [21,63]. It restricts the patient's mobility and provides only indirect, if any, control over the fracture fragments. Generally, no better than fracture "approximation" can be obtained despite meticulous attention to the weight and apparatus. Occasionally, however, skeletal traction proves useful for comminuted fractures or as a temporary measure to stabilize a fracture in order to facilitate care of associated soft tissue injuries. In this situation, one must be careful not to excessively distract

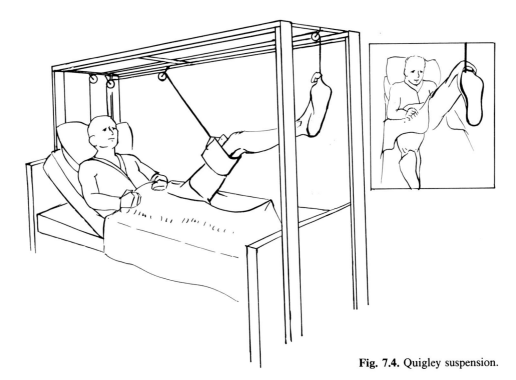

Fig. 7.4. Quigley suspension.

the talus from the articular surface of the tibia [21].

Vertical Transarticular Pin Fixation

For certain unstable ankle injuries, where satisfactory reduction cannot be maintained by closed means and internal fixation is not possible, vertical transarticular pinning is a viable alternative

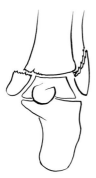

Fig. 7.5. Quigley suspension is contraindicated as treatment for supracollicular (basal) fractures of the medial malleolus since there is no bony buttress to prevent overreduction.

provided satisfactory reduction can be achieved by manipulation. Various techniques have been described [22,33,36,110].

Using local or general anesthesia, the fracture is reduced with the ankle in slight equinus position [22]. A Kirschner wire is then drilled proximally through the calcaneus for approximately 4 in. into the dome of the talus. The wire should penetrate the calcaneus 1 in. proximal to the calcaneocuboid joint and should point toward the center of the tibia with the fracture in reduced position. Radiographs are obtained in two planes, and if the Kirschner wire placement is satisfactory, it is used as a guide for insertion of a $\frac{7}{64}$-in. smooth Steinmann pin across the talocalcaneal and tibiotalar joints into the metaphysis of the distal tibia. The original Kirschner wire is then removed. The protruding Steinmann pin is cut off 1 in. from the plantar surface of the foot and bent to a right angle. A short leg cast is applied with care not to incorporate the pin. Weight bearing is prohibited until the pin is removed 5–6 weeks later (Fig. 7.6).

Childress has recommended this technique for patients with unstable ankle fractures when open reduction and internal fixation is prohibited due to coexisting local or systemic conditions [22].

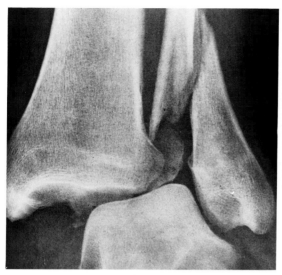

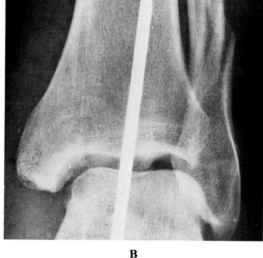

A   **B**

Fig. 7.6. Vertical transarticular pin fixation. **A** Unstable ankle fracture in a young athlete. **B** Treated by open reduction, repair of the deltoid ligament, and stabilization with a vertical transarticular pin. Courtesy of Dr. Harold M. Childress.

It may also be used as a supplement in conjunction with formal open reduction–internal fixation procedures (Fig. 7.7). Complications with this technique have been few. Joint violation by the fixation pin has not apparently caused any adverse effect.

Percutaneous Pin Fixation

Closed reduction combined with percutaneous pin fixation [54,75,93] has also been recommended for treatment of unstable injuries about the ankle. Provided adequate reduction can be obtained by manipulation, many fractures can be secured quickly and atraumatically with this technique (Fig. 7.8). A power driver and image intensifier are particularly helpful in this regard.

Rigid fixation, however, is seldom achieved, so that some form of external immobilization is usually required; also, repair of ligaments and removal of joint debris are not possible with this technique. Percutaneous pinning, like vertical transarticular pin fixation, is well suited for unstable fractures occurring in patients who are not candidates for open reduction and internal fixation because of systemic illness or associated injuries.

External Skeletal Fixation

Another alternative for reduction and stabilization of severe ankle injuries, when internal fixation is impractical or hazardous, involves external skeletal fixation. Vidal et al. have coined the term "ligamentotaxis" to refer to fracture reduction and maintenance via distraction forces acting through capsular and ligamentous structures (Fig. 14.7) [126].

A similar effect can be achieved using pins incorporated into circumferential plaster, as described by Laskin [74]; or, without circumferential plaster, the pins can be connected externally, using plaster or methylmethacrylate bone cement [57,122]. Pins in plaster or methylmethacrylate, however, provide less rigid fixation than the formal external fixators, and they do not readily permit adjustments of fracture position. External skeletal fixation techniques are frequently useful in the treatment of comminuted fractures of the tibial plafond (Chapter 14).

Open Fractures

An open fracture at any site represents a challenging surgical problem. This is especially true

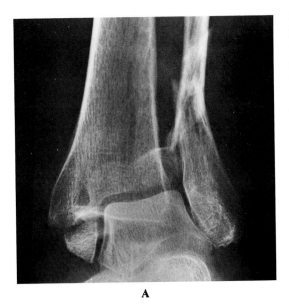

A

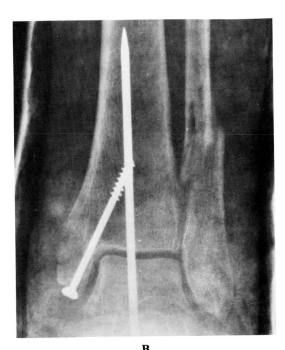

B

Fig. 7.7. A Unstable ankle fracture in an elderly, debilitated patient with circulatory insufficiency. **B** Treated with vertical transarticular pin fixation in conjunction with open reduction and screw fixation of the medial malleolus.

when the fracture involves a weight-bearing joint since accurate reduction is required for optimal restoration of function.

The subcutaneous location of the malleoli should make the ankle particularly susceptible to violation of the integument; yet, only 5% or less of ankle fractures are complicated by open wounds [11,13,76,87]. Since most ankle fractures are secondary to indirect violence, associated wounds are usually caused by laceration of skin tented over malleolar prominences or jagged fracture surfaces. Under these circumstances, wounds are from "inside out" [8] and generally are oriented transversely [58]. In the less common situation, where ankle fractures are caused by direct trauma, wound appearance is quite variable. Although the wound introduces another variable and is likely to complicate treatment, the primary objective of restoring a stable, painless, mobile articulation should not be abandoned or even relegated to a secondary concern. Wheelhouse and Rosenthal [133], as well as Joy et al. [60], have demonstrated that open fractures properly reduced and treated have as good a chance of successful result as closed injuries.

General Principles

Besides wound cultures [97,98], tetanus prophylaxis [26,58], and broad spectrum antibiotics [40,58,97,98], initial treatment should include prompt, meticulous wound exploration with thorough debridement of bone and soft tissue [10,44,123,125]. This is intended to reduce contamination as well as remove foreign material and devitalized tissue that, left alone, would serve as a "pabulum" for bacterial growth [45]. Copious wound irrigation, especially with a pulsatile system, is necessary and helpful, but it will not remove devitalized tissue or bacteria that have already migrated below the surface of exposed tissues. For this, only surgical debridement will suffice. Only after the wound has been properly cared for should attention be directed to treatment of the fracture itself.

Fracture Treatment

Since open fractures frequently represent unstable injuries, it is often difficult or impossible to maintain satisfactory reduction by closed means. Although many of these unstable injuries can be satisfactorily controlled using traction or external skeletal fixation techniques, there remains a group where satisfactory restitution can only

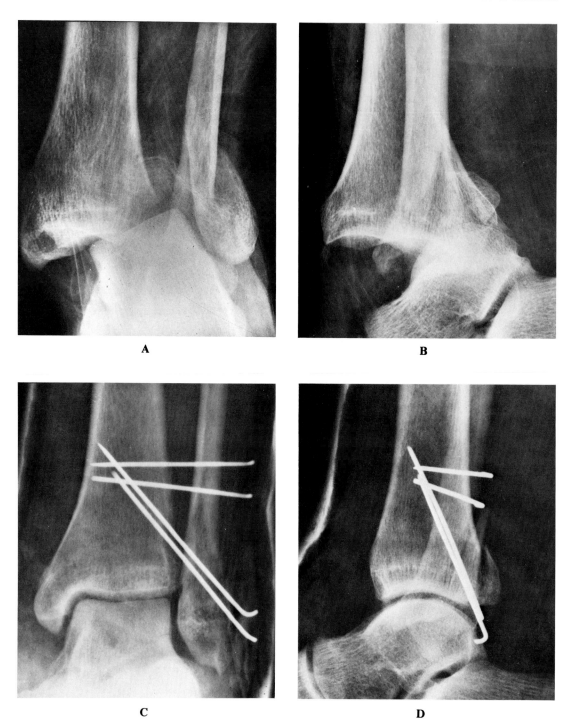

Fig. 7.8. A and B Displaced supination-external rotation fracture, stage IV. C and D After treatment by closed reduction and percutaneous pin fixation.

be achieved and maintained by use of primary metallic fixation. Unfortunately, internal fixation of open fractures has traditionally been associated with an increased incidence of wound sepsis [23,117,127] and the conventional surgical approach has been to omit internal fixation in open fractures [19,46,63,127] or, at least, defer it until primary wound healing has occurred [10,52,118]. Frequently, however, by the time soft tissue healing has progressed to the state where internal fixation can be safely accomplished, the soft tissues have contracted and the fracture elements are demineralized and have fibrosed or even healed in less than ideal position [8,82,84]. Under these circumstances, fixation is more difficult and the ultimate result is frequently less than ideal. Also, the surgeon, in his zest to secure early soft tissue healing so as to permit internal fixation without too much delay, may be tempted originally to preserve devitalized skin or close a wound that really should be packed open.

Lane contributed immensely to our present methods of fracture treatment by emphasizing the importance of restoring skeletal elements to their original form. The crude and mismatched metallic implants of his era, however, were subject to frequent corrosion, and Lane assumed that the inflammatory reaction they induced represented infection [53]. As a result, Hicks noted that "a firm teaching based upon a fear of infection has grown up banning internal fixation as a routine treatment for compound fractures" [53]. The clinical data commonly recruited to support this axiom is surprisingly scant and does not specifically refer to ankle fractures or other joint injuries, where little dissection and minimal metal insertion are required to obtain fixation [23,29,42,43,117].

Metal in vitro does not foster or support bacterial growth [41], and it is unlikely that properly manufactured and employed metal has any effect on bacterial colonization or wound infection in vivo [62]. One might still properly argue that the additional soft tissue dissection and periosteal stripping required for insertion of metal into wounds might predispose to infection [10,20, 53,62]; however, the unstable fractures most in need of internal fixation will usually have had most of their exposure accomplished at the time of injury or debridement [109]. Provided minimal or no additional exposure is required to introduce metallic implants, primary metallic fixation

should not be particularly hazardous [19,20,45]. On the other hand, if considerable additional exposure is required to introduce the implants, one should seriously question the advisability of employing internal fixation; under these circumstances [2,10,19], limited internal fixation combined with external immobilization or external skeletal fixation is often a better alternative.

One must also consider the nature of the wound when deciding whether to employ metallic internal fixation. The wound classification of Gustilo and Anderson [2,42] (Table 7.1) which relates to the degree of energy absorption, is helpful in this regard. As might be expected, type III injuries are complicated by infection in a high percentage of cases.

Table 7.1. Classification of Open Fractures. (Gustilo and Anderson)

Type I:	Open fractures with clean wounds less than 1 cm long.
Type II:	Open fractures with lacerations more than 1 cm long without extensive soft tissue damage, flaps, or avulsions.
Type III:	Either an open segmental fracture, an open fracture with extensive soft tissue damage, or a traumatic amputation. Special categories include gunshot injuries, farm injuries, and open fractures with associated vascular injury requiring repair.

From ref. 2.42.

Recent literature suggests that the judicious use of primary metallic fixation in conjunction with careful wound care not only ensures better fracture reduction but also protects soft tissues and facilitates wound care [85,90,118], with a resultant decrease in the infection rate [20, 62,109,123]. Cautious use of metallic fixation seems especially justified in the treatment of open joint fractures since accurate reduction is highly desirable and little additional surgical trauma is usually required to expose and stabilize the fracture [19,20,125]. When primary metallic fixation is employed, debridement and fixation should be performed in separate stages using different gowns, gloves, drapes, and instruments [62,123].

An alternative scheme is to defer metallic internal fixation for 5–14 days after initial debridement [44,97]. A delay of this magnitude is not likely to jeopardize fracture reduction or fixation, and is warranted if one expects that the condition of the soft tissues will improve sufficiently to permit introduction of metallic implants with a greater margin of safety.

Wound Closure or Coverage

Because skin and soft tissue about the ankle are sparse, Cave [14] went so far as to state that bone stock and fracture position should be sacrificed if necessary to preserve skin coverage. This approach necessarily relegates fracture reduction to a secondary role and is likely to result in painful instability or arthrosis. If, despite these measures and sacrifices, delayed soft tissue healing or infection occurs, the patient's problem will be compounded even further.

Lucas-Championniere [78,79], and later Dehne [32], demonstrated that joints as well as fractures could be left open without necessarily incurring undesirable consequences. This experience has been echoed by other clinical investigators [20]. It is often better to leave a wound open temporarily than to close the skin under tension or over devitalized and/or contaminated tissues [20,45,46,58,62,123]. This is particularly true when primary metallic internal fixation has been employed [2,19,40]. Delayed primary closure, split thickness skin grafts, or one of the more sophisticated plastic procedures can be performed when conditions permit [19,118]. Rather than being contraindicated, internal fixation is most advantageous when there is a significant soft tissue defect that will require such plastic procedures [84].

In 1808, fractures accompanied by wounds of the integument not infrequently resulted in amputation or fatal gangrene [102]. At the present time, these complications can generally be avoided and a considerable degree of function restored in many patients with even the most severe bone and soft tissue injury about the ankle. Although advances and improvements in antimicrobial drugs, metallic fixation, and skin coverage techniques have furthered our capabilities considerably, the emphasis should remain on prompt, meticulous surgical care of the open wound. When this basic aspect of wound care is neglected, the efficacy of our technology is reduced and the ultimate result is likely to be compromised.

References

1. Allgöwer M, Spiegel PG: Internal fixation of fractures: Evolution of concepts. Clin Orthop Rel Res 138:26, 1979.
2. Anderson JT, Gustilo RB: Immediate internal fixation in open fractures. Orthop Clin North Am 11:569, 1980.
3. Arimoto HK, Forrester DM: Classification of ankle fractures. An algorithm. Am J Roentgenol 135:1057, 1980.
4. Berridge FR, Bonnin JG: The radiographic examination of the ankle joint including arthrography. Surg Gynecol Obstet 79:383, 1944.
5. Black J: Biomaterials for internal fixation. In Heppenstall RB (ed): Fracture Treatment and Healing. Philadelphia, Saunders, 1980.
6. Bohler L: The Treatment of Fractures, 5th ed. New York, Grune & Stratton, 1956.
7. Bolin H: The fibula and its relationship to the tibia and talus in injuries of the ankle due to forced external rotation. Acta Radiol 56:439, 1961.
8. Bonnin J: Injuries to the Ankle. New York, Grune & Stratton, 1950.
9. Braunstein W, Wade PA: Treatment of unstable fractures of the ankle. Ann Surg 149:217, 1959.
10. Brav EA: Open fractures. Fundamentals of management. Postgrad Med 39:11, 1966.
11. Brodie IAOD, Denham RA: The treatment of unstable ankle fractures. J Bone Joint Surg 56B:256, 1974.
12. Burgess E: Fractures of the ankle. J Bone Joint Surg 26:721, 1944.
13. Burwell HN, Charnley AD: Treatment of displaced fractures at the ankle by rigid internal fixation and early joint movement. J Bone Joint Surg 47B:634, 1965.
14. Cave EF (ed): Ankle injuries. In: Fractures and Other Injuries. Chicago, Year Book Medical, 1958.
15. Cave EF: Complications of the operative treatment of fractures of the ankle. Clin Orthop Rel Res 42:13, 1965.
16. Cedell C-A: Outward rotation-supination injuries of the ankle. Clin Orthop 42:97, 1965.
17. Cedell C-A: Supination-outward rotation injuries of the ankle. Acta Orthop Scand (Suppl) 110:1, 1967.
18. Cedell C-A: Ankle lesions. Acta Orthop Scand 46:425, 1975.
19. Chapman MW: The use of immediate internal fixation in open fractures. Orthop Clin North Am 11:579, 1980.
20. Chapman MW, Mahoney M: The role of early internal fixation in the management of open fractures. Clin Orthop Rel Res 138:120, 1979.
21. Charnley J: The Closed Treatment of Common Fractures, 3rd ed. Baltimore, Williams & Wilkins, 1972.
22. Childress HM: Vertical transarticular pin fixation for unstable ankle fractures. Impressions

after 16 years of experience. Clin Orthop Rel Res 120:164, 1976.

23. Claffey T: Open fractures of the tibia. J Bone Joint Surg 42B:407, 1960.

24. Close R: Some applications of the functional anatomy of the ankle joint. J Bone Joint Surg 38A:761, 1956.

25. Cochrane WA: Fractures in the neighborhood of the ankle joint. IV. Manipulative treatment. Lancet 1:93, 1926.

26. Committee on Trauma of the American College of Surgeons: A guide to prophylaxis against tetanus in wound management. Bull Am Coll Surg 57:32, 1972.

27. Cox FJ, Laxson WW: Fractures about the ankle joint. Am J Surg 83:674, 1952.

28. Dabezies E, D'Ambrosia RD, Shoji H: Classification and treatment of ankle fractures. Orthopedics 1:365, 1978.

29. Dahl-Iversen E: On the frequency and the duration of ostitis after osteosynthesis, illustrated by 274 cases and re-examination of 66 cases of operatively treated fractures. Acta Chir Scand 63:41, 1928.

30. Danis R: Les fractures malleolaire. In: Theorie et Pratique de l'Osteosyntheses. Paris, Masson, 1947.

31. Danis R: The aims of internal fixation. Translated by Steven M. Perren. Clin Orthop Rel Res 138:23, 1979.

32. Dehne E, Torp RP: Treatment of joint injuries by immediate mobilization. Based upon the spinal adaptation concept. Clin Orthop Rel Res 77:218, 1971.

33. Dieterle J: The use of Kirschner wire in maintaining reduction of fracture-dislocations of the ankle joint. J Bone Joint Surg 17:990, 1935.

34. Eventov I, Salama R, Goodwin DRA, Weissman SL: An evaluation of surgical and conservative treatment of fractures of the ankle in 200 patients. J Trauma 18:271, 1978.

35. Fairbank HAT: The operative treatment of ankle fractures. III. Lancet 2:92, 1926.

36. Gallagher JTF: Transarticular pin fixation in fracture dislocations of the ankle. Am J Surg 79:573, 1950.

37. Gaston SR, McLaughlin HL: Complex fracture of the lateral malleolus. J Trauma 1:69, 1961.

38. Giblin MM: Ruptured tibialis posterior tendon associated with a closed medial malleolar fracture. Aust NZ J Surg 50:59, 1980.

39. Golterman AFL: Diagnosis and treatment of tibiofibular diastasis. Arch Chir Neerl 16:185, 1964.

40. Gregory CF: Open fractures. In Rockwood CA Jr, Green DP (eds): Fractures. Philadelphia, Lippincott, 1975.

41. Gristina AG, Rovere GD: An in vitro study of the effects of metals used in internal fixation on bacterial growth and dissemination. J Bone Joint Surg 45A:1104, 1963.

42. Gustilo RB, Anderson JT: Prevention of infection in the treatment of 1025 open fractures of long bones. J Bone Joint Surg 58A:453, 1976.

43. Gustilo RB, Simpson L, Nixon R, Ruiz A, Indeck W: Analysis of 511 open fractures. Clin Orthop Rel Res 66:148, 1969.

44. Hampton OP: Reparative surgery of compound battle fractures in the Mediterranean theater of operations. Ann Surg 122:289, 1945.

45. Hampton OP Jr: Basic principles in management of open fractures. JAMA 159:417, 1955.

46. Harrelson JM: Fractures and dislocations. General principles. In Sabiston DC Jr (ed): Davis-Christopher Textbook of Surgery, 11th ed. Philadelphia, Saunders, 1977.

47. Harvey JP Jr: Fractures of the ankle. A clinical survey of 181 cases. Clin Orthop 42:57, 1965.

48. Hedström Ö, Sundgren R: Missed concomitant ankle injuries in patients with fractures of shaft of the lower leg bones. Acta Orthop Scand 36:338, 1965.

49. Heikel H: Open or closed reduction of ankle joint injuries? Acta Orthop Scand 36:338, 1965.

50. Henderson MS: Fractures of the ankle. Wisc Med J 31:684, 1932.

51. Henderson MS, Stuck WG: Fractures of the ankle: recent and old. J Bone Joint Surg 15:882, 1933.

52. Hey Groves EW: On Modern Methods of Treating Fractures, 2nd ed. Bristol, Wright, 1921.

53. Hicks JH: The relationship between metal and infection. Proc Roy Soc Med 50:842, 1957.

54. Hoffer MM: Percutaneous lateral malleolar transtibial pin fixation of unstable ankle fractures. J Trauma 16:374, 1976.

55. Hughes J: The medial malleolus in ankle fractures. Orthop Clin North Am 11:649, 1980.

56. Hughes JL, Weber H, Willeneger H, Kuner EH: Evaluation of ankle fractures: Non-operative and operative treatment. Clin Orthop Rel Res 138:111, 1979.

57. Inoue D, Ichida M, Imai R, Suzu F, Ohashi K, Sakakida K: External skeletal fixation using methyl methacrylate technique and indications with clinical report. Int Orthop (Sicot) 1:64, 1977.

58. Jergesen F: Open reduction of fractures and dislocations of the ankle. Am J Surg 98:136, 1959.

59. Jones R: Crippling due to fractures. Br Med J 1:909, 1925.

60. Joy G, Patzakis M, Harvey JP Jr: Precise evaluation of the reduction of severe ankle fractures. Technique and correlation with end results. J Bone Joint Surg 56A:979, 1974.

61. Kaye JJ, Bohne WHO: A radiographic study of the ligamentous anatomy of the ankle. Radiology 125:659, 1977.

62. Ketenjian AY, Shelton ML: Primary internal fixation of open fractures. A retrospective study of the use of metallic internal fixation in fresh open fractures. J Trauma 12:756, 1972.

63. Key JA, Conwell HE: Injuries in the region of the ankle. In: The Management of Fractures,

Dislocations and Sprains, 6th ed. St. Louis, Mosby, 1956.

64. Kleiger B: The mechanism of ankle injuries. J Bone Joint Surg 38A:59, 1956.

65. Kleiger B: Treatment of oblique fractures of the fibula. J Bone Joint Surg 43:969, 1961.

66. Kleiger B: Mechanisms of ankle injury. Orthop Clin North Am 5:127, 1974.

67. Klossner O: Late results of operative and non-operative treatment of severe ankle fractures. A clinical study. Acta Chir Scand (Suppl) 293:1, 1962.

68. Kristensen TB: Treatment of malleolar fractures according to Lauge-Hansen's method. Preliminary results. Acta Chir Scand 97:362, 1949.

69. Lambert KL: The weight-bearing function of the fibula. A strain gauge study. J Bone Joint Surg 53A:507, 1971.

70. Lambotte A: The operative treatment of fractures. Br Med J 4:1530, 1912.

71. Lane W: The operative treatment of simple fractures. Surg Gynecol Obstet 8:344, 1909.

72. Lane WA: Method of procedure in operations on simple fractures. Br Med J 4:1532, 1912.

73. Lane WA: The Operative Treatment of Fractures. Medical Publishing Company, London, 1914.

74. Laskin RS: Steinmann pin fixation in the treatment of unstable fractures of the ankle. J Bone Joint Surg 56A:549, 1974.

75. Lee HG, Horan TB: Internal fixation in injuries of the ankle. Surg Gynec Obstet 76:593, 1943.

76. Lindsjo U: Operative treatment of ankle fractures. Acta Orthop Scand (Suppl) 189:1, 1981.

77. Lucas HK: Ankle fractures in association with fractures of tibial shaft. J Bone Joint Surg 54B:556, 1972.

78. Lucas-Championniére J: The Principles, Modes of Application and Results of the Lister Dressing. Translated and edited by FH Gerrish. Portland, Loring, Short and Harmon, 1881.

79. Lucas-Championniére J: Precis du Traitment des Fracture. Paris, Steinheil, 1910.

80. Magnusson R: On the late results in non-operated cases of malleolar fractures. III. Fractures by supination together with a survey of the late results in non-operatively treated malleolar fractures. Acta Chir Scand 92:259, 1945.

81. Malka JS, Taillard W: Results of non-operative and operative treatment of fractures of the ankle. Clin Orthop Rel Res 67:159, 1969.

82. Mast JW, Teipner WA: A reproducible approach to the internal fixation of adult ankle fractures. Rationale, technique and early results. Orthop Clin North Am 11:661, 1980.

83. McLaughlin HL: Trauma. Philadelphia, Saunders, 1960.

84. McLaughlin HL, Ryder CT Jr: Open reduction and internal fixation for fractures of the tibia and ankle. Surg Clin North Am 29:1523, 1949.

85. McNeur JC: The management of open skeletal trauma with particular reference to internal fix-

ation. J Bone Joint Surg 52B:54, 1970.

86. Mears DC: Materials and Orthopaedic Surgery. Baltimore, Williams & Wilkins, 1979.

87. Mendelsohn HA: Nonunion of malleolar fractures of ankle. Clin Orthop 42:103, 1965.

88. Meyer TL Jr, Kumler KW: A.S.I.F. technique and ankle fractures. Clin Orthop Rel Res 150:211, 1980.

89. Mitchell CL, Fleming JL: Fractures and fracture-dislocations of the ankle. Postgrad Med 26:773, 1959.

90. Mitchell WG, Shaftan, GW, Sclafani S: Mandatory open reduction: Its role in displaced ankle fractures. J Trauma 19:602, 1979.

91. Müller ME, Allgöwer M, Schneider R, Willenegger H: Manual of Internal Fixation. New York, Springer-Verlag, 1979.

92. Nahigian SH, Oh I, Zahrawi FB: Wire-loop fixation of the lateral malleolus in ankle fractures. In Bateman JE, Trott AW (eds): The Foot and Ankle. New York, Thieme-Stratton, 1980.

93. Neufeld AJ: Ankle joint fractures and their treatment. Clin Orthop 42:91, 1965.

94. Pankovich AM: Fracture-dislocation of Ankle. Trapping of posteromedial ankle tendons and neurovascular bundle in the tibiofibular interosseous space. A case report. J Trauma 16:927, 1976.

95. Pankovich AM: Adult ankle fractures. JCE Orthop 7:17, 1979.

96. Parker HG, Reitman HK: Changing patterns in fracture management emphasizing early motion and function. Surg Clin North Am 56:667, 1976.

97. Patzakis MJ, Dorr LD, Ivler D, Moore TM, Harvey J Jr: The early management of open joint injuries. J Bone Joint Surg 57A:1065, 1975.

98. Patzakis MJ, Harvey JP Jr, Ivler D: The role of antibiotics in the management of open fractures. J Bone Joint Surg 56A:532, 1974.

99. Phillips RS, Monk CJE, Balmer GA: Lateral rotation fracture of the fibular malleolus. J Bone Joint Surg 50B:879, 1968.

100. Phillips WA, Spiegel PG: Evaluation of ankle fractures, non-operative vs. operative. Clin Orthop Rel Res 138:17, 1979.

101. Platt H: Introduction to a discussion on fractures in the neighborhood of the ankle joint. Lancet 1:33, 1926.

102. Pott P: Remarks on fractures and dislocations. In: Chirurgical Works of Pott. London, Wood & Innes, 1808.

103. Purvis GD: The unstable oblique distal fibular fracture. Clin Orthop Rel Res 92:330, 1973.

104. Quigley TB: Indications and contraindications for the plaster of Paris walking boot. Am J Surg 83:281, 1952.

105. Quigley TB: A simple aid to the reduction of abduction—external rotation fracture of the ankle. Am J Surg 97:488, 1959.

106. Quigley TB: Analysis and treatment of ankle injuries produced by rotatory, abduction and

adduction forces. Instructional Course Lectures. Am Acad Orthop Surg 19:172, 1970.

107. Ramsey P, Hamilton W: Changes in tibiotalar area of contact caused by lateral talar shift. J Bone Joint Surg 58A:356, 1976.

108. Riede U, Willenegger H, Schenk R: Experimenteller Beitrag zur Erklärung der sekundären Arthrose bei Frakturen des oberen Sprunggelenks. Helv Chir Acta 36:343, 1969.

109. Rittmann WW, Schibli M, Matter P, Allgöwer M: Open fractures. Clin Orthop Rel Res 138:132, 1979.

110. Rowe MJ, Sutherland R: Fracture fixation by transarticular pin. A technique for control of severe ankle fractures. Am J Surg 74:24, 1947.

111. Rüedi TP, Allgöwer M: Fractures of the lower end of the tibia into the ankle-joint. Injury 1:92, 1969.

112. Sarkisian JS, Cody GW: Closed treatment of ankle fractures. A new criterion for evaluation. A review of 250 cases. J Trauma 16:323, 1976.

113. Schouwenaars B, Mulier JC: The conservative treatment of ankle fractures. Arch Orthop Traumatic Surg 94:161, 1979.

114. Sisk TD: In Edmonson AP, Crenshaw AH (eds): Campbell's Operative Orthopaedics, 6th ed. St. Louis, Mosby, 1980.

115. Solonen KA, Lauttamus L: Treatment of malleolar fractures. Acta Orthop Scand 36:321, 1965.

116. Solonen KA, Lauttamus L: Operative treatment of ankle fractures. Acta Orthop Scand 39:223, 1968.

117. Soto-Hall R, Horwitz T: The treatment of compound fractures of the femur. JAMA 130:128, 1946.

118. Spiegel PG: Early internal fixation in open fractures. Clin Orthop Rel Res 138:20, 1979.

119. Staples OS: Injuries to the medial ligaments of the ankle. J Bone Joint Surg 42A:1287, 1960.

120. Stören G: Conservative treatment of ankle fractures. Follow-up of 99 fractures treated conservatively. Acta Chir Scand 128:45, 1964.

121. Svend-Hansen H, Bremerskov U, Baekgaard N: Ankle fractures treated by fixation of medial malleolus alone. Late results in 29 patients. Acta Orthop Scand 49:211, 1978.

122. Taylor WH: The open treatment of fractures. NY Med J May 13, 1911.

123. Varma BP, Rao YPC: An evaluation of the results of primary internal fixation in the treatment of open fractures. Injury 6:22, 1974.

124. Vasli S: Operative treatment of ankle fractures. Acta Chir Scand (Suppl) 226:1, 1957.

125. Veliskakis K: Primary internal fixation in open fractures of the tibial shaft. The problem of wound healing. J Bone Joint Surg 41B:342, 1959.

126. Vidal J, Buscayret C, Connes H: Treatment of articular fractures by "ligamentotaxis" with external fixation. In Brooker AF Jr, Edwards CC (eds): External Fixation. The Current State of the Art. Baltimore, Williams & Wilkins, 1979.

127. Wade PA, Campbell RD Jr: Open versus closed methods in treating fractures of the leg. Am J Surg 95:599, 1958.

128. Wade PA, Lance EM: The operative treatment of fracture-dislocation of the ankle joint. Clin Orthop Rel Res 42:37, 1965.

129. Walheim T: Intra-articular malleolar fractures. A survey. Acta Chir Scand 79:166, 1937.

130. Walsh WM, Hughston JC: Unstable ankle fractures in athletes. Am J Sports Med 4:173, 1976.

131. Weber BG: Die Verletzungen des oberen Sprunggelenkes. In: Aktuelle Probleme in der Chirurgie. Bern, Verlag Hans Huber, 1966.

132. Weber BG: Lengthening osteotomy of the fibula to correct a widened mortise of the ankle after fracture. Int Orthop 4:289, 1981.

133. Wheelhouse WW, Rosenthal RE: Unstable ankle fractures. Comparison of closed versus open treatment. South Med J 73:45, 1980.

134. Wilson FC Jr, Skilbred LA: Long-term results in the treatment of displaced bimalleolar fractures. J Bone Joint Surg 48A:1065, 1966.

135. Yablon IG, Heller FG, Shouse L: The key role of the lateral malleolus in displaced fractures of the ankle. J Bone Joint Surg 59A:169, 1977.

136. Yablon IG, Wasilewski S: Isolated fractures of the lateral malleolus. Orthopedics 4:301, 1981.

137. Yde J, Kristensen KD: Ankle fractures. Supination-eversion fractures—stage II. Primary and late results of operative and non-operative treatment. Acta Orthop Scand 51:695, 1980.

138. Yde J, Kristensen KD: Ankle fractures. Supination-eversion fractures—stage IV. Acta Orthop Scand 51:981, 1980.

Chapter 8   Supination-Adduction Injuries

WILLIAM C. HAMILTON

In Supination-adduction injuries, the starting position of the foot is one of **supination** (plantarflexion, adduction, inversion). The pathologic talar motion is that of **adduction** (medial rotation of the talus about its longitudinal axis, frequently associated with some degree of internal rotation and/or medial translation of talus) (Fig. 8.1).

Stages (Fig. 8.2B)
I   Transverse fracture of the lateral malleolus or rupture of the lateral collateral ligaments (Fig. 8.2A).
II   Vertical fracture of the medial malleolus (Fig. 8.2B).

Mechanism

Lauge-Hansen noted experimentally that, when a supinated foot was forcibly adducted, the initial

injury occurred laterally in the form of a transverse, avulsion-type fracture of the lateral malleolus or avulsion of the lateral ligaments from their malleolar origin or their talar/calcaneal insertion (stage I) (Fig. 8.2A) [12,14]. The transverse fracture, when present, was usually located

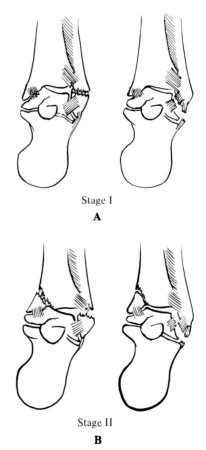

Stage I

A

Stage II

B

Fig. 8.2. Supination-adduction injury. **A** Stage I, characterized by lateral malleolar avulsion fracture or rupture of lateral collateral ligament. **B** Stage II, characterized by vertical fracture of the medial malleolus.

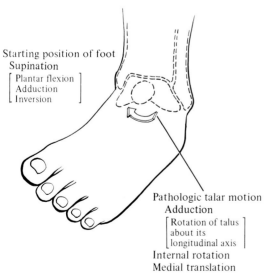

Starting position of foot
Supination
$\begin{bmatrix} \text{Plantar flexion} \\ \text{Adduction} \\ \text{Inversion} \end{bmatrix}$

Pathologic talar motion
Adduction
$\begin{bmatrix} \text{Rotation of talus} \\ \text{about its} \\ \text{longitudinal axis} \end{bmatrix}$
Internal rotation
Medial translation

Fig. 8.1. Supination-adduction injury.

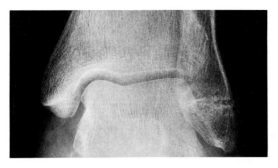

A

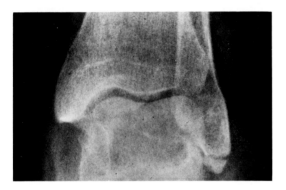

B

Fig. 8.3. Stage I injuries. **A** Nondisplaced avulsion-type fracture of lateral malleolus. **B** Ligamentous avulsion of a small fragment from the tip of the lateral malleolus.

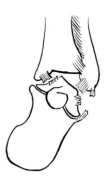

Fig. 8.4. Atypical supination-adduction injury observed by Lauge-Hansen.

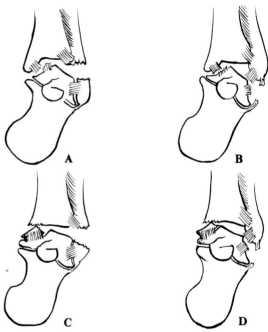

Fig. 8.5. Theoretical atypical supination-adduction variants.

at or distal to the tibial plafond (Fig. 8.3A) [5, 9,11,18]. Ligamentous avulsion sometimes occurred with a small fragment of bone (Fig. 8.3B). With continued force, the talus subluxated medially producing a near vertical fracture of the medial malleolus (stage II); the fracture line originated in the angle where the articular surfaces of the tibial plafond and medial malleolus meet (mortise angle) (Figs. 8.2B and 8.17) [5,8,9].

Variants

Rupture of the Deltoid Ligament Rather than Fracture of the Medial Malleolus

In one of the Lauge-Hansen's eight experimental trials, the talus adducted and rotated about its longitudinal axis after stage I, resulting in rupture of the deltoid ligament, rather than fracture of the medial malleolus (Fig. 8.4). No satisfactory explanation was given for this development, but Lauge-Hansen implied that it should be considered a rare clinical occurrence with this particular mechanism of injury [12]. Theoretically, this type of medial injury could be characterized by ligament rupture or avulsion fracture of the medial malleolus; also, it could be associated with fracture or ligament rupture on the lateral side, such that four different injuries would be theoretically possible in the end stage (Fig. 8.5).

Concomitant Damage to the Tibiofibular Syndesmosis

Lauge-Hansen believed that supination-adduction injury could not be associated with damage to the tibiofibular ligaments, since the lateral malleolus fracture occurs below the level of their insertion (Fig. 8.2A) [12]. As pointed out by Magnusson [15,16], however, if the fibular avulsion fracture occurs more proximally through or above the insertion of the anterior and/or posterior inferior tibiofibular ligaments, and the mal-leolar fragment is displaced medially a sufficient distance, then rupture of one or both of these tibiofibular ligaments might occur (Fig. 8.6). Since the posterior inferior tibiofibular ligament inserts higher on the fibula than the anterior ligament, it is much less likely to be violated under these circumstances. If the posterior tibiofibular ligament is ruptured by this mechanism, however, one can assume that the anterior ligament is torn as well. Even under the most unusual circumstances, however, when both the anterior and posterior inferior tibiofibular ligaments are torn, the interosseous ligament and interosseous membrane remain intact, so that the proximal fibular fragment maintains its normal position in the fibular incisura. Therefore, this injury can be associated with a partial syndesmosis lesion at most; complete ligamentous diastasis cannot occur [16].

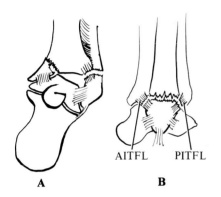

AITFL   PITFL

A   B

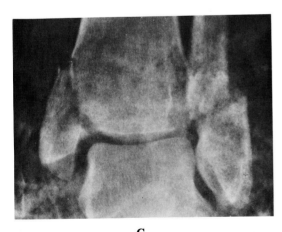

C

Fig. 8.6. Supination-adduction injury with associated ligamentous injury of the syndesmosis [15,16]. **A** and **B** If the fibular avulsion fracture occurs proximal to the insertion of the anterior and/or posterior inferior tibiofibular ligaments and the fragment is displaced medially to a sufficient degree, then rupture of one or both of these ligaments will occur. **C** Radiograph demonstrating supination-adduction fractures of the lateral and medial malleoli. At surgery both the anterior and posterior inferior tibiofibular ligaments were found to be ruptured.

Avulsion Fracture of Lateral Malleolus with Concomitant Damage to Lateral Collateral Ligaments

If, in the unusual situation described above (i.e., avulsion fracture of the lateral malleolus proximal to the anterior and/or posterior inferior tibiofibular ligaments), the deforming force persists but the tibiofibular ligaments resist further medial displacement of the lateral malleolus, damage can occur to the lateral ligamentous structures, resulting in both lateral malleolus fracture and some degree of lateral collateral ligament injury (Fig. 8.7) [7].

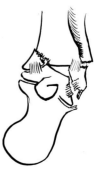

Fig. 8.7. Avulsion fracture of the lateral malleolus **and** rupture of the lateral collateral ligament.

Supination-Adduction Fracture of the Medial Malleolus Without Prior Injury to the Lateral Side

Burwell and Charnley [5] reported three patients with medial malleolar fractures of the supination-adduction type who did not demonstrate fracture of the lateral malleolus or clinical evidence of lateral ligamentous injury (Fig. 8.8A). They concluded that the medial malleolus had fractured in stage I rather than stage II. Possibly, these individuals had excessive lateral ligamentous laxity [9,22], on a constitutional basis or secondary to prior injury, that permitted adduction and medial subluxation of the talus without significant acute damage to the lateral side of the ankle

(Fig. 8.8B). Another explanation is that Burwell and Charnley were dealing with a stage I injury of the pronation-dorsiflexion type, (Chapter 14) which can occasionally simulate a supination-adduction fracture of the medial malleolus (Fig. 14.2A).

Associated Fracture of the Posterior Margin of the Tibia

According to Lauge-Hansen's original description [12], fracture of the posterior tibial margin did not occur as a result of the supination-adduction mechanism. Bonnin [3] stated that this occurred rarely. Klossner [10] reported three such instances and Burwell and Charnley [5] reported two other examples. Probably, this fracture is caused by posterior subluxation of the talus, either by direct pressure on the posterior tibial margin or by avulsion via the tibial periosteum. Yde [25] reported a "few" cases where the posterior tibial margin and medial malleolus were found to be included in a single fracture fragment (Figs. 8.9 and 13.2).

Clinical Significance

Supination-adduction is the most frequent mechanism of ankle injury. Because stage I injuries are frequently characterized by soft tissue involvement only, they may escape recognition, and hence the true frequency of this injury is difficult to ascertain. When all ankle injuries characterized by fracture, however, are analyzed, the supination-adduction mechanism explains

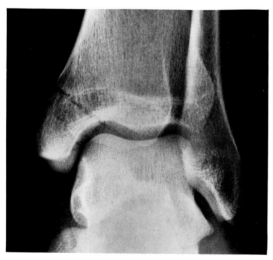

A

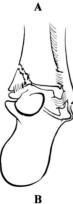

B

Fig. 8.8. A Oblique fracture of the medial malleolus without radiographic or clinical evidence of injury to the lateral ankle. **B** This can occur as a result of the supination-adduction mechanism when there is preexisting laxity of the lateral collateral ligaments.

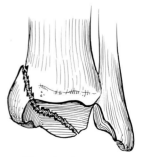

Fig. 8.9. In stage II supination-adduction injuries, the medial fracture may include the posteromedial margin of the tibia.

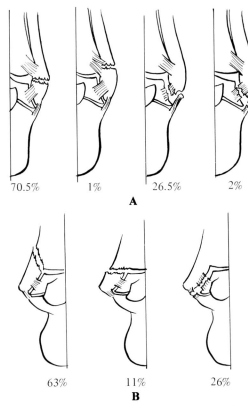

70.5%   1%   26.5%   2%

A

63%   11%   26%

B

Fig. 8.10. Distribution of stage II supination-adduction lesions (Yde) [25]. **A** Lateral side. **B** Medial side.

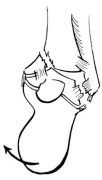

Fig. 8.11. Typical supination-adduction mechanism (adduction and medial translation of the talus).

two instances of combined lateral and medial collateral ligament injury.

Our own cadaver experiments may help to explain the observation of Ashhurst and Bromer [1] and Magnusson [15]. There are apparently two varieties of supination-adduction injury due to slightly different mechanisms:

1. Adduction with medial translation of the talus producing the typical vertical or oblique fracture of the medial malleolus associated with medial subluxation of the talus (Fig. 8.11).
2. Adduction with rotatory subluxation of the talus resulting in an avulsion-type injury on the medial as well as lateral side of the ankle, such that one observes avulsion-type fracture of the medial malleolus or deltoid ligament rupture, rather than the typical vertical or oblique fracture (Fig. 8.12). In this situation, medial dislocation of the talus will be prevented if the medial injury is ligamentous or if the avulsion fracture occurs below the level of the tibial plafond.

The key to the diagnosis of supination-adduction injuries is the typically transverse fracture of the lateral malleolus at or below the tibiotalar joint line and to a lesser extent the near vertical (or occasionally transverse) fracture of the medial malleolus.

Isolated avulsion fracture of the lateral malleolus (stage I) is not usually associated with subluxation or displacement of the talus, and generally demonstrates minimal displacement (Fig. 8.13). Treatment with simple support will usually suffice until healing is complete. The treatment of

approximately 10–20% of injuries [2,13,14, 17,20,23–25]. Of these, 80% are limited to stage I and 20% progress to stage II. Yde [25], in a detailed review of 98 supination-adduction injuries, found the distribution of lesions outlined in Fig. 8.10.

The relatively high incidence of transverse fractures and "avulsion-type" injuries of the medial side, observed by Yde, is somewhat surprising. Ashhurst and Bromer [1] as well as Magnusson [15] also observed that the medial malleolar fracture line in supination injuries could be horizontal or vertical. They noted that medial dislocation of the talus did not occur with the transverse-type fracture, but occurred quite regularly with the vertical- or sagittal-type fracture. Possibly, the variation noted by Lauge-Hansen [14], characterized by rotatory dislocation of the talus about its longitudinal axis with avulsion-type injury to the medial ankle, is more common than previously thought. In a series of 105 surgically explored ankle sprains, Brostrom [4] encountered

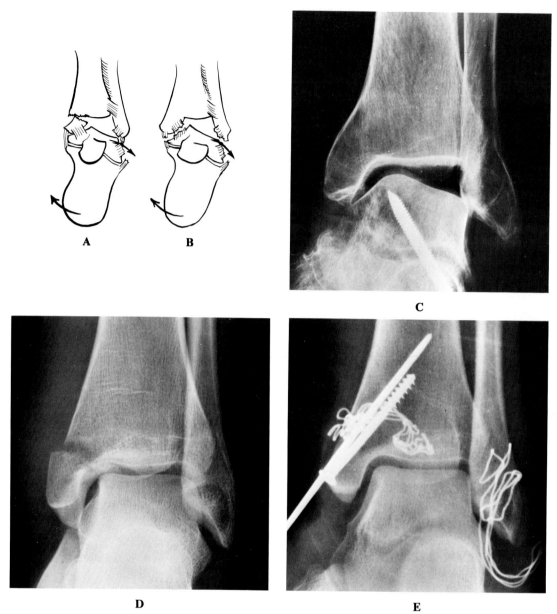

Fig. 8.12. Atypical supination-adduction mechanism (adduction and rotatory subluxation of the talus) may result in various injuries. **A** Medial malleolus avulsion. **B** Deltoid ligament rupture. **C** Experimentally, adduction and rotatory subluxation of the talus was observed to generate tension within the fibers of the deep deltoid ligament. **D** and **E** Avulsion-type fracture of the medial malleolus with lateral soft tissue swelling and tenderness. Patient was found, at surgery, to have complete rupture of the lateral collateral ligaments.

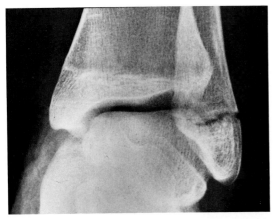

Fig. 8.13. Isolated avulsion fracture of the lateral malleolus with no associated medial soft tissue swelling or tenderness. This represents a stable injury and can be effectively treated with simple support.

stage I ligament injuries will be discussed in Chapter 9.

Stage II supination-adduction injuries may represent unstable situations requiring formal closed reduction or open reduction with internal fixation or ligament repair to restore normal anatomy and function (Fig. 8.14).

Apparently "isolated" lateral malleolus avulsion, or ligament rupture when associated with medial soft tissue swelling or tenderness, should suggest the possibility of an atypical stage II injury with deltoid ligament avulsion, rather than the usual vertical/oblique fracture of the medial malleolus. Frequently, under these circumstances, stress radiographs will be necessary to ascertain the true nature of the injury (Fig. 8.15).

Supination-Adduction Injuries: Closed Reduction (Lauge-Hansen) [13]

Reduction should be performed immediately.
General or spinal anesthesia is required.
Knee should be flexed to 90° to relax gastrocnemius muscle.
An assistant is required.
Immobilization is achieved in a short leg walking cast.

Technique

With counterpressure applied to the distal tibia, the hindfoot is grasped at the heel and the foot

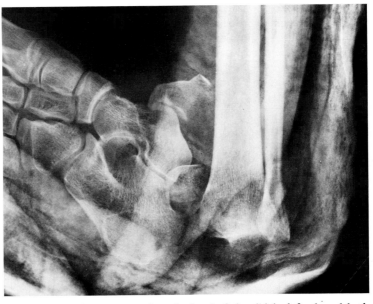

Fig. 8.14. Obviously unstable supination-adduction injury, stage II. Because of rotation, the distal fibular fragment appears small. The fibular avulsion, however, occurred at the level of the tibial plafond, and both the anterior and posterior inferior tibiofibular ligaments were ruptured.

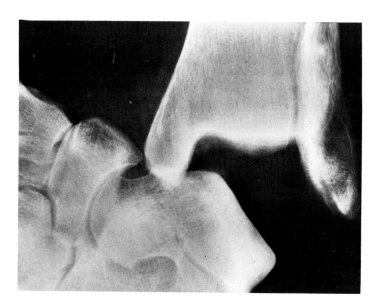

Fig. 8.15. "Bimalleolar ankle sprain."

is moved ventrally and laterally and simultaneously abducted and dorsiflexed to a right angle (Fig. 8.16).

Magnusson [15] has emphasized that in those rare instances where rupture of the anterior and/or posterior inferior tibiofibular ligaments has occurred with this injury, the foot should not be dorsiflexed excessively since this may contribute to widening of the malleolar fork.

Supination-Adduction Injuries: Open Reduction–Internal Fixation

In general, when open reduction is deemed necessary for ankle injuries, it is usually best to repair

as many elements of the injury as possible [24]. Whether lateral ligament injury, either isolated (stage I) or associated with medial injury (stage II), should be treated by closed or operative measures will be discussed in Chapter 9.

Because the typical medial malleolus fracture encountered with this mechanism is caused by direct talar impact, articular comminution at the mortise angle may occur (Fig. 8.17) [9]. It is especially important, in this situation, to explore the joint for evidence of osteocartilaginous loose bodies.

When both sides of the joint are to be repaired, it matters little which side is fixed first. In general, however, fracture fixation will have a protective

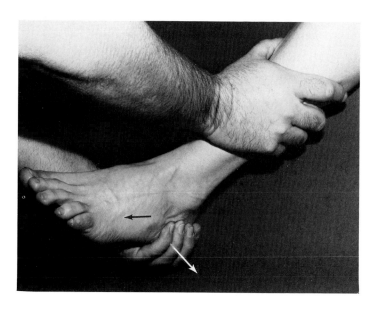

Fig. 8.16. Supination-adduction injuries: closed reduction technique [13].

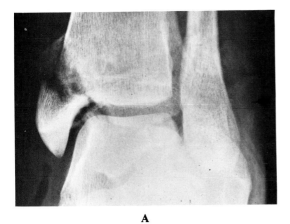

A

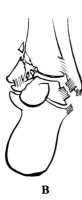

B

Fig. 8.17. A and B Comminution of the mortise angle.

effect on ligament repair. In supination-adduction injuries, characterized by lateral malleolar fracture, lateral fixation will have an especially protective effect on the medial repair, because the lateral fracture occurs earlier in the sequence of injury. If indicated, the lateral collateral and/or deltoid ligament should be approximated with interrupted nonabsorbable sutures; generally, these are not tied until the end of the procedure when some degree of stabilization has been achieved.

In the exceptional supination-adduction injury, characterized by high lateral malleolus avulsion and damage to the anterior and/or posterior inferior tibiofibular ligaments, the interosseous ligament and interosseous membrane remain intact (Fig. 8.6). If the fibular fracture is treated surgically, the syndesmotic ligaments should be explored and repaired, but tibiofibular fixation is not usually necessary.

Supination-adduction injury with posteromedial dislocation of the talus may be associated

with a large posterior tibial margin fracture. The fragment arises from the posteromedial corner of the tibia and may even remain in continuity with the medial malleolus (Fig. 8.9). If the fragment involves more than 25–35% of the articular surface and/or permits subluxation of the talus, open reduction and internal fixation is indicated (see Chapter 13).

Supination-Adduction: Fixation Techniques

Avulsion Fracture of Lateral Malleolus

Figure-of-Eight Tension Band

Since the fibular fracture occurring by this mechanism is usually transverse and the result of tensile forces, it is well suited for tension band fixation (Fig. 8.18) [21]. A 2-mm hole is drilled from front to back through the proximal fibular fragment 1 cm above the fracture site, and a strand of 20-gauge wire is passed through this hole. After the fracture site is inspected and debrided of clot, soft tissue, and bony spicules, the fracture is held reduced as two parallel 1.25-mm smooth Kirschner wires are drilled from the tip of the lateral malleolus proximally across the fracture site into the medullary canal of the fibula. The ends of the 20-gauge wire are crossed over the

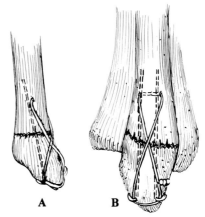

A   **B**

Fig. 8.18. A and B Figure-of-eight tension band for lateral malleolus avulsion fractures.

lateral aspect of the fracture and the anterior wire is passed under the protruding Kirschner wires at the tip of the lateral malleolus. The ends of the wire are tightened and twisted with care to locate the "knot" posterior to the fibula, where soft tissue coverage is better. The ends of the Kirschner wires are then cut, bent over, and impacted into the lateral malleolus to avoid creating an irritating prominence.

Intramedullary Fixation

Various intramedullary devices, including screws, have been used to fix fractures of this type (Fig. 8.19) [6]. These devices will maintain axial alignment, but they cannot be relied upon to neutralize forces tending to rotate, shorten, or distract at the fracture site. Bonnin stated that a vertical screw obtained a poor grip in the medullary canal of the fibula and, instead, preferred a bone peg [3].

Axial Screw (A-O Modification)

Another alternative is the axial screw technique as modified by the A-O group (Fig. 8.20) [21]. The fracture site is reduced under direct vision and the bone is drilled from the anterolateral tip of the lateral malleolus, across the fracture site, through the posteromedial cortex of the proximal fibular fragment. After overdrilling of

the distal fragment (and if necessary, tapping of the far cortex), a 5- to 8-cm screw is inserted and tightened to compress the fracture. This differs from intramedullary fixation in that the screw engages the cortex of the proximal fragment, such that a greater degree of compression is possible. Other than interdigitation at the fracture site, however, there is still nothing to prevent the distal malleolar fragment from rotating about the screw.

Plate

If the fracture is located sufficiently proximal, a carefully contoured one-third tubular or small fragment plate can be employed to fix fibular injuries of this type. Violation of the fibular articular surface (Fig. 8.21) by the distal screws is undesirable and can usually be avoided by fixing the distal plate with malleolar screws that do not require bicortical purchase.

Lateral Ligament Rupture or Small Avulsion Fracture of the Lateral Malleolus

Small apical avulsion fragments that will not accommodate a lag screw or tension band wire can generally be repaired by direct suture to the periosteum or through drill holes in the proximal fibular fragment. Exploration and repair of inju-

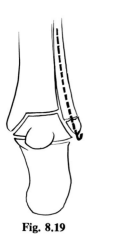

Fig. 8.19

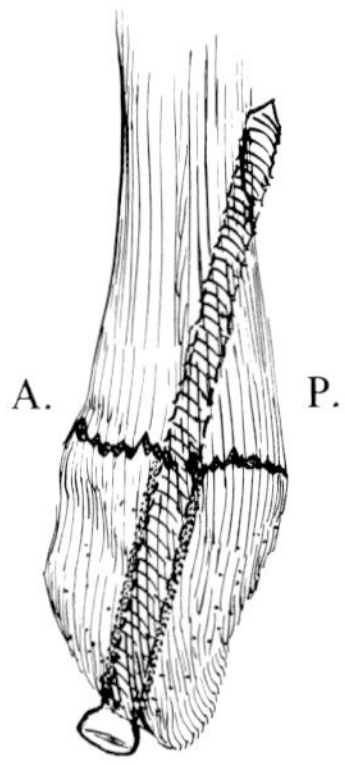

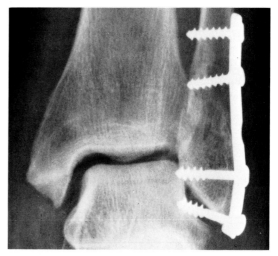

Fig. 8.20

Fig. 8.19. Avulsion fracture of the lateral malleolus, stabilized with an intramedullary device (Rush rod).

Fig. 8.20. Axial screw (A-O modification) for avulsion fracture of lateral malleolus.

Fig. 8.21. Although a small plate can be employed to fix avulsion fractures of the lateral malleolus, care should be taken so that the distal screws do not violate the articular surface of the lateral malleolus or the talus.

ries through the substance of the lateral ligaments is discussed in Chapter 9.

Oblique or Transverse Fracture of the Medial Malleolus

Lag Screw Fixation

Generally, these are large fragments that lend themselves well to lag screw fixation. Usually two or more screws can be employed. If it is comminuted, the mortise angle is not a helpful guide to the adequacy of reduction, so it is especially important that the proximal limit of the fracture on the medial aspect of the distal tibial metaphysis be well visualized and reduced anatomically. With the atypical avulsion-type fracture of the medial malleolus, the technique of lag screw fixation is identical to that employed for avulsion-type fractures caused by external rotation (Fig. 10.37). With the usual shear or oblique fracture of the medial malleolus, one needs to be careful that compression screws inserted at an angle to the fracture site do not result in proximal migration of the medial malleolar fragment (Fig. 8.22B) [19]. This can usually be avoided if one is aware of the possibility (Fig. 8.22A). Mast and Teipner have recommended inserting one screw perpendicular to the fracture site and then one screw perpendicular to the external surface of the bone in order to avoid this complication (Fig. 8.23B) [17].

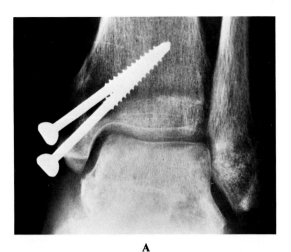

A

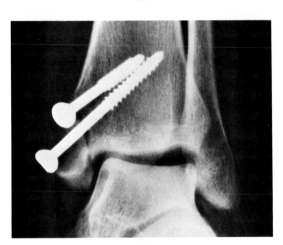

B

Fig. 8.22. Lag screw fixation of oblique fractures of the medial malleolus. **A** Satisfactory reduction achieved. **B** Medial malleolus has been permitted to migrate proximally.

Figure-of-Eight Tension Band

This technique is suitable for transverse fractures of the medial malleolus (Fig. 8.24A,B), but should be avoided for the shear-type fractures that usually characterize this injury (Fig. 8.24C). The technique for transverse fractures is identical to that described for external rotation injuries in Chapter 10.

Buttress Plate

Rarely, if the medial malleolar fragment is comminuted, a small buttress plate may be required to maintain reduction [17]. The distal screws should not be allowed to violate the articular surface of the medial malleolus.

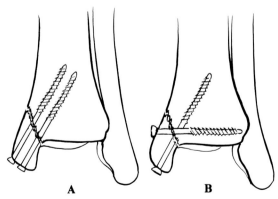

A   **B**

Fig. 8.23. Alternative screw fixation techniques for oblique fracture of the medial malleolus. **A** Standard technique. **B** If fragment is large enough, screws can be inserted at an angle to each other to prevent proximal migration of the medial malleolar fragment.

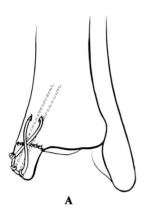 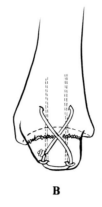 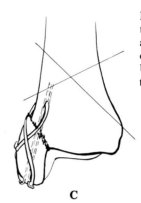

A   B   C

Fig. 8.24. Figure-of-eight tension band. **A** and **B** Suitable for transverse fractures of the medial malleolus. **C** Unsuitable for oblique fractures.

Hook Plate

Another alternative for fixation of comminuted medial malleolar fragments employs the hook plate of Zuelzer (Fig. 10.40). This technique is described in Chapter 10.

References

1. Ashhurst PC, Bromer RS: Classification and mechanism of fractures of the leg bones involving the ankle. AMA Arch Surg 4:51, 1922.
2. Bohler L: The Treatment of Fractures, 5th ed. New York, Grune & Stratton, 1956.
3. Bonnin JG: Injuries to the Ankle. New York, Grune & Stratton, 1950.
4. Brostrom L: Sprained ankles. I. Anatomic lesions in recent sprains. Acta Chir Scand 128:483, 1964.
5. Burwell HN, Charnley AD: Treatment of displaced fractures at the ankle by rigid internal fixation and early joint movement. J Bone Joint Surg 47B:634, 1965.
6. Dabezies E, D'Ambrosia RD, Shoji H: Classification and treatment of ankle fractures. Orthopedics 1:365, 1978.
7. Golterman AFL: Diagnosis and treatment of tibiofibular diastasis. Arch Chir Neerl 16:185, 1964.
8. Henderson MS: Fractures of the ankle. Wisc Med J 31:684, 1932.
9. Kleiger B: Mechanisms of ankle injury. Orthop Clin North Am 5:127, 1974.
10. Klossner O: Late results of operative and non-operative treatment of severe ankle fractures. Acta Chir Scand (Suppl) 293:1, 1962.
11. Kristensen T: Treatment of malleolar fractures according to Lauge-Hansen's method. Preliminary results. Acta Chir Scand 97:362, 1949.
12. Lauge-Hansen N: Fractures of the ankle. II.

Combined experimental-surgical and experimental-roentgenologic investigations. Arch Surg 60:957, 1950.
13. Lauge-Hansen N: Fractures of the ankle. IV. Clinical use of the genetic roentgen diagnosis and genetic reduction. AMA Arch Surg 64:488, 1952.
14. Lauge-Hansen N: Fractures of the ankle. III. Genetic roentgenologic diagnosis of fractures of the ankle. Am J Roentgenol 71:456, 1954.
15. Magnusson R: On the late results in non-operated cases of malleolar fractures. III. Fractures by supination together with a survey of the late results in non-operatively treated malleolar fractures. Acta Chir Scand 92:259, 1945.
16. Magnusson R: Ligament injuries of the ankle joint. Acta Orthop Scand 36:317, 1965.
17. Mast JW, Teipner WA: A reproducible approach to the internal fixation of adult ankle fractures: rationale, technique and early results. Orthop Clin North Am 11:661, 1980.
18. McLaughlin HL: Trauma. Philadelphia, Saunders, 1960.
19. Mitchell CL, Fleming JL: Fractures and fracture-dislocations of the ankle. Postgrad Med 26:773, 1959.
20. Mitchell WG, Shafton GW, Sclafani S: Mandatory open reduction. Its role in displaced ankle fractures. J Trauma 19:602, 1979.
21. Müller ME, Allgöwer M, Schneider R, Willenegger H: Manual of Internal Fixation, 2nd ed. Translated by J. Schatzker. New York, Springer-Verlag, 1979.
22. Pankovich AM: Adult ankle fractures. JCE Orthop 7:17, 1979.
23. Sarkisian JS, Cody GW: Closed treatment of ankle fractures. A new criterion for evaluation. A review of 250 cases. J Trauma 16:323, 1976.
24. Solonen KA, Lauttamus L: Operative treatment of ankle fractures. Acta Orthop Scand 39:223, 1968.
25. Yde J: The Lauge-Hansen classification of malleolar fractures. Acta Orthop Scand 51:181, 1980.

Chapter 9 Lateral Ligamentous Injuries of the Ankle

JEROME M. COTLER

The most frequent injury of the musculoskeletal system is the lateral ankle sprain. One would suppose that, for such a common injury, a uniform assessment and treatment scheme would be available and accepted. However, this is not the case. Treatment recommendations range from almost neglect to early surgical repair.

Vulnerability of structures is, to some degree, a function of age. Thus, ligamentous injuries of the ankle are most frequently observed in the young adult period, a physiologic era subsequent to epiphyseal closure and prior to the onset of osteopenia.

Anatomy

The structures of primary concern on the lateral aspect of the ankle include the ankle capsule and the three fasciculi of the lateral collateral ligament: the anterior talofibular ligament, posterior talofibular ligament, and calcaneofibular ligament (Fig. 1.10). The reader is referred to Chapter 1 for a detailed review of these structures.

The ankle capsule originates at the cartilage-bone junction of the tibia and fibula and extends to the cartilage-bone junction of the talus. The capsule with its accompanying synovial lining is loose and willowy anteriorly and posteriorly (Fig. 1.1). The anterior and posterior talofibular ligaments present as reinforcement of the capsule; the calcaneofibular ligament is a discreet extra-capsular structure.

As discussed in Chapter 2, the anterior talofibular ligament, because of its spatial orientation, is well suited to resist internal rotation, anterior subluxation, and plantarflexion of the talus; it is not well situated to resist adduction. The calcaneofibular ligament, on the other hand, is ideally

situated to resist adduction of the talus and the calcaneus, but poorly placed to restrict plantarflexion or internal rotation of these bones (Fig. 2.11). The exact function of the posterior talofibular ligament is uncertain. This ligament, however, is well designed to limit the separation of the fibula and talus necessarily associated with extreme degrees of lateral talar tilt; also, its short anterior fibers probably assist the anterior talofibular ligament in limiting internal rotation of the talus within the ankle mortise.

Our own cadaver studies, performed several years ago, suggested the following scheme:

1. The anterior talofibular ligament appeared to be the primary restraint to excessive internal rotation and plantarflexion of the talus. Rupture or sectioning of this structure and the adjacent anterolateral capsule permitted the lateral talus to migrate anteriorly out of the ankle mortise about a medial tether provided by the intact deltoid ligament. Radiographs obtained in this position frequently suggested anterior translation of the body of the talus, but in fact only the lateral border was displaced anteriorly [2], producing what has been referred to as anterolateral rotatory instability (Fig. 9.1A) (Chapter 4). Anterior translation of the entire body of the talus required violation of the superficial and deep deltoid ligament, as well as the anterior talofibular ligament and anterolateral capsule (Fig. 9.1C). Further degrees of anterior or anterolateral instability were made possible by section or rupture of the anterior fibers of the posterior talofibular ligament. The calcaneofibular ligament appeared to offer little, if any, resistance to anterior or anterolateral displacement of the talus.

2. With the talus in neutral position in the tibiofibular mortise, the lateral malleolus

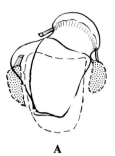
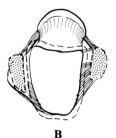
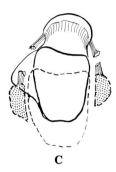

Fig. 9.1. A Anterolateral rotatory instability of the talus. **B** Normal talar-malleolar relationship. **C** Straight anterior instability of the talus.

A	**B**	**C**
Anterolateral rotatory instability of the talus	Normal talar-malleolar relationship	Straight anterior instability of the talus

provided a firm bony restraint to excessive adduction (or lateral tilt) of the talus (Fig. 9.2A). With plantarflexion and internal rotation of the talus, this bony restraint was reduced and pathologic talar tilt was restricted primarily by soft tissue structures. With excessive anterior or anterolateral translation of the talus (as permitted by sectioning of the anterior talofibular and anterior fibers of the posterior talofibular ligaments), this bony restraint was removed entirely and only the calcaneofibular ligament and posterior fibers of the posterior talofibular ligament

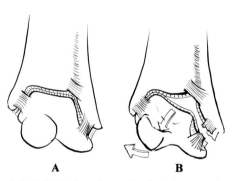

A	B

Fig. 9.2. A With the talus maintained in neutral position, the lateral malleolus provides a restraint to excessive adduction or lateral tilt. **B** Sectioning of the anterolateral capsule, anterior talofibular ligament, and anterior fibers of the posterior tibiofibular ligament facilitates plantarflexion and internal rotation of the talus, such that the fibular restraint to lateral tilt of the talus is removed entirely. Only the calcaneofibular ligament and the posterior fibers of the posterior talofibular ligament remain to prevent frank dislocation of the talus.

remained to prevent extreme talar tilt (Fig. 9.2B). Rupture of these structures as well as the anterior talofibular ligament and anterolateral capsule appeared necessary to permit significant adduction instability of the talus.

3. Isolated sectioning of the posterior talofibular and/or calcaneofibular ligaments, in our experience, produced little talar instability since the anterior talofibular ligament and anterolateral capsule prevented escape of the lateral talus from the bony constraints of the ankle mortise. We concluded that violation of all three lateral fasciculi was necessary, but violation of no single fasciculus was sufficient to produce significant talar instability in the coronal plane (talar tilt).

Mechanism of Injury

Considerable controversy surrounds any attempt to relate mechanism of injury to the site or degree of lateral ligamentous damage. Injury can be produced by single forces or, more commonly, by some combination of forces tending to adduct, internally rotate, and/or plantarflex the talus [5,18].

The mutually protective function of the lateral ligaments prevents complete disruption at any one site without some degree of damage to related structures. Yet, distinct clinical syndromes can be produced depending on the specific mechanism of injury and the site of maximal damage.

Clinical Syndromes

The typical ankle sprain is caused by internal rotation, plantarflexion, and to a lesser degree, adduction of the talus beyond its physiologic limit. The anterior talofibular ligament and adjacent anterolateral capsule are ruptured most consistently; with persistent force, secondary restraints including the posterior talofibular and calcaneofibular ligaments are injured resulting in an extreme degree of talar instability.

When plantarflexion forces predominate, the capsular injury is liable to extend dorsally across the ankle, resulting clinically in an inordinate amount of discomfort and anterior soft tissue swelling. There may be an associated avulsion fracture from the dorsal navicular or anterior aspect of the distal tibia (Fig. 13.16). This injury generally has little destabilizing effect, but acute symptoms are severe and recovery is frequently protracted because of the extent of hemorrhage, edema, and subsequent soft tissue organization that temporarily limit ankle motion.

When adduction forces predominate, the origin and insertion of the calcaneofibular ligament are most vulnerable. The resultant injury is frequently characterized by avulsion fracture of the distal fibula, as already described under supination-adduction injuries (Chapter 8). Calcaneofibular ligament avulsion from the fibula is manifested by localized tenderness and swelling at the tip of the lateral malleolus. Calcaneofibular ligament avulsion from its insertion on the calcaneus is apparently uncommon, although its true frequency might be underestimated since local findings in this area can be obscured by the overlying peroneal tendons.

Injury to the lateral ligaments of the ankle may be associated with rupture or contusion of the extensor digitorum brevis muscle. This is not likely to complicate the problem, but may serve to make the injury appear more serious than it actually is.

Clinical Evaluation

Since radiographic findings are usually minimal, assessment of lateral ankle injuries relies heavily on clinical observation [8–10,12,18–20,26,29]. A review of the circumstances culminating in injury is most valuable, including the terrain, task at hand, position of the foot at impact, as well as any sensation perceived by the patient at the moment of injury. Did the patient recognize a transient or fixed deformity of the foot or ankle? Was the patient able to continue the activity at hand or immediately disabled? Where was the initial site of swelling and how quickly did it develop? Was it confined to the anterolateral capsule or did it develop simultaneously about the periphery of the fibula?

Evaluation is most rewarding when performed early after the injury before soft tissue swelling and tenderness have become diffuse. The initial examiner is usually in the best position to accurately observe and record the extent of injury. Examination should include careful inspection for swelling and/or deformity, as well as palpation to determine areas of maximal tenderness. This should include the entire lower extremity, ankle, and foot if associated tibiofibular or deltoid ligament injuries are to be recognized.

Initial evaluation should also include at least a clinical assessment of stability in the coronal (adduction instability of the talus), sagittal (anterior drawer phenomenon), and horizontal (anterolateral rotatory instability) planes [4,6]. If performed early, an anesthetic is frequently unnecessary. Later, the development of painful soft tissue swelling and reflex protective muscle spasm will frequently conspire to obscure the true degree of instability. Adequate general or regional anesthesia will then be necessary to avoid inflicting unnecessary pain as well as to permit the examiner to ascertain the degree of hypermobility without causing further soft tissue disruption.

Radiography

To confirm or document suspected instability, radiographs should be obtained under strain conditions as described in Chapter 4. Plain films should have already been performed to exclude associated fractures of the malleoli, calcaneus, and base of the fifth metatarsal. These should also be carefully studied for the presence of osteochondral fractures of the talus (Chapter 16). Further investigation, employing conventional or axial tomography, may be necessary if occult injury of the talar articular surface is suspected. Arthrography [3,16,17] has been described and discussed already (Chapter 4). Although it is helpful as an investigative tool, the many arthrographic variants of normal as well as the poor correlation between dye extravasation and clinical instability limit the usefulness of this study in clinical practice.

Grading of Injuries

Injuries to the lateral ankle can be graded according to the site and/or degree of injury. Injuries can theoretically be classified according to whether one, two, or all three fasciculi of the lateral collateral ligament are involved. Also, any given fascicular sprain can be described as follows:

Grade I: Mild—a stretch, partial ligamentous fibrillar fault, or tear with overall structural integrity maintained

Grade II: Moderate—a greater degree of ligamentous disruption with overall continuity maintained

Grade III: Severe—complete loss of ligamentous continuity

By this scheme, the mildest form of damage consists of a stretch injury of the anterior talofibular ligament, whereas the most severe form of injury is characterized by complete rupture of the calcaneofibular and both talofibular ligaments. Although the extremes of this spectrum can usually be recognized clinically, intermediate grades of injury can only be accurately determined at this time by surgical exploration. Hence, grading of injuries in this manner has only limited applicability.

Our own practice has been to grade injuries according to the specific fascicular injury. When tenderness or soft tissue swelling is demonstrable, corresponding to two or more fascicular regions, stress testing in three planes under radiographic control is performed.

Treatment

The management of lateral ligament injuries of the ankle is probably as protean and provincial as any subject in orthopedic surgery. No uniform approach appears valid for this injury and management will necessarily depend on many variables.

Absolute immobilization intervals to protect ligament injuries are not available. Complicating factors include patient's age, specific area and degree of injury, speed of healing response, and individual joint demands. Most would agree that the minimum care necessary for the common ankle sprain (partial tear of the anterior talofibular ligament) is immobilization in a neutral position to restrict plantarflexion, adduction, and internal rotation of the talus. This can be accomplished with a Jones-type dressing, gel cast, adhesive strapping, or short leg plaster.

In addition, we need to know when healing collagen reaches such milestones as 25%, 50%, 75%, and 100% of normal strength, and if the latter figure ever truly occurs. A more fundamental question is, what percentage of maximum collagen strength sustains normal activities of daily living? Questions such as what degree of collagen strength is adequate for normal gait, and will such a degree of stress strengthen, weaken, or have no effect upon the functioning ankle, are indeterminate. In practical terms, rest and support to the area appear indicated until pain, soreness, and tenderness are no longer elicited. This usually requires anywhere from 3 to 8 weeks.

Technique (Adhesive Strapping)

The extremity is shaved from mid-calf to toes, allowed to dry, and then coated with tincture of benzoin. The foot is positioned in neutral (Fig. 9.3) dorsiplantarflexion and in slight valgus-eversion attitude. This position can be maintained with a length of muslin or adhesive positioned at the base of the toes and held by the patient (Fig. 9.3A). For the typical adult, 2-in. wide strips of strong adhesive are employed. The initial strip is similar to a stirrup. It begins on the medial aspect of the distal calf and is extended under the heel and then proximally along the lateral calf to maintain a mild degree of valgus positioning of the hindfoot (Fig. 9.3B). A strip of similar length is then started on the plantar aspect of the heel and extended proximally to cross the ankle anteriorly to terminate on the calf in the vicinity of the original strip. A smaller

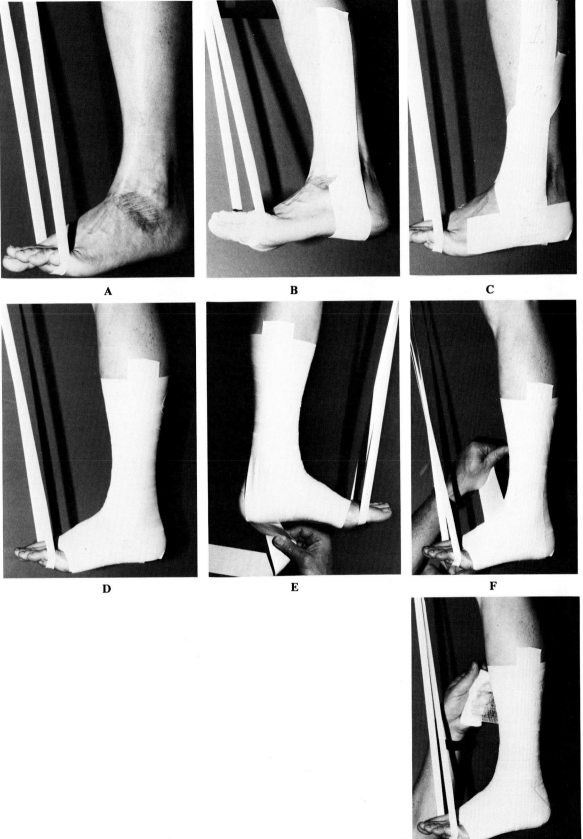

Fig. 9.3. Technique of adhesive strapping.

length of adhesive is then applied around the hindfoot, extending from the base of the first metatarsophalangeal joint to the base of the fifth metatarsophalangeal joint (Fig. 9.3C). Similar alternating strips are then applied with the lateral to medial strips overlapping the midline anteriorly for approximately 2 in. This is continued until the skin is completely covered with adhesive (Fig. 9.3D). An additional two to four strips are then applied, each extending from the medial malleolus under the plantar aspect of the heel to the midline of the dorsum of the foot (Fig. 9.3E,F). The entire support strapping can then be covered with gauze or an Ace bandage for cleanliness and to limit the tendency of the adhesive to roll (Fig. 9.3G).

Whatever form of immobilization is employed, careful monitoring of the distal neurovascular status is necessary in the immediate postinjury stage. Ideally, the extremity is elevated to just above heart level to take advantage of gravitational forces. Application of cold packs tends to decrease local tissue metabolic needs and vascular diapedesis and serves to minimize soft tissue swelling and discomfort. In most instances, 12–36 h of observation will suffice. At this point, the patient is usually sufficiently comfortable to share weight with crutches and in approximately 7–14 days can usually bear weight unprotected. Muscle pumping action appears to decrease local edema as well as strengthen collagen cross-linkage during the reparative process. Strapping or immobilization should be reapplied as loosening is noted.

Upon removal of the external support, the ankle should be reexamined for swelling, tenderness, and stability. Should significant local symptoms persist, further protection is necessary. If only mild soft tissue swelling or tenderness persist, gradual resumption of activity, accompanied by warm soaks and elastic external support for an additional 3 to 6 weeks, is recommended. During this rehabilitative phase, the patient is encouraged to exercise the intrinsic musculature of the foot and ankle and to restore muscular control, motion, strength, and gait.

Patients with this injury should be protected from forced plantarflexion and internal rotation since such movements stress the anterior and posterior talofibular ligaments and predispose to talar subluxation. If the patient is a competitive athlete, the ankle should be strapped and pro-tected for at least the remainder of the season, and probably for 9 to 10 months total.

For complete ligamentous disruption, controversy characterizes therapeutic considerations. Over the years, strong support for primary operative treatment has been voiced by some, whereas others recommend this only occasionally, if ever. Data to absolutely compare both groups are not available at present, thus rendering the selection of treatment subject to individual assumption or bias, albeit sincere. It appears difficult to refute the argument that one is able to obtain a stronger, more durable union of completely disrupted soft tissues by accurate approximation of ligament ends. It is our distinct impression that primary surgical intervention should be considered for active patients with evidence of complete ligamentous disruption of the lateral ankle complex. Our indications for surgical exploration are as follows:

1. Conviction by the examiner of at least double ligamentous disruption allowing for talar tilt (adduction) in excess of 10° compared to the normal uninjured extremity.
2. Patient demonstration of functional instability subsequent to a recent injury.
3. Avulsion fracture of the distal fibula with associated excessive talar tilt in excess of 10° compared to the opposite extremity.
4. Clinically or radiographically demonstrable anterior or anterolateral translation of the talus.

Operative Repair

Repair of the lateral ankle structure is best accomplished through the lateral inferior approach as described by Kocher (Chapter 3). One should avoid damaging by incision or retraction the intermediate branch of the superficial peroneal nerve anteriorly as well as the sural nerve posteriorly. Usually, hematoma is encountered directly below subcutaneous tissues; this must be carefully evacuated to allow assessment of the soft tissue disruption as well as intraarticular inspection for cartilage damage or osteochondral fragments. The anterolateral capsule, anterior talofibular ligament, and proximal portion of the calcaneofibular ligament can easily be visualized through this approach. The distal portion of the calcaneofibular ligament and its attachment to the calcaneus, however, are obscured by the overlying peroneal tendons. If necessary, the incision can be extended proximally and the peroneal tendons reflected anteriorly by incising the peroneal retinaculum; if so, these tendons should be carefully replaced and the retinaculum repaired or reconstructed at the end of the procedure to avoid the syndrome of peroneal subluxation.

The ends of the ruptured posterior talofibular ligament may be readily visualized in extreme degrees of instability that permit adduction of the talus. With lesser degrees of instability, the integrity of this ligament can be ascertained by palpation with an instrument passed into the posterior talofibular interval.

The anterior talofibular ligament, synovium, and adjacent capsule should be repaired [27] as a single tissue mass with interrupted nonabsorbable sutures. The calcaneofibular ligament represents a distinct extracapsular structure and is repaired separately [2]. The posterior talofibular ligament does not lend itself well to direct surgical repair because of its location and short length. Reduction of the talus and repair of the anterior talofibular and calcaneofibular ligaments, however, will necessarily guarantee that the ends of the posterior talofibular ligament are in optimal position for healing.

Midsubstance ligament ruptures are generally repaired end to end, but if any evidence of elongation is present, plication is advisable. If failure has occurred at the bone-ligament interface, with or without a small bony avulsion, the ligament should be repaired directly to bone using drill holes. The avulsed fragment may be excised or retained to enhance the holding power of sutures. Large displaced avulsion fractures of the lateral malleolus should be reduced and fixed internally, as described in Chapter 8.

Following ligamentous repair, the patient should be immobilized in a short leg cast, positioned in neutral dorsiplantarflexion with the hindfoot in valgus, for at least 6 weeks to allow soft tissue healing. Subsequently, the repair should be protected from excessive tensile forces for at least 3 to 9 months, depending on the nature of the injury and the adequacy of repair.

Occasionally, even with subacute injury (greater than 3 weeks duration), sufficient soft tissue structures are still present to allow for adequate primary repair. These circumstances are unusual since by this time ligamentous and capsular contraction frequently preclude surgical approximation. However, if this circumstance is present, the problem is simplified and offers a better repair than that available through most reconstructive procedures. Brostrom [7] suggested that primary repair may be possible even several years after the original injury, but this view is not widely accepted.

Chronic Lateral Ligamentous Insufficiency

Posttraumatic lateral instability of the ankle has been recognized for some time. Complaints include recurrent sprains, a chronic sense of ankle instability, frequent giving way, intermittent discomfort, and recurrent swelling and tenderness. Although antecedent trauma without adequate ligament healing is responsible for this syndrome in most instances, other causative and/or contributory factors need be considered.

Freeman and Wyke [14] reported abnormal articular reflexes in the cat ankle and suggested this as a mechanism of faulty ankle function in humans. Other experiments involving denervation of alternative support areas and assessment of reciprocal muscle group function by electromyography have demonstrated normal or dissociated muscle responses. Over the years, by following a large number of patients with "weak ankles," the author has observed a tendency for many of these patients to demonstrate varying degrees of S-1 nerve root dysfunction. This is not to suggest that all or many of these patients ultimately demonstrate a full-blown sciatic syndrome requiring surgical decompression; many experience a chronic waxing and waning syndrome with vague degrees of back, hip, and leg complaints, characterized by pain, ache, numbness, muscle weakness, and paresthesias, as well as giving way of the ankle. This observation has included a lack of synchronous and balanced function between the posterior tibial and peroneal muscle groups. Unbridled posterior tibial function is capable of initiating all the forces necessary to foster adduction, internal rotation, and/or plantarflexion of the talus, associated with lateral ankle instability, particularly when these moments are reinforced by body weight. A similar mechanism has been reported by Abraham [1], in an instance of neglected rupture of the peroneal tendons, predisposing to repetitive ankle sprain.

Congenital ligamentous laxity offers still another circumstance predisposing to recurrent ankle sprains or "giving way." Patients with these alterations in collagen fibers and cross-linkage notoriously offer complaints suggestive of limited tether to the lateral malleolus. Also, patients with excessive internal tibial torsion, either isolated or in association with clubfoot deformity or cerebral palsy, frequently offer complaints of chronic lateral ankle instability. Finally, old trauma with osteophyte formation on opposing tibial or talar surfaces has been demonstrated to block motion and produce a clinical syndrome of lateral ankle instability.

For sedentary patients who experience a repetitive tendency to uncontrolled varus instability of the ankle, a shoe with a reverse Thomas heel and/or outer heel flange of $\frac{3}{16}$ to $\frac{3}{8}$ in. can offer great assistance.

For more active patients with disabling or annoying symptoms, exercises to improve ankle strength and proprioception, as recommended by Freeman [14], when combined with prophylactic strapping and custom orthoses, many times are quite beneficial.

Young active patients with disability refractory to these measures should be considered for lateral ligamentous reconstruction. Toward this end, many different procedures have been devised. Most techniques are designed to replace either the anterior talofibular ligament or calcaneofibular ligament; some procedures provide for reconstruction of both structures. Usually, autogenous tendon is employed, although autogenous fascia, allografts of fascia or tendon and artificial ligament have been recommended by some authors. Some modifications specify the use of free grafts, but most employ local tissue with an attachment maintained proximally or distally in the hopes of preserving blood supply and/or innervation.

Procedures for Reconstruction

Table 9.1 and Figures 9.4–9.6 depict reconstructive procedures for the anterior talofibular, calcaneofibular, and anterior talofibular plus calcaneo-

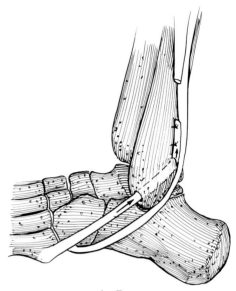

A Evans

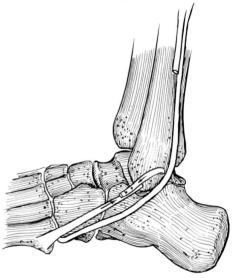

B Ottosson

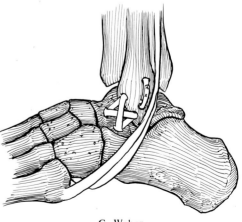

C Weber

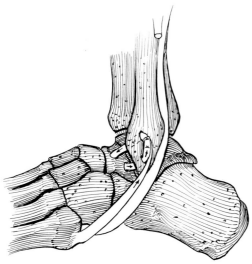

D   Watson Jones

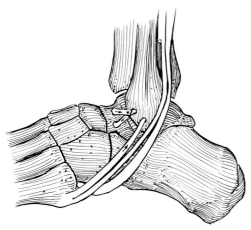

E   Lemberger

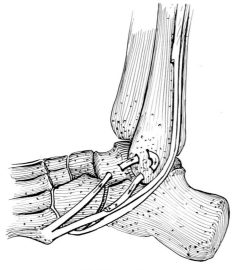

F   McLaughlin

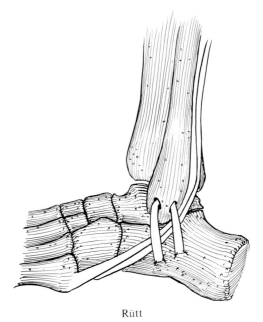

Rütt

Fig. 9.5. The Rütt procedure employs a free fascial graft to reconstruct the calcaneofibular ligament [28].

Table 9.1. Procedures for Lateral Ankle Reconstruction

Anterior Talofibular (Fig. 9.4)
  A.   Evans procedure (distal peroneus brevis) [13]
  B.   Modified Evans (Ottosson) [23]
  C.   Weber (free plantaris tendon) [28]
  D.   Watson-Jones (distal peroneus brevis) [15]
  E.   Lemberger (split distal peroneus brevis) [28]
  F.   McLaughlin (split distal peroneus brevis) [21]
Calcaneofibular (Fig. 9.5)
  A.   Rütt (free fascial graft) [28]
Anterior Talofibular and Calcaneofibular (Fig. 9.6)
  A.   Elmslie (split distal peroneus brevis) [11]
  B.   Viernstein (proximal peroneus brevis) [28]
  C.   Weisbach-Jaeger (lyophilized homograft dura) [28]
  D.   Chrisman (Rechting) (split distal peroneus brevis) [11,26]

fibular ligaments, respectively. Whatever specific technique is utilized, surgery in this area requires the utmost care to avoid complications of skin necrosis and infection. Pain and dysesthesia from cutaneous nerve (sural or superficial peroneal) damage also may contribute to dissatisfaction if

◁
Fig. 9.4. Procedures intended to reconstruct the anterior talofibular ligament.

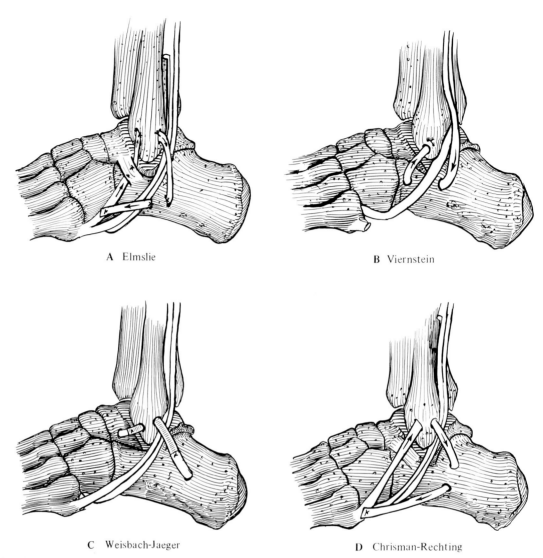

A Elmslie

B Viernstein

C Weisbach-Jaeger

D Chrisman-Rechting

Fig. 9.6. Reconstructive procedures that provide for the anterior talofibular **and** calcaneofibular ligaments.

these structures are not carefully avoided or protected.

Complete immobilization of the reconstructed ankle should be maintained for 6–8 weeks after surgery. As with ligamentous reconstruction at other sites, evidence continues to accumulate that transplanted tissues require significant support and protection for extended periods of time, if they are ever to acquire the strength and mechanical characteristics necessary to truly substitute for the original structure. It is paramount for patients undergoing such procedures to realize the commitment of time and effort necessary to maximize the final clinical result. With careful patient selection, attention to operative detail,

and supervised rehabilitation, good results can be anticipated in 80–90% of patients.

References

1. Abraham E, Stirnaman JE: Neglected rupture of the peroneal tendons causing recurrent sprains of the ankle. Case report. J Bone Joint Surg 61A:1247, 1979.
2. Anderson KL, Lecocq JF: Operative treatment of injury to the fibular collateral ligament of the ankle. J Bone Joint Surg 36A:825, 1954.
3. Arner O, Ekengren K, Hulting B, Lindholm A: Arthrography of the talo-crural joint. Anatomic, roentgenographic, and clinical aspects. Acta Chir Scand 113:253, 1957.

4. Bonnin JG: Injuries to the Ankle. New York, Grune & Stratton, 1950.

5. Bosien WR, Staples OS, Russell SW: Residual disability following acute ankle sprains. J Bone Joint Surg 37A:1237, 1955.

6. Brostrom L: Sprained ankles. I. Anatomic lesions in recent sprains. Acta Chir Scand 128:43, 1964.

7. Brostrom L, Liljedahl SO, Lindvall N: Sprained ankles. IV. Surgical treatment of chronic ligament ruptures. Acta Chir Scand 132:551, 1966.

8. Caro D, Howells JB, Craft IL, Shaw PC: The diagnosis and treatment of injuries of the lateral ligaments of the ankle joint. Lancet 2:720, 1964.

9. Cave EF: Fractures and Other Injuries. Chicago, Year Book Medical, 1958.

10. Charnley J: Sprains and dislocations. Practitioner 164:314, 1950.

11. Chrisman OD, Snook GA: Reconstruction of lateral ligament tears of the ankle. An experimental study and clinical evaluation of seven patients treated by a new modification of the Elmslie procedure. J Bone Joint Surg 51A:904, 1969.

12. Dziob JM: Ligamentous injuries about the ankle joint. Am J Surg 91:692, 1956.

13. Evans DL: Recurrent instability of the ankle. A method of surgical treatment. Proc Roy Soc Med 46:343, 1953.

14. Freeman MAR, Wyke B: Articular reflexes at the ankle joint. An electromyographic study of normal and abnormal influences of ankle joint mechanoreceptors upon reflex activity in the leg muscles. Br J Surg 54:990, 1967.

15. Gillespie HS, Boucher P: Watson-Jones repair of lateral instability of the ankle. J Bone Joint Surg 53A:920, 1971.

16. Glastrup H: Arthrography in acute ankle lesions. Proceedings of the Nordish Ortopedish Forenings. Acta Orthop Scand 36:337, 1965.

17. Gordon RB: Arthrography of the ankle joint. Experience in 107 studies. J Bone Joint Surg 52A:1623, 1970.

18. Hughes JR: Sprain and subluxations of the ankle joint. Proc Roy Soc Med 35:765, 1942.

19. Leonard MH: Injuries of the lateral ligaments of the ankle. J Bone Joint Surg 31A:373, 1969.

20. Makhani JS: Diagnosis and treatment of acute ruptures of the various components of the lateral ligaments of the ankle. Am J Orthop 4:224, 1962.

21. McLaughlin HL: Trauma. Philadelphia, Saunders, 1959.

22. Nilsonne H: Making a new ligament in ankle sprain. J Bone Joint Surg 14:380, 1932.

23. Ottosson L: Lateral instability of the ankle treated by a modified Evans procedure. Acta Orthop Scand 49:302, 1978.

24. Pennal GF: Subluxation of the ankle. Can MAJ 49:92, 1943.

25. Quigley TB: Fractures and ligament injuries of the ankle. Am J Surg 98:477, 1959.

26. Rechting GR, McCarroll JR, Webster DA: Reconstruction for chronic lateral instability of the ankle. A review of 28 surgical patients. Orthopaedics 5:46, 1982.

27. Ruth C: The surgical treatment of injuries of the fibular collateral ligaments of the ankle. J Bone Joint Surg 43A:229, 1961.

28. Rütt A: Surgery of the Lower Leg and Foot. Philadelphia, Saunders, 1980.

29. Staples OS: Ligamentous injuries of the ankle joint. Clin Orthop Rel Res 42:21, 1965.

Chapter 10 External Rotation Injuries

WILLIAM C. HAMILTON

Although supination-adduction is the most common mechanism producing ankle injury, external rotation of the foot with respect to the lower leg is the most common mechanism resulting in ankle fracture [46,47,54]. Lauge-Hansen described two varieties of external rotation fracture, depending on whether the foot was supinated or pronated at the moment of injury (Fig. 10.1). **Supination-external rotation** injuries will be discussed in this chapter, and **pronation-external rotation** injuries will be discussed in Chapter 11.

In supination external rotation injuries [44], the starting position of the foot is that of supination (plantarflexion, adduction, inversion). The pathologic talar motion is that of eversion (external rotation) (Fig. 10.1A). The stages of this type of injury are as follows (Fig. 10.2):

I. Rupture or avulsion of the anterior inferior tibiofibular ligament (AITFL) (Fig. 10.2A).
II. Spiral or oblique fracture of the lateral malleolus (Fig. 10.2B).
III. Rupture or avulsion of the posterior inferior tibiofibular ligaments (PITFL and ITTFL) (Fig. 10.2C).
IV. Rupture of the deltoid ligament or avulsion-type fracture of the medial malleolus (Fig. 10.2D,E).

Mechanism

Lauge-Hansen noted that the deltoid ligament was relaxed when the foot was in the starting position of supination [44,45]. As the foot was externally rotated, the first injury to occur was rupture or avulsion of the anterior inferior tibiofibular ligament (stage I), permitting the anterior syndesmosis to widen 2–3 mm (anterior diastasis) (Fig. 10.2A). If the force was dissipated at this point, the fibula generally recoiled to its normal position. Experimentally, the anterior inferior tibiofibular ligament usually failed via avulsion of the anterior tibial tubercle, but occasionally it

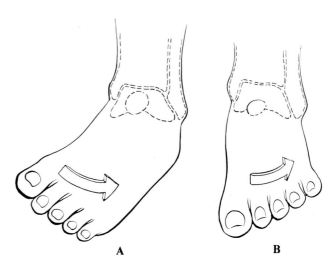

Fig. 10.1. External rotation injuries. **A** Supination-external rotation. **B** Pronation-external rotation.

A   B

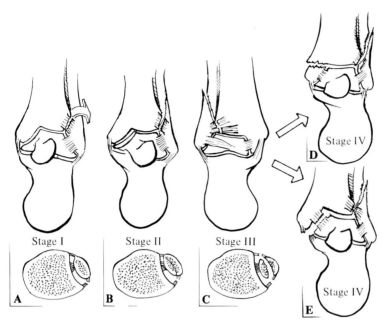

Fig. 10.2. Supination-external rotation (SER) injury—**A** Stage I, **B** Stage II, **C** Stage III, **D** Stage IV with medial malleolus fracture, **E** Stage IV with deltoid ligament rupture.

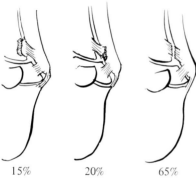

Fig. 10.3. Modes of failure of anterior inferior tibiofibular ligament (relative frequency according to Cedell [18]).

detached from its fibular insertion or ruptured through its substance (Fig. 10.3). Lauge-Hansen believed that this injury explained the Tillaux (anterior tibial tubercle) (Fig. 10.4) as well as the Wagstaffe (anterior fibular tubercle) fractures (Fig. 10.5).

With continued force, the posterior inferior tibiofibular and interosseous ligaments resisted further displacement or rotation of the fibula, and a spiral or oblique fracture of the lateral malleolus (stage II) occurred (Fig. 10.6). The fracture line characteristically began anteriorly on the fibula at or above the insertion of the anterior inferior tibiofibular ligament and ran

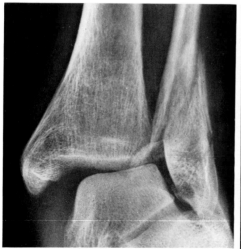

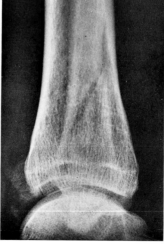

Fig. 10.4. Anteroposterior (**A**) and lateral (**B**) radiographs of SER IV injury characterized by avulsion of the anterior inferior tibial tubercle (Tillaux fracture).

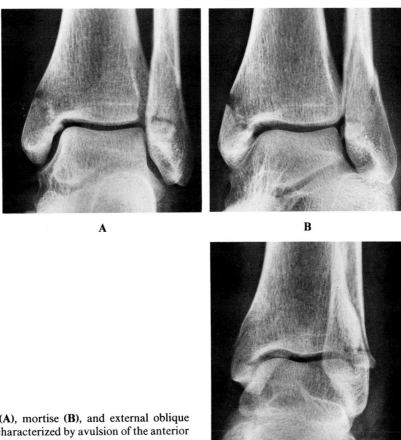

Fig. 10.5. Anteroposterior **(A)**, mortise **(B)**, and external oblique **(C)** views of SER IV injury characterized by avulsion of the anterior fibular tubercle (Wagstaffe type II).

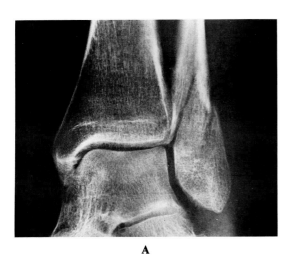

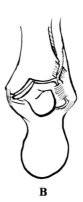

Fig. 10.6. Radiograph **(A)** and schematic **(B)** of supination-external rotation injury, stage II.

posteriorly and proximally a variable distance. The fracture was situated behind the attachment of the interosseous ligament [66], in that interval of the distal fibula which is occupied by the tibiofibular sac and is therefore devoid of ligamentous attachments. The distal fibular fragment remained firmly united to the talus via the lateral collateral ligaments, as well as to the distal tibia via the posterior inferior tibiofibular ligaments (PITFL and ITTFL); the latter ligaments acted initially as a hinge, permitting lateral rotation of the distal fibular fragment with the talus. The proximal fibular fragment remained firmly seated in the fibular groove of the tibia due to the intact interosseous ligament and interosseous membrane (Fig. 10.6B). The proximal fibular fragment subsequently remained undisturbed, since it no longer had any significant connection to the distal fibular fragment.

With continued external rotation, the lateral malleolar fragment not only rotated externally but also displaced laterally, dorsally, and proximally (Fig. 10.7). At this stage, the combination of traction on the distal tibia via the intact posterior inferior tibiofibular ligaments and direct pressure on the dorsal lip of the tibia by the dislocating talus produced rupture of the posterior tibiofibular ligaments, or more commonly, an avulsion fracture of the dorsal tibial margin (stage III). Lauge-Hansen noted that this posterior malleolar fragment remained firmly fixed to the distal fibula via the posterior inferior tibiofibular ligaments (PITFL/ITTFL). This fragment was usually small but could be quite large, and sometimes comprised a significant portion of the distal tibial articular surface.

By this point in the injury, there was frequently some degree of damage to the anterior and anteromedial capsule. With continued force, serving to encourage external rotation of the talus–lateral malleolus, the medial side of the ankle was injured by some combination of traction by the deltoid ligament and/or direct pressure on the posterior aspect of the medial malleolus by the dorsomedial corner of the subluxating talus. This could take the form of a medial malleolar fracture or deltoid ligament rupture or avulsion (Fig. 10.8).

As noted by Pankovich and Shivaram [68,69], since the superficial deltoid ligament originates from the anterior colliculus and the deep deltoid ligament from the posterior colliculus of the me-

dial malleolus, the two components can be injured separately. Therefore, a stage IV injury can be characterized by total ligamentous injury (rupture of superficial and deep deltoid ligament), total bone injury (supracollicular or basal fracture of the medial malleolus), or a combination of bone and ligament injury (most commonly, avulsion fracture of the anterior colliculus with rupture of the deep deltoid ligament) (Fig. 10.9). Furthermore, deltoid failure can occur at its origin, its insertion, or through its substance, such that there are many different modes of medial joint failure.

Variants

Mixed Oblique Fracture of the Lateral Malleolus

As a rare variant (2–4%), the lateral malleolus fracture may commence below the insertion of the anterior inferior tibiofibular ligament, such that this ligament escapes injury [18,91]. This was referred to as the "mixed oblique" fracture by Destot, since the fracture crosses both the articular and nonarticular surface of the distal fibula (Fig. 10.10) [1]. There is no satisfactory explanation for this phenomenon.

Supination-External Rotation Fracture with Rupture of the Interosseous Ligament (in Addition to Rupture of the Anterior and Posterior Inferior Tibiofibular Ligaments)

This fracture is a rare occurrence but should be kept in mind since it denotes complete ligamentous tibiofibular diastasis with all of its implications in terms of tibiofibular instability [18,22,66]. Cedell [18] observed several instances of this phenomenon among the 406 supination-external rotation injuries he treated surgically. Colton [22] described seven such cases, but the actual incidence of this phenomenon cannot be derived from his material.

The injury described by Bosworth (Fig. 6.15) [8] would fall into this category since, prior to fracture, the entire fibula is dislocated posterior to the tibia, implying that all of the distal tibiofibular soft tissues, have been violated. After re-

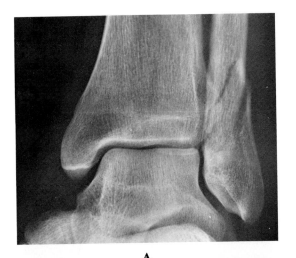

A

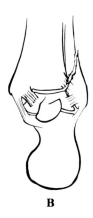

B

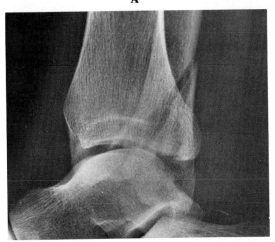

C

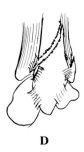

D

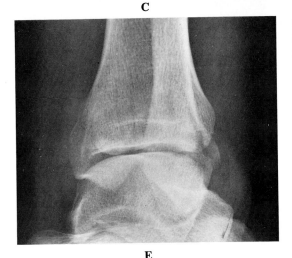

E

Fig. 10.7. SER III injury. Stage I characterized by avulsion of anterior fibular tubercle (**E**). Stage II demonstrated by typical spiral fracture of distal fibula (**A** and **B**). Stage III characterized by minimally displaced nonarticular posterior tibial lip fracture (**C** and **D**).

duction of the fibular dislocation and fixation of the distal fibular fracture, considerable tibiofibular instability may persist.

Supination-External Rotation Fracture of the Proximal Fibula

Pankovich [64] has postulated that supination-external rotation injury, under certain circumstances, may result in spiral fracture of the proximal fibula distinct from the proximal fibular fracture usually encountered with pronation-external rotation injuries. The fracture line in this situation resembles the typical supination-external rotation fracture of the distal fibula in that it extends from anterodistal to posteroproximal, unlike the pronation-external rotation fracture which, according to Pankovich, courses from anteroproximal to posterodistal (Fig. 10.11). At

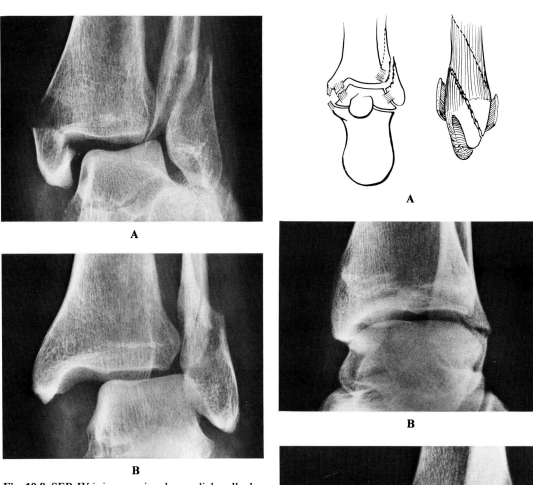

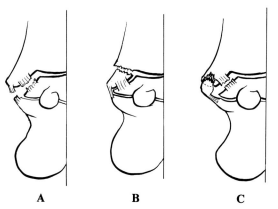

Fig. 10.8. SER IV injury can involve medial malleolus avulsion (**A**) or deltoid ligament rupture (**B**).

Fig. 10.9. Modes of medial joint failure by avulsion (SER IV injury). **A** Rupture of superficial and deep deltoid ligament. **B** Supracollicular avulsion fracture of medial malleolus. **C** Avulsion fracture of anterior colliculus with rupture of deep deltoid ligament.

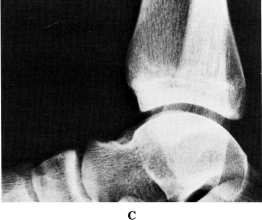

Fig. 10.10. Mixed oblique fracture (Destot) spares the anterior inferior tibiofibular ligament. **A** AP and lateral schematic (dotted line marks location of the "typical" SER fracture of the fibula). **B** 55° External rotation view. **C** Lateral view.

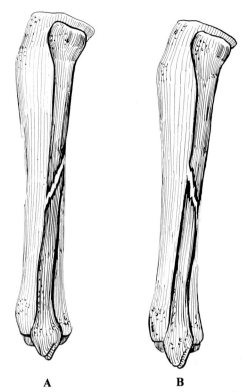

A   **B**

Fig. 10.11. Supramalleolar fractures of the fibula encountered with supination-external rotation (**A**) and pronation-external rotation (**B**) injuries [64].

surgery, Pankovich observed that these atypical supination-external rotation fractures were associated with rupture of the anterior inferior tibiofibular and interosseous ligaments. He apparently was able to reproduce this proximal-type fracture in cadaver limbs by sectioning these ligaments prior to inflicting a supination-external rotation strain.

The interosseous ligament is variable in size and strength. If Pankovich's observations are correct, then individuals with an inadequate interosseous ligament, who incur supination-external rotation injury, might sustain a spiral fracture of the proximal, rather than the distal, fibula. A stage II or III supination-external rotation injury of this type with a proximal fibular fracture would explain the occasional clinical situation characterized by spiral fracture of the proximal fibula, associated with tenderness over the anterior syndesmosis, but without evidence of medial joint injury (Fig. 10.12); this situation is not well explained by Lauge-Hausen's description.

Clinical Significance

The Supination-external rotation mechanism accounts for 40 to 75% of ankle fractures, depending on the series [5,18,46,47,77,79,93]. According to Cedell [18], this type of fracture occurs most commonly in females over age 50; in general, older patients sustain more severe degrees of this injury.

Stage I

Stage I lesions (isolated rupture of the anterior inferior tibiofibular ligament) are relatively uncommon, comprising approximately 5% of supination-external rotation injuries. This has led some investigators to conclude that force sufficient to damage the anterior tibiofibular ligament (stage I) will usually fracture the lateral malleolus (stage II) as well [18]. Isolated rupture or avulsion of the anterior inferior tibiofibular ligament is difficult to demonstrate [78], however, and the true incidence of stage I lesions may be higher than is commonly thought. Even if characterized by bone avulsion from the anterior tibial tubercle, this lesion will only be obvious if radiographs are taken with the anterior tibia thrown into relief (i.e., 55° external rotation view) (Fig. 10.5C) [18]. In the absence of bone involvement plain radiographs are normal, and stress radiographs are not sensitive enough to detect slight openings of the anterior syndesmosis [6,18]. Arthrographic studies, however, by Berridge and Bonnin [3], have demonstrated that isolated injury does exist; and Brostrom [12], in a series of 105 "ankle sprains" studied by arthrography and treated surgically, demonstrated damage to the anterior syndesmosis in 5.7% of patients.

Lauge-Hansen [44] noted experimentally that the anterior inferior tibiofibular ligament usually failed at its origin by avulsion of the anterior tibial tubercle. Since his patients, however, were treated by closed means, he could not confirm this impression with operative findings. Magnusson [48] followed 211 cases of supination-external rotation fracture and in only 75 instances (36%) was able to demonstrate radiographic changes in the anterior tibial tubercle or lateral malleolus consisting of sclerosis, surface defects, or contour changes. Cedell [18] explored 405 supination-ex-

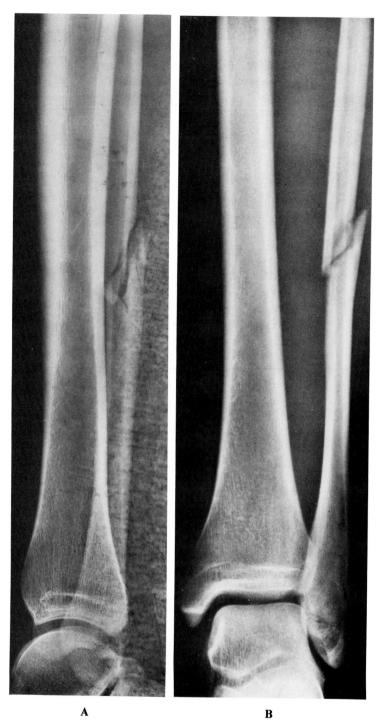

A   **B**

Fig. 10.12. A Supination-external rotation fracture of
mid-fibula associated with anterior syndesmosis tenderness but without evidence of deltoid ligament injury
clinically or by stress examination under anesthesia
(B).

ternal rotation injuries and observed anterior inferior tibiofibular ligament injury in 96% of patients, with rupture through the substance of the ligament representing the most common mode of failure (65%). Avulsion of the fibular attachment was the second most common injury, and avulsion of the anterior tibial tubercle was the least common lesion (Fig. 10.3).

Isolated injury of the anterior inferior tibiofibular ligament (stage I) has been described clinically by McLaughlin [52], who considered it to be a sprain common amongst skiers. The injury can be distinguished from the typical inversion ankle sprain, since tenderness is localized to the anterior syndesmosis and symptoms are aggravated by external rotation and/or dorsiflexion of the ankle, rather than by supination or inversion [18,53]. Ordinarily, the injury is stable and can be treated similar to an inversion sprain [66,74,81].

Incomplete healing of an isolated anterior inferior tibiofibular ligament injury is not likely to produce significant functional instability, but McLaughlin [52] has described a symptom complex due to chronic herniation of synovium through a rent or defect in this ligament that may require herniorrhaphy (Fig. 10.13A). Menelaus [53] has also suggested that this ligament, if torn and interposed between the distal fibula and tibia, might be a source of persistent pain and swelling (Fig. 10.13B). Cedell [18] believed that isolated rupture through the substance of the anterior inferior tibiofibular ligament should have a good prognosis with conservative treatment, but a demonstrable bone fragment from the tibia or fibula should be treated operatively, so as to avoid a painful pseudoarthrosis.

Stage II

Stage II supination-external rotation injury (rupture or avulsion of the anterior inferior tibiofibular ligament associated with spiral fracture of the lateral malleolus) accounts for approximately 34% of supination-external rotation injuries, and explains the commonly encountered spiral fracture of the lateral malleolus (Fig. 10.6A). Although the degree of obliquity is variable, the fracture generally commences at the level of the tibial plafond and extends proximally and posteriorly [18,66]. The fracture in stage II is characterized by little or no displacement, and may only be evident radiographically on the lateral or mortise view (Fig. 10.14). There is no clinical or radiographic evidence of medial joint damage. This injury, which is judged to be stable [1,6], should be treated with simple support [11,87], usually in a weight-bearing plaster [16,23,25, 38,39,52,60,65,66,90,92]. Serial radiographs are necessary, however, to monitor for displacement, which would indicate that the stage or severity of the injury had been underestimated [86].

Stage III

Stage III lesions comprise approximately 23% of supination-external rotation fractures. In addition to injury to the anterior inferior tibiofibular ligament and the distal fibula, there is rupture or avulsion of the posterior inferior tibiofibular ligaments (PITFL and ITTFL). It is important to distinguish this injury from the more benign stage II injury. Generally, the stage III injury will be characterized by greater initial disability and soft tissue tenderness, especially posteriorly [65]. Radiographs should be carefully reviewed for evidence of lateral malleolus displacement (dorsally, laterally, or proximally) or evidence of avulsion fracture of the posterior tibial tubercle or process (Fig. 10.15) [44]. Generally, stage III injuries will require more aggressive treatment than stage II lesions.

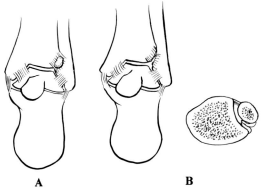

Fig. 10.13. Potential sequelae of anterior inferior tibiofibular ligament rupture. **A** Herniation of synovium through a rent in the ligament [52]. **B** Interposition of ligament in anterior syndesmotic space [53].

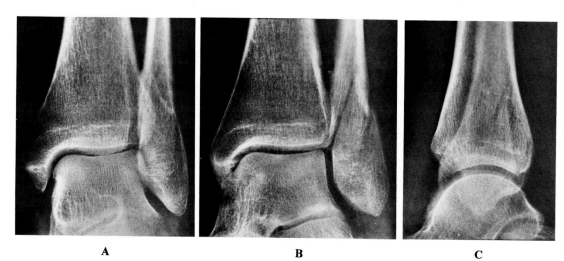

Fig. 10.14. SER II injury. Fibular fracture obvious on mortise view (**B**) but occult on anteroposterior (**A**) and lateral (**C**) views.

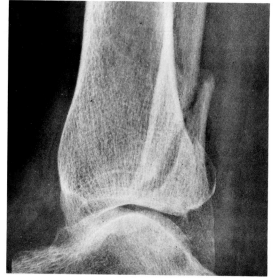

Fig. 10.15. SER III injury characterized by dorsal and proximal displacement of the distal fibular fragment as well as fracture of the posterior tibia.

Stage IV

Stage IV supination-external rotation injury, according to Lauge-Hansen, comprises 40% of external rotation injuries occurring in supination. This stage is characterized by rupture of the del-

toid ligament or avulsion fracture of the medial malleolus and is associated with subluxation or dislocation of the talus in approximately 40% of cases (Fig. 10.30C) [18]. Cedell observed that females were more likely to have medial malleolus fracture (81%) than deltoid ligament rupture (19%), whereas in males the two variations occurred with comparable frequency [18].

The diagnosis of stage IV injury is obvious if the displacement persists or if the medial injury involves fracture. Stage IV injuries, however, which are characterized by deltoid ligament rupture rather than fracture, and which reduce spontaneously prior to radiographic study, may simulate a stage II or stage III supination-external rotation injury. To help make this important distinction, Kleiger [39] has described a clinical test for stability (Fig. 10.16). It is performed with the patient sitting with his knee flexed to 90°. The examiner gently grasps the foot and rotates it externally. If the ankle is unstable, this maneuver will cause pain laterally and medially, and the examiner can frequently perceive that the talus is displacing from the medial malleolus. If there is any question concerning interpretation, the test should be repeated under X-ray or fluoroscopic control; anesthesia may be necessary [3,39,57]. Widening of the medial clear space, between the talus and medial malleolus, in excess of 3–4 mm, suggests complete rupture of the deltoid ligament (Fig. 10.17) [21,29,30,67,69,81, 86,93].

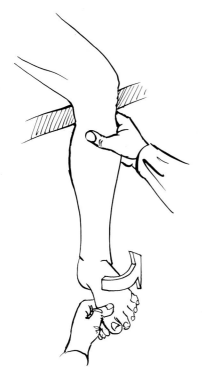

Fig. 10.16. Kleiger test for instability.

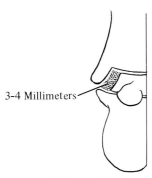

3-4 Millimeters

Fig. 10.17. Increase of the medial clear space between the talus and the medial malleolus in excess of 3–4 mm implies complete rupture of the deltoid ligament.

Supination-External Rotation Injuries: Closed Reduction (Lauge-Hansen) [46]

1. Reduction should be performed immediately.

2. General or spinal anesthesia is required.
3. Knee should be flexed to 90° to relax gastrocnemius muscle.
4. An assistant is required.
5. Immobilization should be achieved by use of a short leg walking cast.

Technique (Fig. 10.18)

1. Foot is supinated and externally rotated—to separate and disimpact fracture surfaces. (Fig. 10.18A)
2. Foot is plantarflexed as traction is applied in the long axis of the limb—to restore fibular length (via lateral collateral ligaments) (Fig. 10.18B).
3. Foot is translated anteriorly—to reduce the dorsal subluxation of the talus and (via ligamentous attachments) dorsal displacement of the lateral malleolus and posterior tibial lip. (Fig. 10.18C)
4. Foot is internally rotated—to correct external rotation of the talus and fibula (via the anterior talofibular ligament). (Fig. 10.18D)
5. Foot is pronated and dorsiflexed to a right angle, with internal rotation maintained. (Fig. 10.18E)
6. As plaster sets, hindfoot is adducted—to prevent valgus tilt of talus and fibular fragment.

Closed reduction of this injury is based on the fact that the talus, lateral malleolus, and posterior tibial lip maintain their normal connections with each other via the lateral collateral and posterior tibiofibular ligaments; therefore they can be moved as a unit (Fig. 10.19) [14]. The talus and the lateral malleolus have been referred to as the "Siamese twins" of ankle injury [7].

Although the anatomic principles underlying this technique are sound, one must seriously question the advisability of using a short leg cast to control rotatory forces at the ankle [74]. Most authors would recommend a long leg cast if the fracture has been displaced sufficiently to require reduction [39,52,73,78,90]. If, for some reason, inclusion of the knee is undesirable or impractical, rotation can be effectively controlled by inserting a pin in the proximal tibia and incorporating it into a short leg cast [6].

Also, early weight bearing is ill-advised when reduction has been necessary [19,38,39,74]. At a later date, when weight bearing is permitted, a cast boot or·rocker heel is preferable to walking

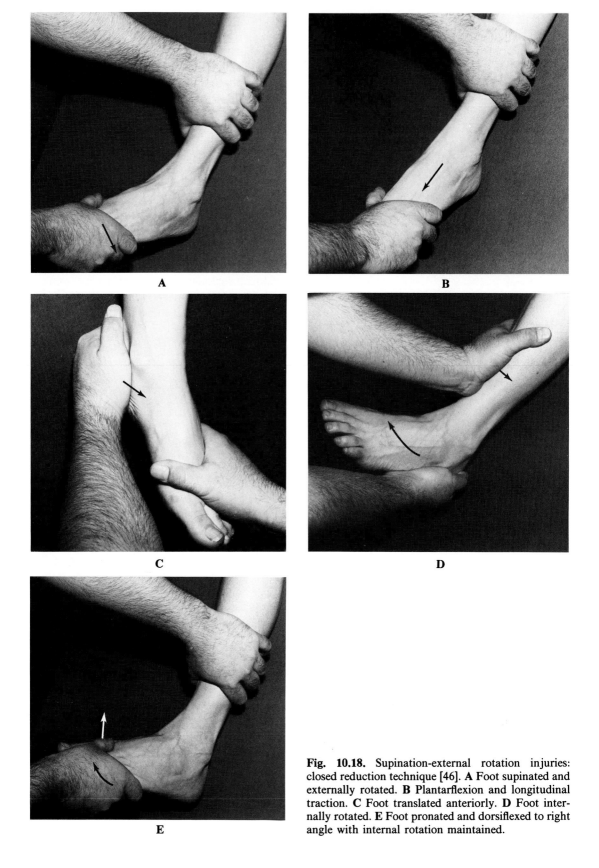

Fig. 10.18. Supination-external rotation injuries: closed reduction technique [46]. **A** Foot supinated and externally rotated. **B** Plantarflexion and longitudinal traction. **C** Foot translated anteriorly. **D** Foot internally rotated. **E** Foot pronated and dorsiflexed to right angle with internal rotation maintained.

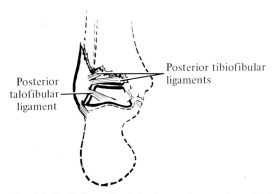

Fig. 10.19. Talus, distal fibula, and posterior tibial fragment firmly connected by stout posterior tibiofibular and talofibular ligaments.

irons, pegs, or other devices that encourage external rotation of the foot with each step [39,74].

The stage IV supination-external rotation injury characterized by fracture of the medial malleolus at the level of the tibial plafond requires special care, lest attempts at reduction result in overcorrection of the deformity with medial displacement of the medial malleolus and talus (Fig. 10.20) [11,40]. With an intact medial malleolus, however, overcorrection is not possible [11].

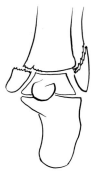

Fig. 10.20. SER IV injuries characterized by basal fracture of the medial malleolus are difficult to reduce by closed means since there is no end point and overreduction is possible.

Supination-External Rotation Injuries: Open Reduction and Internal Fixation

At one time, it was popular to repair the medial side of the ankle (deltoid ligament or medial mal-

leolus) and then treat the lateral malleolus fracture by closed reduction and plaster immobilization [13,16,20,23,33,34,41,51,57,61,74,84]. This necessarily incurred the risks of both closed and operative treatment [10,43,52]. Bonnin [6] stated that if the medial side of the ankle were reduced, the lateral side of the joint would almost always reduce perfectly. This is not necessarily true, however. Even after the medial side has been stabilized, reduction of the lateral side can be quite difficult, due to shortening, impaction, and interposition of soft tissue at the fibular fracture site (Fig. 10.21) [15,83]. The difficulty encountered in restoring fibular length and accurately reducing the lateral malleolus at surgery, let alone by closed means, has been well publicized [17,28,41,50,56,84,89]. Since the ankle functions as a closed ring, if the lateral malleolus is not reduced anatomically, the mortise cannot truly be restored to normal; either the medial reduction is compromised in some way or the lateral collateral ligaments are stretched by efforts to completely correct subluxation of the talus (Fig. 10.22) [49,89]. Even in those situations where satisfactory closed reduction of the lateral malleolus can be accomplished, maintenance will require prevention of external rotation, and this can be quite difficult with plaster immobilization [9,17,49,78].

Since the lateral malleolus fracture occurs before the medial injury in supination-external rotation injuries, it seems more logical in stage IV injuries to repair the lateral side and then treat the medial side by closed means (Fig. 10.23) [50,88]. The reduced lateral malleolus would then have a restorative and protective effect on the medial malleolus fracture or deltoid ligament rupture [56,85,88]. Several authors have documented favorable results with closed treatment of deltoid ligament injuries [7,57,72,80]. Although this approach has been adopted by some clinicians in general [2,10,15,24,58,71,88], or at least in older age groups [35,86], the efficacy of this treatment is jeopardized if there is any soft tissue interposed in the medial malleolus fracture site or medial tibiotalar space that prevents anatomic reduction of the medial side [9,56]. Therefore, if internal fixation of a supination-external rotation injury is undertaken, most authorities would presently recommend simultaneous exploration and repair of both medial and lateral sides of the ankle [9,40,52,55,56,66,72,78]. Even if the

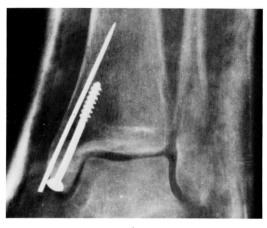 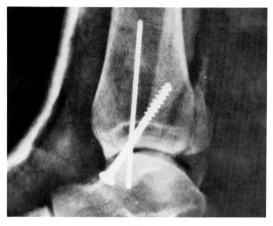

| A | B |

Fig. 10.21. SER IV injury treated by open reduction and internal fixation of medial malleolus with residual fibular shortening (**A**) and posterior displacement of the lateral malleolus (**B**).

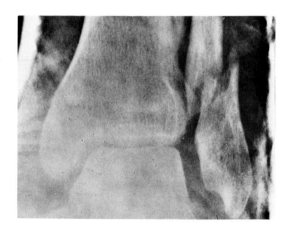

◁

Fig. 10.22. SER IV injury treated by deltoid ligament repair and attempted closed reduction of the lateral malleolus. Immobilization in marked internal rotation succeeded in restoring the medial clear space to normal; however, the position of the fibular fracture remained unchanged. Note the apparent increase in the talofibular clear space, implying that the lateral collateral ligaments have been stretched.

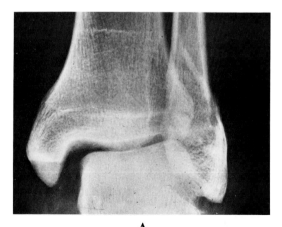 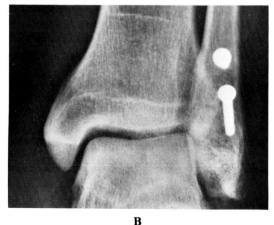

| A | B |

Fig. 10.23. A SER IV injury treated by open reduction and interfragmentary screw fixation of lateral malleolus without exploration or repair of deltoid ligament.

B Intraoperative radiograph was obtained to document that the medial clear space had been restored to normal.

deltoid ligament is not amenable to repair by suture [39], medial exploration will guarantee that there is no interposed tissue preventing concentric reduction and apposition of ligament ends [79]. In the absence of medial exploration, radiographic examination is mandatory to guarantee complete reduction of the talus [58]. It is important to strive for deltoid ligament healing at normal length, since there is no satisfactory reconstructive procedure to correct insufficiency of this structure [86].

With the bilateral approach to stage IV injuries, either side can be exposed initially, but neither side should be repaired until the other is at least visualized. The medial ankle is well exposed by an anteromedial or posteromedial approach, depending on whether one is dealing with a fracture or a deltoid ligament rupture [84]. The joint should be carefully inspected for osteocartilaginous fragments or other debris.

If the medial malleolus has been fractured near its base, interposed soft tissue should be carefully removed from the fracture site and the periosteum on each side of the fracture should be carefully stripped back one-eighth in. to facilitate fracture reduction and prevent soft tissue invagination [24].

If the medial injury is entirely ligamentous in nature, the ligament ends should be identified and approximated carefully. For repair of the deep deltoid ligament, it is advisable to insert and tag sutures prior to fibular fixation when the talus can still be displaced laterally to facilitate visualization of the ligament ends. In order to protect the repair, however, these sutures should not be tied until bony stabilization has been accomplished [56,85].

When the deep deltoid ligament is torn at its origin from the posterior colliculus of the medial malleolus, it should be repaired directly to bone. This can be accomplished by inserting sutures into the substance of the ligament and then bringing them through drill holes in the medial malleolus to be tied over the medial surface of the bone (Fig. 10.24A) [55]. Similarly, if the deltoid ligament is torn at or near its insertion on the talus, sutures can be brought through drill holes and tied over the lateral aspect of the talus in front of the lateral facet (Fig. 10.24B).

When the medial injury is characterized by fracture of the anterior colliculus and rupture of the deep deltoid ligament (Fig. 10.31A), it is necessary to recognize the important, but sometimes occult, deep deltoid rupture as well as the obvious anterior colliculus avulsion [69]. A similar sequence should be followed, i.e., the deep deltoid sutures should be inserted early, but not tied until the lateral malleolus and anterior colliculus have been fixed.

After the medial joint has been explored and the extent of the injury determined, the fibular fracture is exposed and the deformity is gently

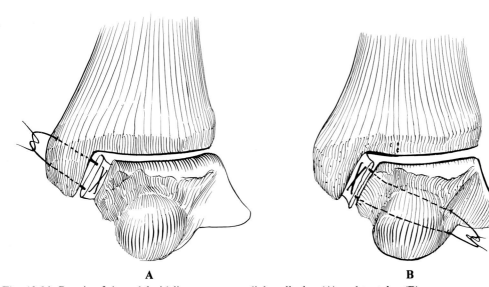

A   **B**

Fig. 10.24. Repair of deep deltoid ligament to medial malleolus (**A**) and to talus (**B**).

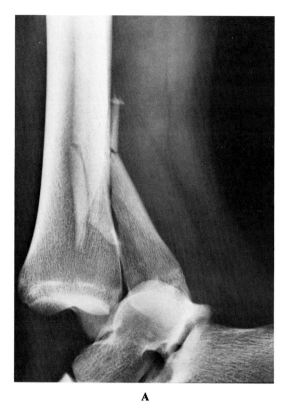

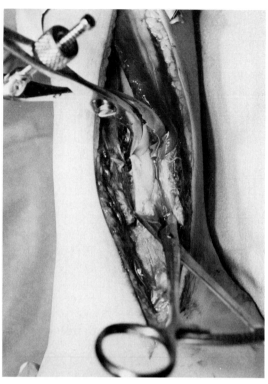

A   B

Fig. 10.25. Small clamps are essential to maintain reduction of fibular fracture as internal fixation is accomplished. **A** Comminuted fracture of the distal fibula.

B At surgery, reduction was temporarily maintained with small clamps until internal fixation could be accomplished.

exaggerated to allow careful removal of interposed soft tissue and/or bone fragments at this site [50]. Traction and internal rotation applied to the distal fibular fragment with a bone hook or clamp will facilitate reduction of the fracture. The reduction is held with clamps as the fracture is fixed internally (Fig. 10.25).

The anterior inferior tibiofibular ligament lesion (rupture or avulsion) should be identified at this stage to be certain that there is no bone or soft tissue interposed between the distal fibula and tibia that might prevent anatomic reduction of the anterior syndesmosis [53]. The anterior inferior tibiofibular ligament should be repaired if at all possible [58,79], or if characterized by large bone avulsion from the fibula or tibia, the fragment should be reduced and fixed with a screw (Fig. 7.3) [58,66,93]. Cedell [17] recommended protecting the anterior syndesmosis with a staple inserted parallel with the fibers of the anterior inferior tibiofibular ligament; this gener-

ally is not necessary, however, if the fibular fracture can be fixed internally.

At this point in the procedure the medial side is protected, and medial repair can be completed by tying the previously inserted deltoid ligament sutures or by approximation and fixation of the medial malleolus fracture.

As already noted, this injury, even in its most severe form, is not ordinarily associated with complete ligament disruption of the tibiofibular syndesmosis [26,44,50,66]. Since the proximal fibular fragment maintains its normal connections with the tibia via the interosseous ligament and membrane (Fig. 10.2D,E) [26], reconstitution of the fibula will restore normal tibiofibular relationship and set the stage for uneventful healing of the anterior and posterior inferior tibiofibular ligaments [36]. Techniques that routinely employ screw fixation of the tibiofibular syndesmosis as a means of stabilizing the fibular fracture should be avoided since they restrict the syndes-

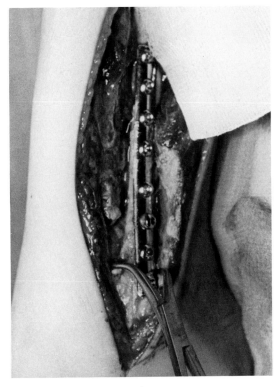

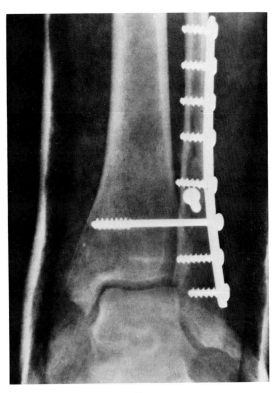

A   B

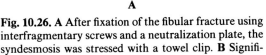

Fig. 10.26. A After fixation of the fibular fracture using interfragmentary screws and a neutralization plate, the syndesmosis was stressed with a towel clip. **B** Significant instability was demonstrated and a tibiofibular positioning screw was employed.

mosis unnecessarily and provide poor fixation of the fibular fracture [15].

Occasionally, however, as with the rare variant already described [66] or due to excessive surgical stripping of the proximal fibular fragment, a supination-external rotation injury can be associated with significant tibiofibular instability [22]. A helpful technique to demonstrate this situation is to test tibiofibular mobility by pulling on the lateral malleolus with a towel clip or bone hook after the fibular fracture has been reduced and fixed (Fig. 10.26). If excessive mobility of the fibula with respect to the tibia (more than 2 mm of play, according to Lindsjo [47]) can be demonstrated, a complete ligamentous tibiofibular diastasis should be presumed to exist and treated with a tibiofibular screw as described for pronation-external rotation injuries (Fig. 10.27) [66].

Damage to the posterior inferior tibiofibular ligaments usually (67%) involves avulsion of a posterior tibial lip fragment of variable size [91].

The only direct connection between the talus and the posterior tibial fragment is the posterior capsule (Fig. 10.28); this is redundant and cannot be relied upon to pull even a small posterior fragment into proper position [15,62]. The posterior tibial lip fragment, however, remains firmly attached to the distal fibula via the stout posterior inferior tibiofibular ligament (Fig. 10.19) [31]. Satisfactory reduction of the distal fibular fracture usually automatically effects reduction of the posterior tibial marginal fragment (Fig. 10.29) unless it is large or unless the reduction is obstructed by interposed soft tissue or bone fragments [24,31,32,58,84,86]. If the posterior marginal fragment is large and remains displaced (Fig. 13.9), then it must be exposed, reduced, and fixed separately, usually prior to fibular fixation. The indications and techniques for internal fixation of posterior tibial lip fragments are outlined in Chapter 13.

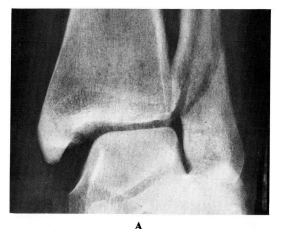

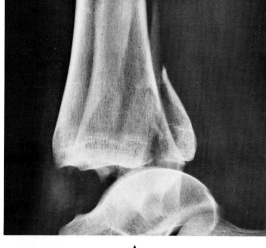

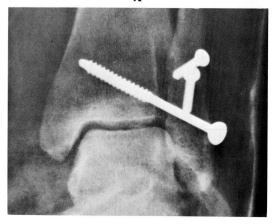

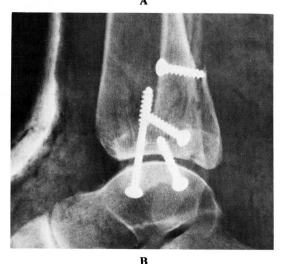

Fig. 10.27. A SER IV injury. **B** Following open reduction and interfragmentary screw fixation of fibular fracture, considerable horizontal tibiofibular instability was observed. Syndesmosis was therefore stabilized with a tibiofibular screw; this was inserted obliquely so as to avoid the fibular fracture site.

Fig. 10.29. Because of stout ligamentous attachments (PITFL/ITTFL) between the lateral malleolus and posterior tibial fragment, reduction and fixation of the fibular fracture will automatically restore a small posterior tibial fragment to normal position. **A** Preoperative. **B** Following open reduction–screw fixation of medial malleolus and fibular fracture.

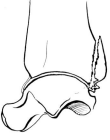

Fig. 10.28. Traction on the lax posterior tibiotalar capsule will not usually effect reduction of a displaced posterior tibial fragment.

Supination-External Rotation Injuries: Fixation Techniques

Long Spiral Fracture of the Distal Fibula

Interfragmentary Compression

With the fracture exposed, reduced anatomically, and stabilized with bone clamps, multiple short

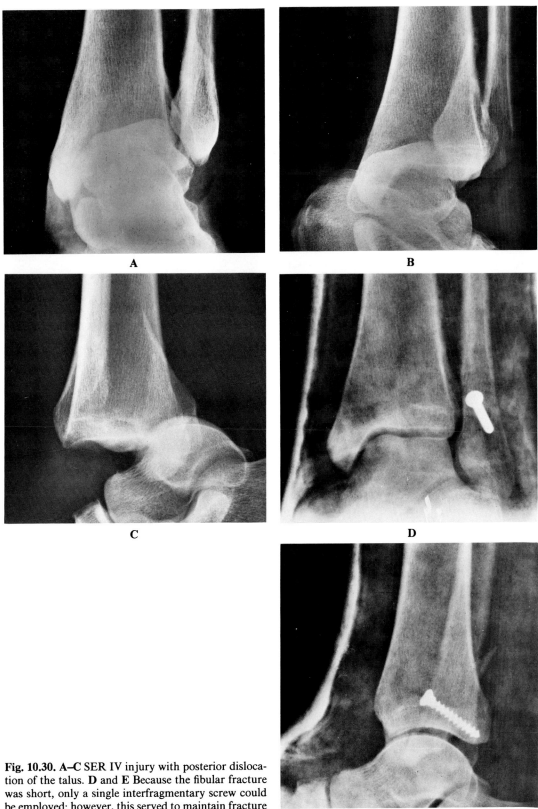

Fig. 10.30. A–C SER IV injury with posterior dislocation of the talus. **D** and **E** Because the fibular fracture
was short, only a single interfragmentary screw could
be employed; however, this served to maintain fracture
position in conjunction with plaster immobilization.

screws are inserted across the fracture site to achieve fixation (Figs. 10.30 and 10.31) [15, 36,58,93]. The fragment adjacent to the screw head should be overdrilled to permit compression at the fracture site. Either 3.5- or 4.5-m screws can be used for this purpose, depending on the size of the bone and the length of the fracture. Generally, a minimum of two or three screws are required (Fig. 10.31), but a single well-placed screw (Fig. 10.30) may suffice if plaster immobilization is planned [36,70].

Interfragmentary Compression and Neutralization Plate

If external immobilization is to be avoided, interfragmentary fixation should be supplemented with a one-third tubular or small fragment neutralization plate (5–6 holes) (Fig. 10.32) [54, 58,88], intended to conduct torsional stresses past the fracture site and protect the underlying interfragmentary fixation [50,56,66].

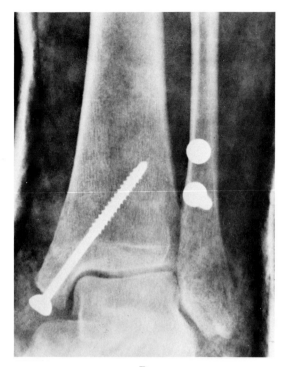

B

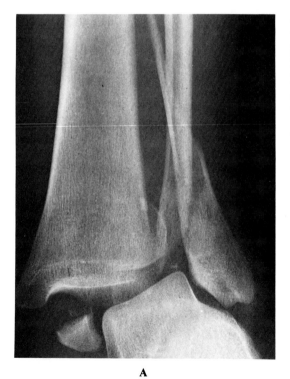

A

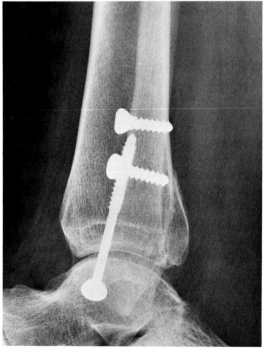

C

Fig. 10.31. SER IV injury. **A** Medial injury included fracture of anterior colliculus and rupture of deep deltoid ligament. **B** and **C** Injury treated by exploration and repair of deep deltoid ligament through drill holes in posterior colliculus, screw fixation of anterior colliculus, and interfragmentary screw fixation of lateral malleolus. Satisfactory reduction was obtained. Plaster immobilization was employed because of medial ligament injury and the degree of fibular fixation.

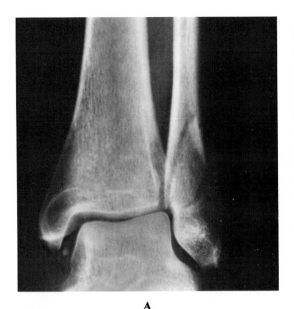

A

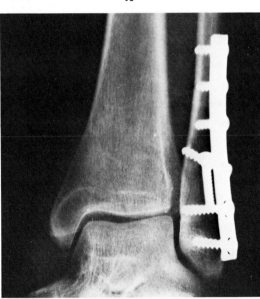

B

Fig. 10.32. Incomplete SER IV injury. **A** Medial injury limited to small avulsion, corresponding to injury of superficial deltoid ligament; deep deltoid ligament intact. **B** Treated by open reduction of fibula, using interfragmentary screws with neutralization plate. External immobilization was avoided and early motion permitted.

Wire-Loop Fixation

With wire-loop fixation, the fibular fracture needs to be exposed only well enough to achieve reduction (Fig. 10.33) [2,59,63,84,88,93]. Using a curved wire passer or aneurysm needle, 18- or 20-gauge wires are passed extraperiosteally about the fibula at the level of the fracture and tightened with a mechanical wire tightener (e.g., Rhinelander). One to three wires are generally employed to span the length of the fracture. To qualify for this form of fixation, the length of the fracture should be at least twice the width of the bone at the level of the fracture site [63]. Proponents of this technique contend that it provides more rigid fixation than interfragmentary screws yet requires less soft tissue dissection [63]. It does not necessarily eliminate the need for external immobilization [2,17,63]. Wire-loop fixation has also been used in conjunction with an intramedullary device for comminuted fractures (Fig. 10.33B) [36,63,85].

Figure-of-Eight Cerclage (Sudman Modification)

Unlike transverse avulsion fractures, oblique fractures of the distal fibula do not lend themselves well to fixation by figure-of-eight cerclage as ordinarily described, since compression may cause shortening at the fracture site (Fig. 10.34A). Sudman [82], however, has reported a modification of the technique that can be effectively utilized for fractures of this type (Fig. 10.34B). It involves placing the proximal fibular drill hole close to the fracture site in an oblique direction, such that the proximal portion of the cerclage wire encircles the distal fibular fragment and prevents telescoping at the fracture site.

Intramedullary Fixation

Various devices have been recommended to provide intramedullary fixation of long oblique distal fibular fractures [10,24,27,29,31,36,61,79]. These include bone pegs [6], Kuntscher rod [42], axial screws [15,36,51,55], Rush pins [9,75,84–86], and Kirschner wires [49].

Intramedullary devices are inserted retrograde from the tip of the lateral malleolus after the fibular fracture has been exposed to permit anatomic reduction (Fig. 10.35). Their advantage is that minimal soft tissue stripping is required. However, they all suffer from the same deficiency, i.e., lack of protection against shortening and external rotation of the distal fibular fragment (Fig. 10.36) [17,24,59].

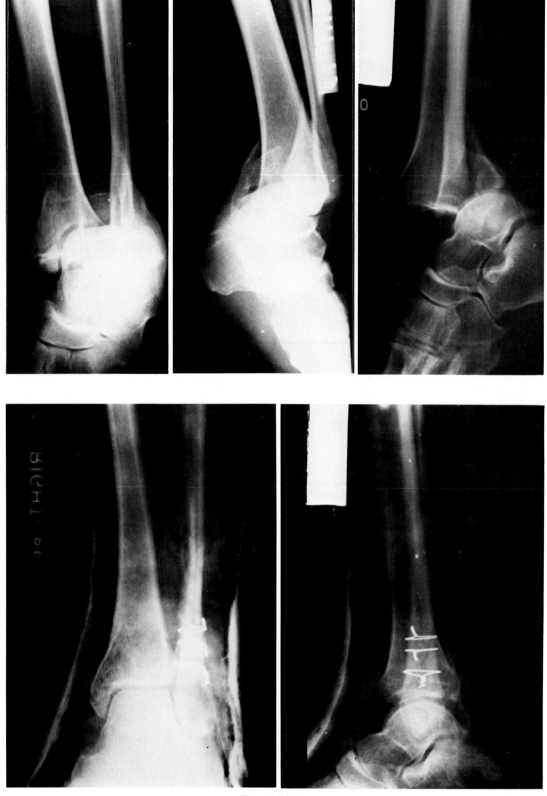

Fig. 10.33A

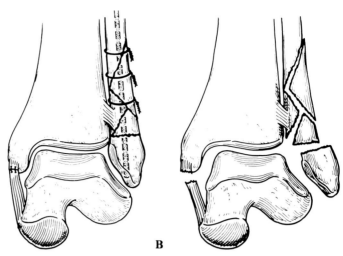

B

Fig. 10.33. A Severe SER IV injury characterized by posterolateral dislocation of the talus. Treated with open reduction and wire-loop fixation of the distal fibular fracture. **B** Wire-loop fixation can also be used in conjunction with intramedullary stabilization for comminuted fractures of the distal fibula. From ref. 59. Reprinted with permission.

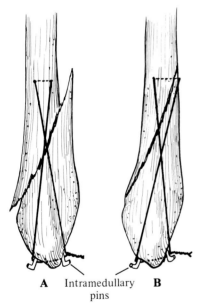

A Intramedullary **B**
pins

Fig. 10.34. Figure-of-eight cerclage for oblique fracture of the lateral malleolus. **A** Standard technique is contraindicated. **B** Sudman technique may be employed satisfactorily.

Axial Screw (A-O Modification)

The A-O group has modified the axial screw technique so that the screw engages the cortex of the proximal fragment (Fig. 8.20) [58]. The screw should penetrate the proximal fibular fragment posteriorly or medially above the tibiofibular syndesmosis. This provides better fracture fixation than an intramedullary screw.

Medial Malleolus

Lag Screw Fixation

The entire fracture site should be visualized and the medial malleolar fragment everted from the talus to facilitate joint debridement, screw placement, and subsequent fracture reduction (Fig. 10.37) [10,13,15,23,24,35,50,54,76]. Through a small vertical incision in the superficial deltoid ligament, the medial malleolus is drilled from its apex toward the visualized fracture site (Fig. 10.37A). This ensures that the joint surface will not be violated by the fixation device. One or two holes can be made in this manner depending on the size of the fragment and how many screws it will accommodate.

The fracture is then reduced, paying particular attention to restoration of the mortise angle, and temporarily stabilized with a towel clip, bone hook, or smooth Kirschner wires passed across the fracture site [15,35]. The drill hole(s) are then extended proximally a short distance into the tibial metaphysis with care to prevent rotation

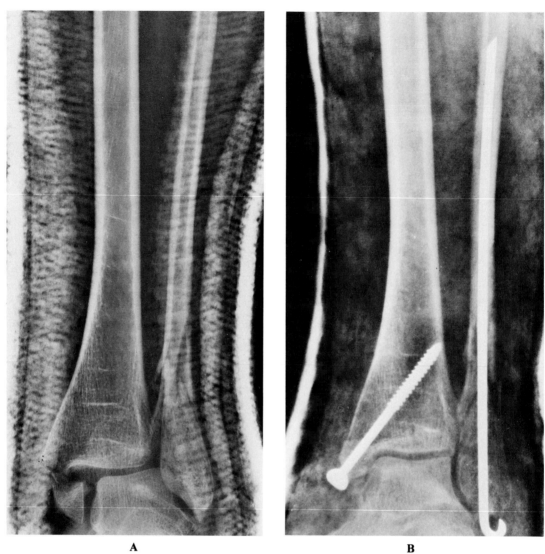

A   **B**

Fig. 10.35. A SER IV injury. Fibular fracture is quite comminuted. **B** Satisfactorily stabilized by screw fixation of medial malleolus and "blind" stabilization of lateral malleolus using a Rush rod.

of the medial malleolar fragment (Fig. 10.37B). Since the metaphyseal bone is soft, there is no need to drill the full length of the proposed screw. Also, there is no need for the screw to penetrate the far cortex of the tibia [24,85] unless the bone is very soft and porotic [35]. To provide compression at the fracture site, the fixation screws should be lagged. With an ordinary cortical screw, this requires overdrilling of the malleolar fragment; if a malleolar screw is employed, overdrilling is not necessary [79]. With this device, however, it is important that the threads are all located in the proximal fragment (metaphysis) and do

not cross the fracture site as this will prevent full compression [41]. A screw (or screws), 4–7 cm long, should be inserted and tightened evenly as the fracture site and mortise angle continue to be observed (Fig. 10.37C). Occasionally, for large fragments involving osteoporotic bone, a cancellous-type screw is preferable [10]. All screws should be countersunk to prevent formation of a painful adventitious bursa [36].

The ideal arrangement for maintaining compression and resisting rotation at the medial malleolar fracture site employs two parallel screws at a distance from each other (Fig. 10.38). If

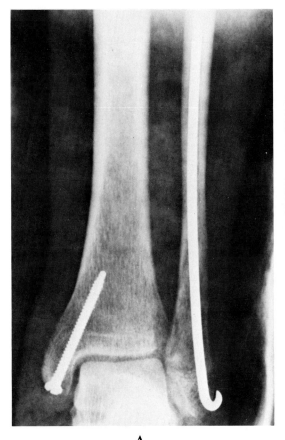

A

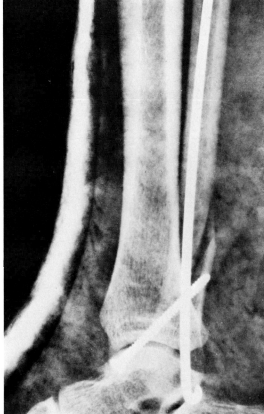

B

Fig. 10.36. SER IV injury. Fixed by single medial malleolar screw and open reduction–internal fixation of lateral malleolus using a Rush rod. Rush rod has permitted recurrent external rotation of the distal fibular fragment, despite satisfactory medial fixation.

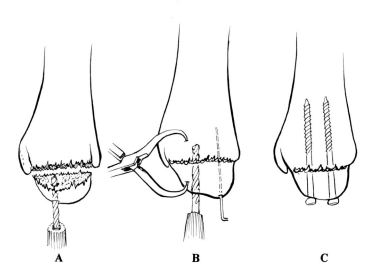

Fig. 10.37. Lag screw fixation of medial malleolus. See text for explanation.

A   **B**   **C**

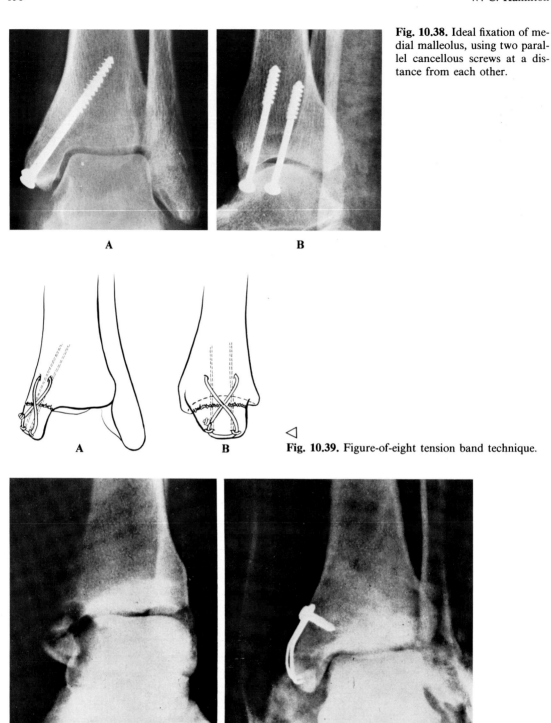

Fig. 10.38. Ideal fixation of medial malleolus, using two parallel cancellous screws at a distance from each other.

A   B

A   B   **Fig. 10.39.** Figure-of-eight tension band technique.

Fig. 10.40. Fixation of comminuted medial malleolus fracture using a Zuelzer plate. From ref. 94. Reprinted with permission.

the fragment is too small to permit two screws, one can use a single screw and a Kirschner wire (Fig. 10.21) [50,56]. Where there is only room for a single screw, one must rely upon bony interdigitation at the fracture site to resist rotation.

Figure-of-Eight Tension Band

For fragments that are small or fractures that involve osteoporotic bone, an alternative technique described by the A-O group employs two parallel Kirschner wires to maintain axial alignment and a figure-of-eight tension band to provide compression (Fig. 10.39) [35,50,54,58]. The tibial hole should be 2 mm in diameter and placed approximately 1 cm proximal to the fracture site. Distally, the wires are passed under the Kirschner wires where they enter the medial malleolus. The knot should be buried, so that it does not create an irritating prominence.

Hook Plate (Zuelzer)

This device was originally fabricated from a Lane plate but now is available commercially (Fig. 10.40) [76,94]. It is useful for fixation of small medial malleolar fragments. After anatomic reduction and temporary stabilization of the medial malleolar fracture, the hook plate is bent to conform to the contour of the bone in this region. The medial malleolus is then predrilled at two sites corresponding to the hooks of the plate. The hooks are impacted into these holes and the plate is affixed to the medial aspect of the distal tibia, usually with one screw.

References

1. Ashhurst APC, Bromer RS: Classification and mechanism of fractures of the leg bones involving the ankle. AMA Arch Surg 4:51, 1922.
2. Bergkvist A, Hultengren N, Lindholm A, Lindvall N: Circumferential wire fixation of the lateral malleolus for fractures at the ankle. Acta Chir Scand 115:476, 1958.
3. Berridge FR, Bonnin JG: The radiographic examination of the ankle joint including arthrography. Surg Gynecol Obstet 79:383, 1944.
4. Bistrom O: Conservative treatment of severe ankle fractures. A clinical and follow-up study. Acta Chir Scand (Suppl) 168:1, 1952.
5. Bohler L: The Treatment of Fractures, 5th ed. New York, Grune & Stratton, 1956.
6. Bonnin JG: Injuries to the Ankle. New York, Grune & Stratton, 1950.
7. Bonnin JG: Injury to the ligaments of the ankle. J Bone Joint Surg 47B:609, 1965.
8. Bosworth DM: Fracture-dislocation of the ankle with fixed displacement of the fibula behind the tibia. J Bone Joint Surg 29:130, 1947.
9. Braunstein PW, Wade PA: Treatment of unstable fractures of the ankle. Ann Surg 149:217, 1959.
10. Brodie IAOD, Denham RA: The treatment of unstable ankle fractures. J Bone Joint Surg 56B:256, 1974.
11. Broomhead R: Discussion on fractures in the region of ankle joint. Proc Roy Soc Med 25:1082, 1932.
12. Brostrom L: Sprained ankles. I. Anatomic lesions in recent sprains. Acta Chir Scand 128:483, 1964.
13. Burgess E: Fractures of the ankle. J Bone Joint Surg 26:721, 1944.
14. Burns BH: Diastasis of the inferior tibio-fibular joint. Proc Roy Soc Med 36:330, 1943.
15. Burwell HN, Charnley AD: Treatment of displaced fractures at the ankle by rigid internal fixation and early joint movement. J Bone Joint Surg 47B:634, 1965.
16. Cave EF (ed): Ankle injuries. In: Fractures and Other Injuries. Chicago, Year Book Medical, 1958.
17. Cedell C-A, Wiberg G: Treatment of eversion-supination fracture of the ankle (second degree). Acta Chir Scand 124:41, 1962.
18. Cedell C-A: Supination-outward rotation injuries of the ankle. Acta Orthop Scand (Suppl) 110:1, 1967.
19. Charnley J: The Closed Treatment of Common Fractures, 3rd ed. Baltimore, Williams & Wilkins, 1972.
20. Childress HM: Vertical transarticular pin fixation for unstable ankle fractures. Impressions after 16 years of experience. Clin Orthop Rel Res 120:164, 1976.
21. Close R: Some applications of the functional anatomy of the ankle joint. J Bone Joint Surg 38A:761, 1956.
22. Colton CL: Fracture-diastasis of the inferior tibio-fibular joint. J Bone Joint Surg 50B:830, 1968.
23. Cox FJ, Laxson WW: Fractures about the ankle joint. Am J Surg 83:674, 1952.
24. Denham RA: Internal fixation for unstable ankle fractures. J Bone Joint Surg 46B:206, 1964.
25. DePalma AF: The Management of Fractures and Dislocations, 2nd ed. Philadelphia, Saunders, 1970.
26. DeSouza Dias L, Foerster TP: Traumatic lesions of the ankle joint. The supination-external rotation mechanism. Clin Orthop Rel Res 100:219, 1974.
27. Eventov I, Salama R, Goodwin DRA, Weissman SL: An evaluation of surgical and conservative treatment of fractures of the ankle in 200 Patients. J Trauma 18:271, 1978.
28. Fairbank HAT: The operative treatment of ankle fractures. III. Lancet 2:92, 1926.
29. Gaston SR, McLaughlin HL: Complex fracture of the lateral malleolus. J Trauma 1:69, 1961.

30. Grath G: Widening of the ankle mortise. A clinical and experimental study. Acta Chir Scand (Suppl) 263:1, 1960.
31. Gristina AG, Rovere GD, Moses TE, Nicasto JF, Poehling GG: Injuries of the ankle syndesmosis: Base slider's ankle fracture. Orthop Rev 8:75, 1979.
32. Hall H: A simplified workable classification of ankle fractures. In Bateman JE, Trott AW (eds): The Foot and Ankle. New York, Thieme-Stratton, 1980.
33. Harvey JP Jr: Fractures of the ankle. A clinical survey of 181 cases. Clin Orthop 42:57, 1965.
34. Henderson MS, Stuck WG: Fractures of the ankle: Recent and old. J Bone Joint Surg 15:882, 1933.
35. Hughes J: The medial malleolus in ankle fractures. Orthop Clin of North Am 11:649, 1980.
36. Jergesen F: Open reduction of fractures and dislocations of the ankle. Am J Surg 98:136, 1959.
37. Joy G, Patzakis MJ, Harvey JP Jr: Precise evaluation of the reduction of severe ankle fractures. Technique and correlation with end results. J Bone Joint Surg 56A:979, 1974.
38. Key JA, Conwell HE: Injuries in the region of the ankle. In: The Management of Fractures, Dislocations and Sprains, 6th ed. St. Louis, Mosby, 1956.
39. Kleiger B: Treatment of oblique fractures of the fibula. J Bone Joint Surg 43:969, 1961.
40. Kleiger B: Mechanisms of ankle injury. Orthop Clin North Am 5:127, 1974.
41. Klossner O: Late results of operative and non-operative treatment of severe ankle fractures. A clinical study. Acta Chir Scand (Suppl) 293:1, 1962.
42. Kuntscher G: Practice of Intramedullary Nailing. Translated by H.H. Rinne. Springfield, Ill., Thomas, 1967.
43. Laros GS, Spiegel PG: Rigid internal fixation of fractures. Clin Orthop Rel Res 138:2, 1979.
44. Lauge-Hansen N: Fractures of the ankle. II. Combined experimental-surgical and experimental-roentgenologic investigations. Arch Surg 60:957, 1950.
45. Lauge-Hansen N: Fractures of the ankle. III. Genetic roentgenologic diagnosis of fractures of the ankle. Am J Roentgenol 71:456, 1954.
46. Lauge-Hansen N: Fractures of the ankle. IV. Clinical use of the genetic roentgen diagnosis and genetic reduction. AMA Arch Surg 64:488, 1952.
47. Lindsjo U: Operative treatment of ankle fractures. Acta Orthop Scand (Suppl) 189:1, 1981.
48. Magnusson R: On the late results in non-operated cases of malleolar fractures. I. Fractures by external rotation. Acta Chir Scand (Suppl) 84:1, 1944.
49. Malka JS, Taillard W: Results of non-operative and operative treatment of fractures of the ankle. Clin Orthop Rel Res 67:159, 1969.
50. Mast JW, Teipner WA: A reproducible approach to the internal fixation of adult ankle fractures: Rationale, technique and early results. Orthop Clin North Am 11:661, 1980.
51. McLaughlin HL, Ryder CT Jr: Open reduction and internal fixation for fractures of the tibia and ankle. Surg Clin North Am 29:1523, 1949.
52. McLaughlin HL: Trauma. Philadelphia, Saunders, 1960.
53. Menelaus MB: Injuries of the anterior inferior tibio-fibular ligament. Aust NZ J Surg 30:279, 1960.
54. Meyer TL Jr, Kumler KW: A.S.I.F. technique and ankle fractures. Clin Orthop Rel Res 150:211, 1980.
55. Mitchell CL, Fleming JL: Fractures and fracture-dislocations of the ankle. Postgrad Med 26:773, 1959.
56. Mitchell WG, Shaftan GW, Sclafani S: Mandatory open reduction: Its role in displaced ankle fractures. J Trauma 19:602, 1979.
57. Monk CJE: Injuries of the tibiofibular ligaments. J Bone Joint Surg 51:330, 1969.
58. Müller ME, Allgöwer M, Schneider R, Willenegger H: Manual of Internal Fixation, 2nd ed. Translated by J. Schatzker. New York, Springer-Verlag, 1979.
59. Nahigian SH, Oh I, Zahrawi FB: Wire-loop fixation of the lateral malleolus in ankle fractures. In Bateman JE, Trott AW (eds): The Foot and Ankle. New York, Thieme-Stratton, 1980.
60. Neer CS II: Injuries of the ankle joint—evaluation. Connecticut State Med J 17:580, 1953.
61. Neufeld AJ: Ankle joint fractures and their treatment. Clin Orthop 42:91, 1965.
62. Nyström G: A contribution to the treatment of fractures of the posterior border of the tibia by malleolar fractures. Acta Radiol 25:672, 1944.
63. Oh I, Nahigian SH, Salas AS, Zahrawi FB: Cerclage of the lateral malleolus in displaced fracture of the ankle. Orthopaedics 1:374, 1978.
64. Pankovich AM: Maisonneuve fracture of the fibula. J Bone Joint Surg 58A:337, 1976.
65. Pankovich AM: Fractures of the fibula proximal to the distal tibiofibular syndesmosis. J Bone Joint Surg 60A:221, 1978.
66. Pankovich AM: Fractures of the fibula at the distal tibiofibular syndesmosis. Clin Orthop Rel Res 143:138, 1979.
67. Pankovich AM: Adult ankle fractures. JCE Orthop 7:17, 1979.
68. Pankovich AM, Shivaram MS: Anatomical basis of variability in injuries of medial malleolus and the deltoid ligament. I. Anatomical studies. Acta Orthop Scand 50:217, 1979.
69. Pankovich AM, Shivaram MS: Anatomical basis of variability in injuries of medial malleolus and deltoid ligament. II. Clinical studies. Acta Orthop Scand 50:225, 1979.
70. Patrick J: A direct approach to trimalleolar fractures. J Bone Joint Surg 47B:236, 1965.
71. Proctor H: Lateral rotation fracture-dislocation of ankle. J Bone Joint Surg 36B:148, 1954.
72. Purvis GD: The unstable oblique distal fibular fracture. Clin Orthop Rel Res 92:330, 1973.
73. Quigley TB: Management of ankle injuries sus-

tained in sports. JAMA 169:1431, 1959.
74. Quigley TB: Analysis and treatment of ankle injuries produced by rotatory, abduction and adduction forces. Instructional Course Lectures. Am Acad Orthop Surg 19:172, 1970.
75. Rush LV: Atlas of Rush Pin Technics. A System of Fracture Treatment. Meridian, Miss., Berivon, 1955.
76. Rütt A: Surgery of the Lower Leg and Foot. Translated by G. Stiasny. Philadelphia, Saunders, 1980.
77. Sarkisian JS, Cody GW: Closed treatment of ankle fractures. A new criterion for evaluation. A review of 250 cases. J Trauma 16:323, 1976.
78. Solonen KA, Lauttamus L: Treatment of malleolar fractures. Acta Orthop Scand 36:321, 1965.
79. Solonen KA, Lauttamus L: Operative treatment of ankle fractures. Acta Orthop Scand 39:223, 1968.
80. Staples OS: Injuries to the medial ligaments of the ankle. J Bone Joint Surg 42A:1287, 1960.
81. Staples OS: Ligamentous injuries of the ankle joint. Clin Orthop 42:21, 1965.
82. Sudman E: Compression osteosynthesis of lateral malleolar fractures with the figure-of-eight cerclage. Acta Chir Scand 140:37, 1974.
83. Svend-Hansen H, Bremerskov U, Baekgaard N: Ankle fractures treated by fixation of medial malleolus alone. Late results in 29 patients. Acta Orthop Scand 49:211, 1978.
84. Vasli S: Operative treatment of ankle fractures. Acta Chir Scand (Suppl) 226:1, 1957.
85. Wade PA, Lance EM: The operative treatment of fracture-dislocation of the ankle joint. Clin Orthop Rel Res 42:37, 1965.
86. Walsh WM, Hughston JC: Unstable ankle fractures in athletes. Am J Sports Med 4:173, 1976.
87. Watson-Jones R: Fractures and Other Joint Injuries, 4th ed. Baltimore, Williams & Wilkins, 1955.
88. Yablon IG, Heller FG, Shouse L: The key role of the lateral malleolus in displaced fractures of the ankle. J Bone Joint Surg 59A:169, 1977.
89. Yablon IG, Wasilewski S: Management of unstable ankle fracture. In Bateman JE, Trott AW (eds): The Foot and Ankle. New York, Thieme-Stratton, 1980.
90. Yablon IG, Wasilewski S: Isolated fractures of the lateral malleolus. Orthopedics 4:301, 1981.
91. Yde J: The Lauge-Hansen classification of malleolar fractures. Acta Orthop Scand 51:181, 1980.
92. Yde J, Kristensen KD: Ankle fractures: Supination-eversion fractures, stage II. Acta Orthop Scand 51:695, 1980.
93. Yde J, Kristensen KD: Ankle fractures: Supination-eversion fractures, stage IV. Acta Orthop Scand 51:981, 1980.
94. Zuelzer WA: Fixation of small but important bone fragments with a hook plate. J Bone Joint Surg 33A:430, 1951.

Chapter 11   Pronation-External Rotation Injuries

William C. Hamilton

The starting position of the foot in pronation-external rotation injuries [26] is that of pronation (dorsiflexion, abduction, eversion). The pathologic talar motion is that of eversion (external rotation) (Fig. 11.1).

The stages of pronation-external rotation injuries are as follows [26]:

I. Rupture of deltoid ligament or avulsion fracture of the medial malleolus (Fig. 11.2A,B).

II. Rupture or avulsion of the anterior inferior tibiofibular ligament (AITFL), interosseous membrane (IOM), and interosseous ligament (IOL) (Fig. 11.2C).

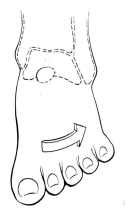

Fig. 11.1. Pronation-external rotation mechanism.

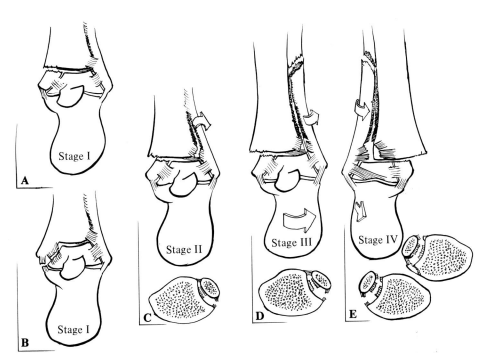

Fig. 11.2. Pronation-external rotation injury. **A** Stage I with medial malleolus fracture, **B** Stage I with deltoid ligament rupture, **C** Stage II with medial malleolus fracture, **D** Stage III with medial malleolus fracture, **E** Stage IV posterior view.

III. Spiral fracture of the fibula at a variable distance above the syndesmosis (Fig. 11.2D).

IV. Rupture or avulsion of the posterior inferior tibiofibular ligaments (PITFL and ITTFL) (Fig. 11.2E).

Mechanism

Lauge-Hansen observed that with the foot in a pronated attitude, the deltoid ligament was taut [26,28]. When the talus was rotated externally with the foot in this position, tension developed initially within the deltoid ligament, resulting in either ligament rupture or avulsion fracture of the medial malleolus (stage I) (Fig. 11.2A,B).

With continued force, he observed a simultaneous rupture or avulsion of the anterior inferior tibiofibular ligament, interosseous membrane, and interosseous ligament, permitting up to 2 cm of anterior diastasis of the tibiofibular syndesmosis (stage II). This occurred as the talus rotated laterally and simultaneously abducted about its longitudinal axis (Fig. 11.2C). If the deforming force was discontinued at this point, the fibula usually recoiled to its normal position in the fibular groove.

Further external rotation of the talus beyond this stage caused torsion of the fibula about its longitudinal axis, producing a spiral fracture of the fibula proximal to the syndesmosis (stage III) (Fig. 11.2D). Usually, the fibular fracture occurred where the rupture of the interosseous ligament and interosseous membrane ceased; i.e., the line of injury passed proximally through soft tissue, then through bone (Fig. 11.3A,B). The fibular fracture in Lauge-Hansen's experience was spiral, usually located 8–9 cm or more above the tip of the lateral malleolus. The distal fibula was displaced posteriorly with the talus so that the fibular fracture angulated with the apex anteriorly (Fig. 11.3C).

With persistent force tending to laterally rotate and displace the foot, Lauge-Hansen noted that the talus impinged on the dorsolateral corner of the tibia and simultaneously the tension within the intact posterior inferior tibiofibular ligaments (PITFL and ITTFL) increased, resulting in either rupture of these ligaments or avulsion of a bony fragment of variable size from the postero-

lateral margin of the tibia (stage IV) (Figs. 11.2E and 11.3).

As an extreme degree of this injury, the talus dislocated proximally and centrally between the distal tibia and fibula (Fig. 11.4). Lauge-Hansen stated that the talus dislocated proximally into the anterior syndesmosis during stage III, when the dorsal tibiofibular ligaments were still intact. This situation could also occur at or after stage IV, when all continuity between the distal tibia and fibula has been lost.

Of the five mechanisms described by Lauge-Hansen, the pronation-external rotation injury is probably the most controversial. Pankovich [40] has recently questioned the validity of this mechanism as well as the specific sequence of events leading up to the stage III and stage IV injury. Walsh and Hughston [53] however have published a photograph of a football player sustaining an injury analogous to that described by Lauge-Hansen (Fig. 11.5).

Clinical Significance

Pronation-external rotation accounts for 7–19% of ankle fractures [3,27,28,30,32,36,48]. Stages III and IV of the pronation-external rotation mechanism correspond to the injury frequently referred to as a "Maisonneuve fracture."

In the early stages (I and II), it is impossible to clearly distinguish between injuries caused by pronation-external rotation and those due to pronation-abduction (Chapter 12), since both are characterized initially by fracture of the medial malleolus or rupture of the deltoid ligament (stage I) associated with incomplete ligamentous injury of the syndesmosis (stage II) (Fig. 11.6). For this reason, the true incidence of pronation-external rotation as well as pronation-abduction injuries cannot be ascertained with assurance.

Stage I

Stage I pronation-external rotation injury—isolated fracture of the medial malleolus or rupture of the deltoid ligament (identical to stage I pronation-abduction injury)—is generally considered to be a rare clinical occurrence [13,14,25,33, 44,49]. Grath [20] and Yablon [55,56] demon-

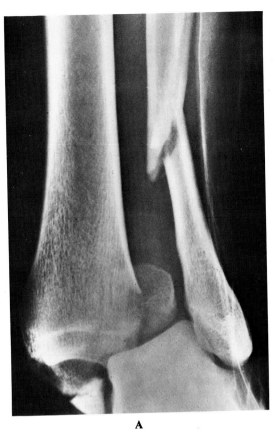

A

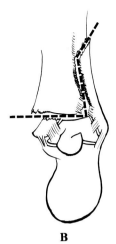

B

Fig. 11.3. A PER IV injury with posterolateral dislocation of talus. **B** Line of injury travels proximally from the ankle through the syndesmosis to the level of the fracture. **C** With the distal fibula displaced posteriorly with the talus, the fracture is angulated with the apex anteriorly. Note the large shell of bone from the posterior aspect of the tibia remaining in association with the distal fibula.

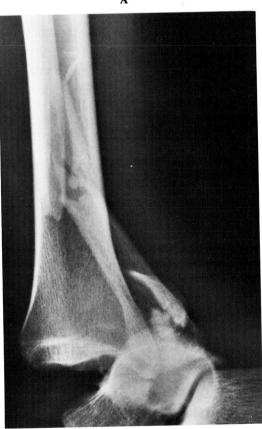

C

strated that the lateral malleolus has a protective effect on the deltoid ligament. Without lateral malleolus fracture or tibiofibular ligament injury, Yablon could not demonstrate any talar instability after division of the entire deltoid ligament; and only 10° of external rotation of the talus was permitted after resection of the medial malleolus. Golterman [19] did not think isolated deltoid rupture could occur. Brostrom [8,9], however, did demonstrate isolated deltoid ligament damage by arthrography in 2–3% of ankle sprains; and apparently "isolated" fractures of the medial malleolus are occasionally encountered in clinical practice (Fig. 11.7), suggesting that isolated medial injury, although rare, is indeed possible [49]. In most clinical situations, however, there is probably a chronologic overlap between stage I and stage II injuries, such that some degree of tibiofibular ligament damage occurs simultaneously with the stage I lesion.

Stage II

Stage II lesions (Fig. 11.2C) comprise 60% of pronation-external rotation injuries according to Lauge-Hansen [28]. As noted, however, this in-

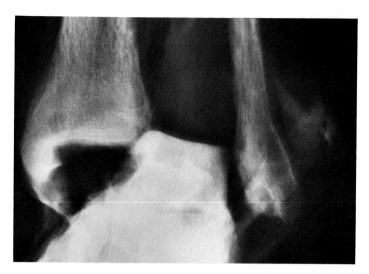

Fig. 11.4. Pronation-external rotation injury with proximal dislocation of the talus.

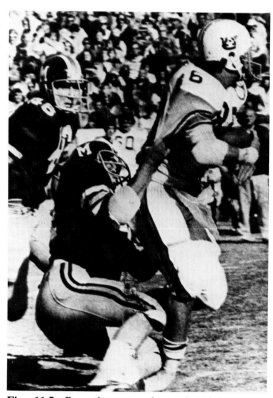

Fig. 11.5. Pronation-external rotation injury. Reprinted with permission from Walsh WM, Hughston JC: Unstable ankle fractures in athletes. Am J Sports Med 4:177, 1976. The Williams & Wilkins Co., Baltimore.

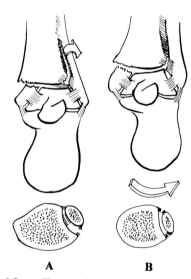

A   B

Fig. 11.6 Stage II pronation-external rotation (**A**) and pronation-abduction (**B**) injuries differ pathologically, but are not distinguishable clinically.

jury cannot be clinically distinguished from pronation-abduction stage II injuries; moreover, the frequency of both stage II pronation-external rotation and pronation-abduction injuries is proba-

bly underestimated since radiographic changes may be subtle or absent entirely if the medial injury is ligamentous and the lateral malleolus and talus recoil to normal position after the pathologic forces are dissipated. Clinically the patient will demonstrate tenderness over the tibiofibular syndesmosis in association with fracture of the medial malleolus or tenderness over the deltoid ligament. The stress test of Kleiger (Fig. 10.16) is useful if this injury is suspected; external rotation stress radiographs will generally demon-

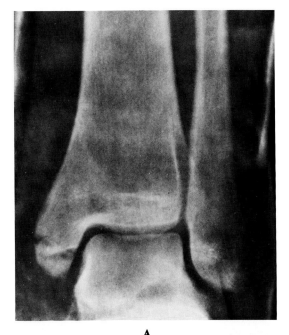

A

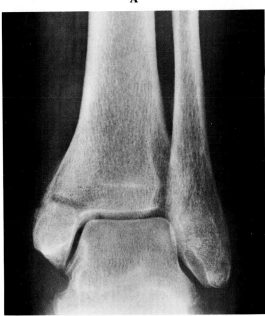

B

Fig. 11.7. Apparently isolated avulsion fractures of medial malleolus. No clinical or radiographic evidence of associated injury. **A** Isolated anterior colliculus fracture. **B** Isolated supracollicular fracture.

strate widening of the medial clear space and/or tibiofibular syndesmosis [28].

Stage III

Stage III pronation-external rotation injuries (fracture of the fibular shaft) account for 20–25% of pronation-external rotation injuries. The fibular lesion usually consists of a spiral or oblique fracture located a variable distance above the syndesmosis. The length of the fracture is quite variable also. When it is short and located near the syndesmosis, it suggests that abduction forces were in part responsible for the injury (see Chapter 12); this distinction is more theoretical than practical, however. This fracture must be distinguished from the relatively innocuous transverse or comminuted fractures of the fibular shaft caused by direct trauma (Fig. 11.8). Clinically the diagnosis of stage III pronation-external rotation injury should at least be suspected whenever there is evidence of a proximal fibular fracture

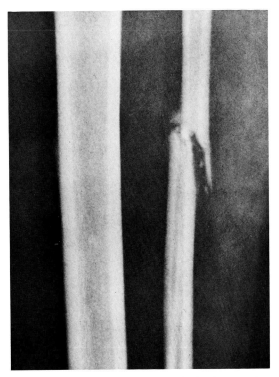

Fig. 11.8. Transverse, comminuted fibular fracture due to direct trauma. Usually the distal fragment is displaced medially. (Courtesy of Dr. Donald M. Qualls) [43].

associated with ankle injury. Since patients can be distracted by their ankle injury, the proximal injury can be easily overlooked, unless one combines examination of the ankle with clinical and radiographic examination of the entire lower leg (Fig. 11.9) [40].

Stage IV

Stage IV injury, accounting for approximately 14% of pronation-external rotation injuries, is reached when the posterior inferior tibiofibular ligaments rupture or avulse with a fragment of bone from the posterior tibia. This constitutes a total tibiofibular ligamentous diastasis and represents a very unstable and serious injury. At this stage, the talus may dislocate laterally, posterolaterally (Fig. 11.3A), or proximally and centrally between the tibia and fibula (Fig. 11.4). In the absence of gross displacement of the distal fibula, the key to diagnosis is the fracture of the posterior tibia. If the posterior inferior tibiofibular ligaments (PITFL/ITTFL) fail through their substance, however, this valuable radiographic finding is absent and one must rely upon stress radiographs or operative exploration to ascertain the true degree of injury (Fig. 11.10). The sever-

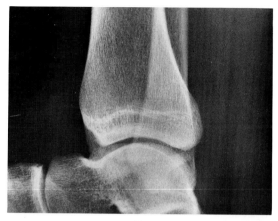

B

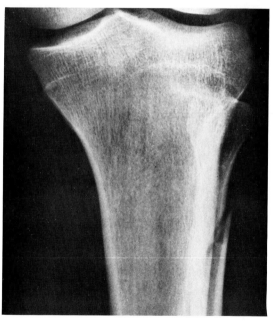

C

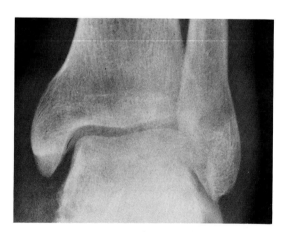

A

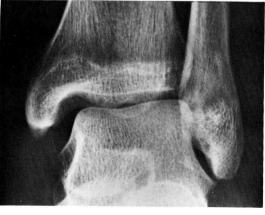

D

Fig. 11.9. Pronation-external rotation injury, stage III. **A** and **B** Initial radiographs demonstrated bimalleolar soft tissue swelling but no fracture. **C** Because of tenderness over the proximal fibula, a radiograph of this area was obtained. **D** Subsequent stress evaluation under anesthesia revealed widening of the medial clear space compatible with deltoid ligament rupture. There was no clinical, radiographic, or intraoperative evidence of posterior syndesmosis damage.

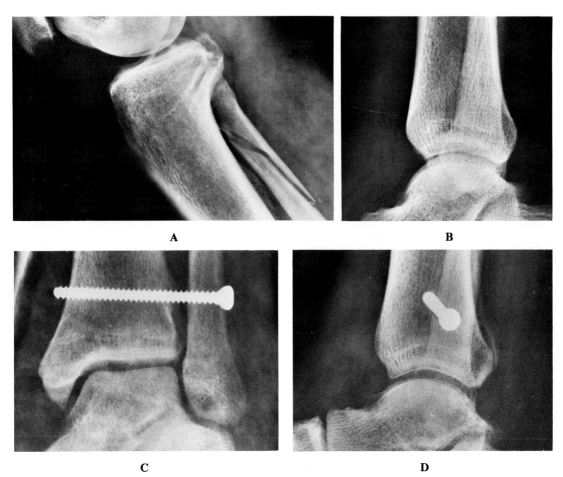

C   D

Fig. 11.10. Pronation-external rotation injury, stage IV. **A** The patient complained of ankle pain and demonstrated tenderness over the proximal fibula. **B** There was no radiographic evidence of posterior syndesmotic injury but operative exploration revealed complete ligamentous diastasis. **C** The syndesmosis was stabilized with a positioning screw to protect repair of the syndesmotic ligaments. **D** Lateral radiographs obtained 8 weeks later, prior to screw removal, demonstrated dystrophic calcification at the site of injury of the posterior syndesmosis.

ity of stage III or stage IV pronation-external rotation injuries, characterized by deltoid ligament rupture rather than medial malleolus fracture, in which the distal fibula recoils into normal relationship with the distal tibia, can be easily underestimated. Unless one realizes that the presence of a spiral supramalleolar fracture of the fibula implies coexisting damage to the medial ankle and at least the anterior portion of the tibiofibular syndesmosis [4,28], the full extent of ankle injury will not be appreciated. Even if one questions the reproducibility of the specific sequence of injuries outlined by Lauge-Hansen [57], a fibular fracture of this type should at least prompt the performance of stress examination

or radiography [1,4], wherein the true degree of instability will be demonstrated (Fig. 11.11).

Pronation-External Rotation Injuries: Closed Reduction (Lauge-Hansen) [27]

1. Reduction should be done immediately.
2. General or spinal anesthesia is required.
3. The knee should be flexed to 90° to relax the gastrocnemius muscle.
4. An assistant is required.

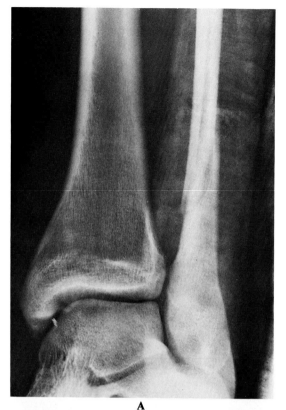

A

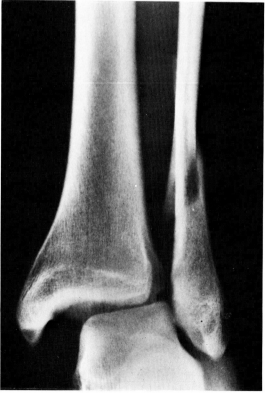

B

5. Immobilization should be obtained by use of a short leg walking cast.

Closed reduction technique (Fig. 11.12) is identical to that employed for supination-external rotation fractures, except for step 1 where the foot is pronated and externally rotated instead of being supinated and externally rotated.

1. Foot is pronated and everted—to separate fracture surfaces. (Fig. 11.12A)
2. Foot is plantarflexed as traction is applied in the long axis of limb—to restore fibular length (via lateral collateral ligaments) and correct proximal displacement of posterior tibial lip fragment (via posterior inferior tibiofibular ligaments). (Fig. 11.12B)
3. Foot is translated anteriorly—to reduce the dorsal subluxation of the talus and (via ligamentous attachments) the dorsal displacement of the lateral malleolus and posterior tibial lip. (Fig. 11.12C)
4. Foot is internally rotated—to correct external rotation of the talus and fibula (via the anterior talofibular ligament). (Fig. 11.12D)
5. Foot is pronated and dorsiflexed to a right angle—with internal rotation maintained. (Fig. 11.12E)
6. As plaster sets, the hindfoot should be adducted—to prevent valgus tilt of the talus and fibular fragment.

When the fibular fracture is short and oblique in orientation, it is easier to regain fibular length and secure reduction than with a long oblique fracture. Because of the extent of soft tissue damage, however, this injury is potentially unstable, and reduction is frequently difficult to maintain by closed means [14]. Again, one must seriously question the advisability of immobilizing this fracture in a short leg walking cast. If one is fortunate enough to obtain satisfactory reduction following this injury, the plaster should be extended above the knee to better control rotation.

◁
Fig. 11.11. A Spiral supramalleolar fracture of fibula. **B** During application of external rotation stress under anesthesia.

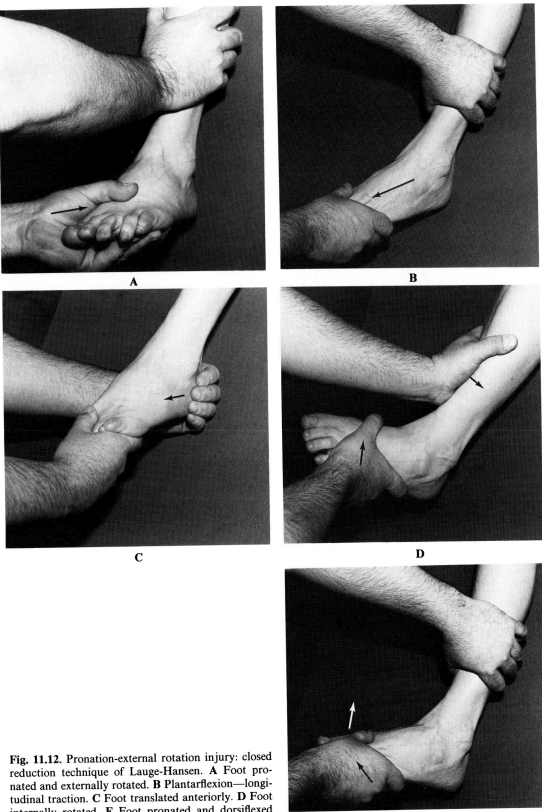

Fig. 11.12. Pronation-external rotation injury: closed reduction technique of Lauge-Hansen. **A** Foot pronated and externally rotated. **B** Plantarflexion—longitudinal traction. **C** Foot translated anteriorly. **D** Foot internally rotated. **E** Foot pronated and dorsiflexed to a right angle with internal rotation maintained.

Pronation-External Rotation Injuries: Open Reduction and Internal Fixation

Internal fixation of pronation-external rotation injuries differs from that of supination-external rotation fractures in two important respects:

1. The fibular fracture is located above the syndesmosis and the interosseous ligament is ruptured. Tibiofibular ligament damage is significant in stage III (AITFL/IOL) and complete in stage IV (AITFL/IOL/PITFL/ITTFL) lesions.
2. Medial joint injury occurs early in the sequence (stage I) rather than as a terminal event.

   Again, both sides of the joint should be exposed simultaneously and interposed soft tissue should be removed from the ankle joint and fracture sites. If the medial injury is characterized by deltoid ligament rupture, sutures should be inserted but not tied.

For fibular fractures located in the distal half of the bone, reduction and fixation will facilitate accurate restoration of the tibiofibular syndesmosis [4]. When the fracture, however, is located in the proximal fibula, considerable tibiofibular instability will persist after fibular fixation, so there is little to be gained by fibular repair except for guaranteed restoration of fibular length.

For stage III injuries, where the posterior inferior tibiofibular ligaments and part of the interosseous ligament remain intact (anterior diastasis), fixation of the fibular fracture and debridement of the tibiofibular syndesmosis will frequently restore a normal and stable distal tibiofibular relationship, permitting satisfactory and secure repair of the anterior inferior tibiofibular ligament [18,41]. The interosseous ligament (IOL), because of its short span and location, does not lend itself to repair by suture, but restoration of normal tibiofibular relationships will permit satisfactory healing of this structure provided external rotation and lateral displacement of the talus can be temporarily prevented [37]. After fibular fixation and tibiofibular reduction, the integrity of the syndesmosis should be tested under direct vision by applying traction to the distal fibula with a bone clamp or hook (as described for supination-external rotation injuries). If significant tibiofibular instability persists, then tibiofibular fixation should be employed [41,42].

With stage IV pronation-external rotation injuries (complete ligamentous diastasis), all of the tibiofibular ligaments have been torn or avulsed, so that considerable tibiofibular mobility will invariably persist after fibular fixation. Under these circumstances, it is frequently difficult and sometimes impossible to maintain satisfactory tibiofibular reduction by closed means. Satisfactory repair of the deltoid and tibiofibular ligaments can be relied upon to facilitate but not necessarily maintain the normal relationship between the distal tibia and fibula. If less than anatomic reduction is tolerated, the deltoid and tibiofibular ligaments will heal in an elongated state, permitting instability and permanent widening of the syndesmosis. Unfortunately, there is no entirely satisfactory reconstructive procedure to correct either deltoid or tibiofibular ligamentous insufficiency [2,5]. Therefore, adequate primary treatment assumes great importance, and temporary tibiofibular fixation is usually necessary [7,16,21].

Over the years, stabilization of the tibiofibular syndesmosis, with a transfixion screw or other device [22], has been characterized by conflicting opinions concerning its value and possible adverse effects [3,11,14–16,21,24,25,37,39,42, 47,51,53]. Many of the problems previously encountered with tibiofibular fixation, however, have been due to faulty techniques. These difficulties can be minimized if the following principles are understood and observed.

1. Tibiofibular fixation should be employed only if necessary. Where possible and practical, the fibular fracture should be stabilized initially. This will frequently restore stability to the syndesmosis since the proximal fibular fragment maintains its ligamentous association with the tibia in all supination-adduction injuries, most supination-external rotation injuries, and many pronation-abduction injuries. Pronation-external rotation fibular fractures are usually associated with rupture of the interosseous ligament, but even so, up to stage IV, the posterior tibiofibular ligaments, binding the distal fibula to the posterior tubercle of the tibia, are intact; once the fibular fracture is stabilized, only an anterior diastasis remains [11]. Tibiofibular screw fixation employed merely as a means of stabi-

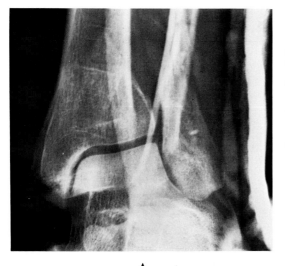
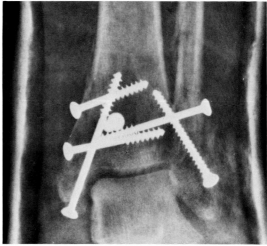

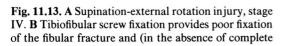

| A | B |

Fig. 11.13. A Supination-external rotation injury, stage IV. **B** Tibiofibular screw fixation provides poor fixation of the fibular fracture and (in the absence of complete ligamentous diastasis) immobilizes the syndesmosis unnecessarily.

lizing a fibular fracture (Fig. 11.13) [10,29] provides poor stabilization of the fracture and immobilizes the syndesmosis unnecessarily [11].

2. Some degree of tibiofibular motion is physiologic and necessary for normal ankle function [20]. Therefore, to permit full recovery, any tibiofibular fixation device should be removed after it has performed its function [4,6,16,21,23,24,30–32,35,38,45,47,50,52]. Failure to remove the device will disturb ankle function until the device loosens or breaks [3,6,12,21,23,46].

3. Tibiofibular fixation can be relied upon only to maintain normal tibiofibular relationship *after* reduction has been achieved under direct vision by exploration of the tibiofibular syndesmosis. Since tibiofibular fixation is only a temporary internal splint, ruptured tibiofibular ligaments should be approximated as best as possible so that they will heal at normal length and assume their stabilizing function when the tibiofibular fixation device is removed.

4. Of the various devices available, a screw is best suited since it will perform the necessary function, and yet can be easily removed when the time comes [4,10,23].

5. Since the tibiofibular screw serves only to maintain the already restored tibiofibular relationship, there is no need to compress these two bones with a compression or lag device [38]. If a normal tibiofibular relationship has been restored, compression is unnecessary. If normal relationship has not been restored, compression is inadequate (Fig. 11.14).

6. In terms of tibiofibular reduction, one needs to think in more than one plane. To date, the width of the tibiofibular syndesmosis has received much attention. It is just as important, however, to correct fibular shortening and malrotation [11]. Tibiofibular fixation with the two bones in anything less than anatomic position is liable to be worse than no fixation at all (Fig. 11.15) [48].

7. If a tibiofibular transfixion screw is employed, placement is important. It should not be located in immediate proximity to the ankle joint where the distal tibia and fibula are in intimate contact (Fig. 11.16), since any bony fragments generated in this interval by screw insertion are liable to cause problems. If inserted too close to the ankle joint, the screw may have a deleterious effect on the articular cartilage [48]. Nor should the screw be located too far posteriorly or anteriorly, such that it creates a rotatory distortion of the fibula with respect to the tibia.

8. Since the purpose of the screw is to hold the fibula in the fibular incisura of the tibia,

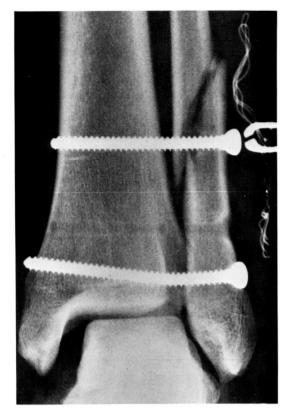

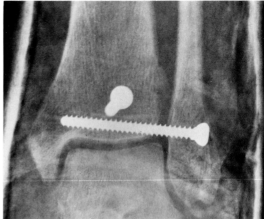

Fig. 11.16. Transfixion screw placed too low.

◁

Fig. 11.14. Tibiotalar and tibiofibular relationships should be restored prior to tibiofibular screw fixation. Otherwise, no amount of screw compression will effect satisfactory reduction.

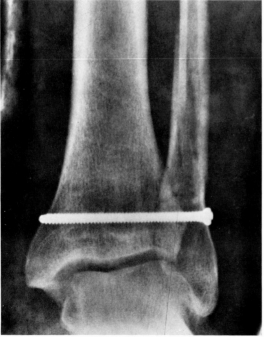

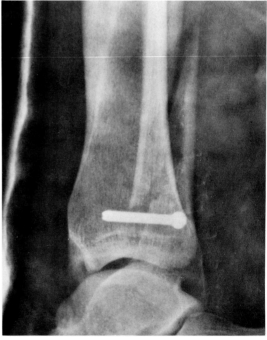

A   B

Fig. 11.15. A and **B** Distal tibia and fibula transfixed with residual shortening and posterior displacement of the distal fibula.

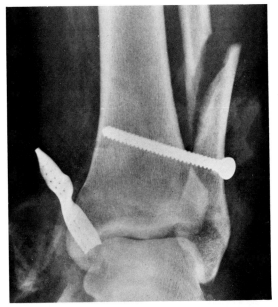

Fig. 11.17. In the absence of prior tibiofibular stabilization an oblique tibiofibular screw may distort both the fibular fracture and the distal tibiofibular relationship.

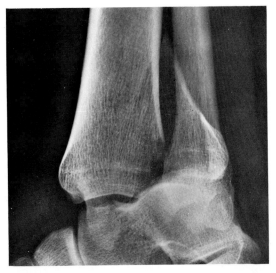

A

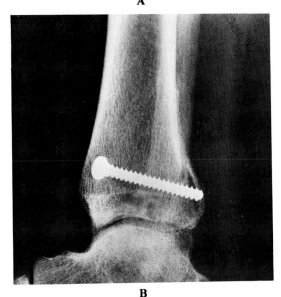

B

Fig. 11.18. A Pronation-external rotation injury, stage IV, with large posterior tibial fragment. **B** Following reduction and screw fixation of this fragment, only an anterior diastasis remained.

the ideal position for the screw is horizontal [1,14,17,23,34,38,45,51,54]. There is little rationale for inserting the screw obliquely. When an oblique tibiofibular screw is used in the absence of prior fibular stabilization, it may serve to distort the relationship between the fibular fragments and, therefore, between the distal tibia and fibula (Fig. 11.17).

9. If the tibiofibular ligament injury is characterized by large bony avulsions anteriorly and/or posteriorly that can be reduced and fixed with screws, then tibiofibular fixation is unnecessary (Fig. 11.18).

Pronation-External Rotation Injuries: Fixation Techniques

Spiral Fracture of the Fibula Above the Syndesmosis

If long enough, this fracture can be fixed with interfragmentary screws or wire loops as described for supination-external rotation injuries (Fig. 11.19). If the fracture is short or comminuted, or if external immobilization is to be avoided, then the fracture site should be protected with a neutralization (semitubular or small compression) plate (Fig. 11.20) [32,38,41].

Fracture of the Medial Malleolus

Since this fracture is caused by avulsion forces, fixation techniques are identical to those outlined in Chapter 10 for supination-external rotation injuries.

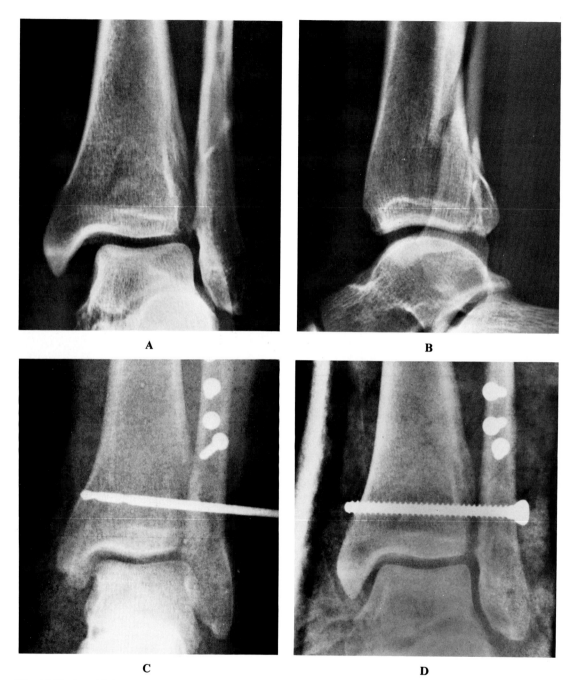

Fig. 11.19. A and **B** Pronation-external rotation injury, stage IV. **C–E** Treated with interfragmentary screw fixation of the fibula, open reduction of the distal tibiofibular syndesmosis, repair of the anterior inferior tib- iofibular ligament, and stabilization of the syndesmosis with a transverse positioning screw. The posterior tibial fragment assumed normal position after the fibular fracture was reduced and stabilized.

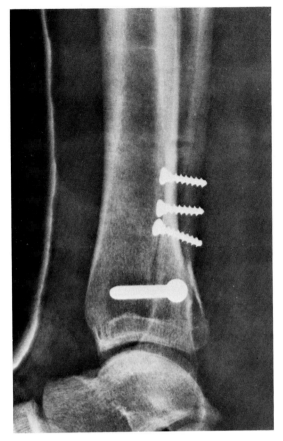

Fig. 11.19E

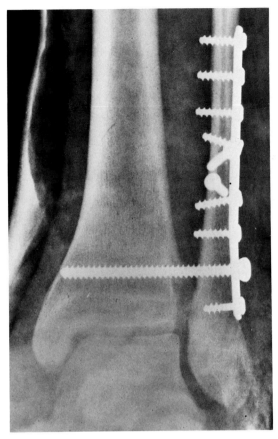

Fig. 11.20. Pronation-external rotation injury, stage IV. Treated with open reduction and fixation of fibular fracture using interfragmentary screws and neutralization plate, open reduction of tibiofibular syndesmosis, and stabilization with a transverse positioning screw.

Fig. 11.21. Tibiofibular screw transfixion without prior fibular fixation (Weber). **A** After reduction of the syndesmosis under direct vision, a smooth pin is inserted transversely, just above the site of the proposed positioning screw, to temporarily immobilize the syndesmosis. **B** The positioning screw is inserted approximately 3 cm above the tibial plafond. This screw is intended only to *maintain* tibiofibular position, and therefore should not be lagged or compressed. The temporary pin is then removed or replaced with a second tibiofibular screw (**C**) to better control rotation in the sagittal plane.

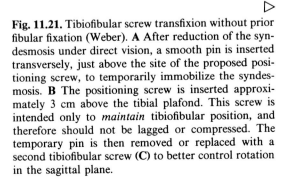

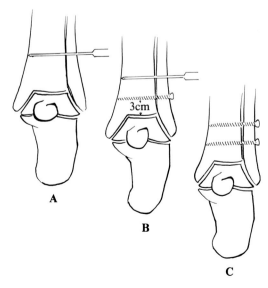

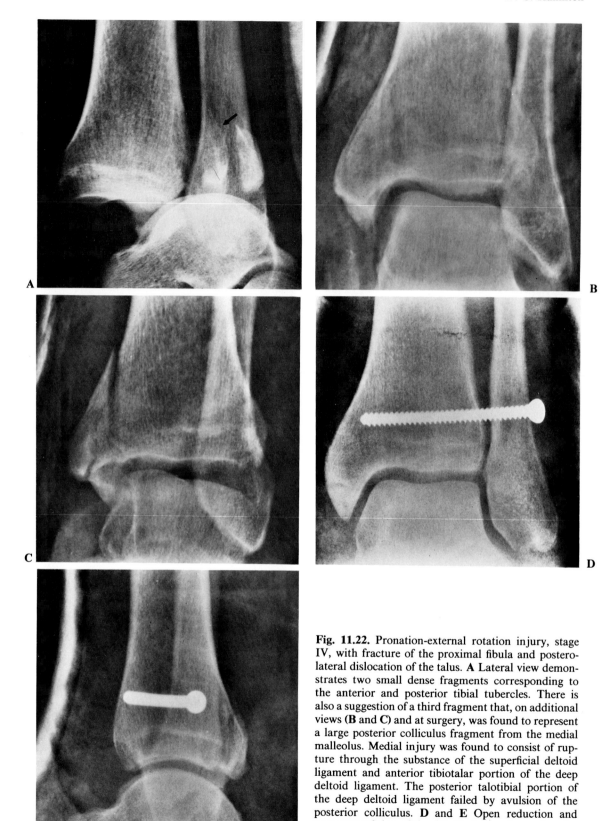

Fig. 11.22. Pronation-external rotation injury, stage IV, with fracture of the proximal fibula and postero-lateral dislocation of the talus. A Lateral view demonstrates two small dense fragments corresponding to the anterior and posterior tibial tubercles. There is also a suggestion of a third fragment that, on additional views (B and C) and at surgery, was found to represent a large posterior colliculus fragment from the medial malleolus. Medial injury was found to consist of rupture through the substance of the superficial deltoid ligament and anterior tibiotalar portion of the deep deltoid ligament. The posterior talotibial portion of the deep deltoid ligament failed by avulsion of the posterior colliculus. D and E Open reduction and screw transfixion of the tibiofibular syndesmosis satisfactorily reduced all fracture components.

Syndesmosis Injury

Tibiofibular transfixion should not be performed until the fibular fracture and tibiofibular syndesmosis have been reduced. This is best accomplished by internal fixation of the fibular fracture, but in situations where this is not feasible, the fibular fracture should be held temporarily in the reduced position prior to tibiofibular transfixion.

Tibiofibular Screw Fixation (Positioning Screw) With Prior Fibular Fixation

After fixation of the fibula and reduction of the tibiofibular syndesmosis and medial clear space, a guide wire or drill is inserted horizontally through the fibula into the tibia approximately 3 cm above the ankle joint [14,32]. A radiograph should be obtained at this point to verify wire location as well as reduction of the syndesmosis and medial joint space (Fig. 11.19C). If satisfactory, the guide wire is removed and the guide pin track is drilled through both cortices of the tibia and fibula; a threaded screw (tapped if necessary) is then inserted across both bones to engage all four cortices (Fig. 11.19D). This screw should not be lagged since this is not necessary if normal tibiofibular relationship has already been restored [38]. The screw should be tightened with the ankle in neutral or slight dorsiflexion, in the event that it does have a slight compressive effect. If the fibula has been fixed with a plate that extends to the level of the syndesmosis, one of its holes can be used for placement of the positioning screw (Fig. 11.20).

Tibiofibular Screw Transfixion Without Prior Fibular Fixation (Indirect Method of Weber)

If it is not practical or feasible to fix the fibula fracture first, then the syndesmosis should be reduced manually prior to tibiofibular stabilization [11]. This can usually be accomplished with a towel clip by applying traction and internal rotation to the distal fibula. Once the syndesmosis is reduced, it can be temporarily stabilized by inserting a smooth tibiofibular pin just above the level of the proposed positioning screw (Fig. 11.21A). After the positioning screw is inserted, the guide pin can be removed, retained, or re-

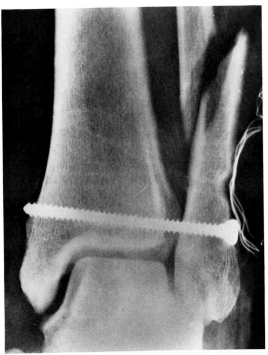

Fig. 11.23. Displacement of the fibular fracture implies that the distal tibiofibular relationship is distorted.

placed by a second positioning screw [37,38] for added stability to control rotation of the distal fibular fragment in the sagittal plane (Fig. 11.21C). Fixation of the syndesmosis should not distort the position of the fibular fracture, since this implies that the distal tibia and fibula have been fixed in an unnatural or unphysiologic position (Figs. 11.23) [11,32,48,51].

References

1. Alldredge RH: Diastasis of the distal tibiofibular joint and associated lesions. JAMA 115:2136, 1940.
2. Anderson KJ, LeCocq JF: Operative treatment of injury to the fibular collateral ligament of the ankle. J Bone Joint Surg 36A:825, 1954.
3. Bohler L: The Treatment of Fractures, 5th ed. New York, Grune & Stratton, 1956.
4. Bonnin JG: Injuries to the Ankle. New York, Grune & Stratton, 1950.
5. Bonnin JG: Injury to the ligaments of the ankle. J Bone Joint Surg 47B:609, 1965.
6. Braunstein PW, Wade PA: Treatment of unstable fractures of the ankle. Ann Surg 149:217, 1959.
7. Brodie IAOD, Denham RA: The treatment of

unstable ankle fractures. J Bone Joint Surg 56B:256, 1974.

8. Brostrom L: Sprained ankles. I. Anatomic lesions in recent sprains. Acta Chir Scand 128:483, 1964.

9. Brostrom L, Liljedahl S-O, Lindvall N: Sprained ankles. II. Arthrographic diagnosis of recent ligament ruptures. Acta Chir Scand 129:485, 1965.

10. Burgess E: Fractures of the ankle. J Bone Joint Surg 26:721, 1944.

11. Burwell HN, Charnley AD: Treatment of displaced fractures at the ankle by rigid internal fixation and early joint movement. J Bone Joint Surg 47B:634, 1965.

12. Cave EF (ed): Ankle injuries. In: Fractures and Other Injuries. Chicago, Year Book Medical, 1958.

13. Cedell C-A: Rupture of the posterior talotibial ligament with avulsion of a bone fragment from talus. Acta Orthop Scand 45:454, 1974.

14. Cedell C-A: Ankle lesions. Acta Orthop Scand 46:425, 1975.

15. Charnley J: The Closed Treatment of Common Fractures, 3rd ed. Baltimore, Williams & Wilkins, 1972.

16. Close R: Some applications of the functional anatomy of the ankle joint. J Bone Joint Surg 38A:761, 1956.

17. Cox FJ, Laxson WW: Fractures about the ankle joint. Am J Surg 83:674, 1952.

18. Dabezies E, D'Ambrosia RD, Shoji H: Classification and treatment of ankle fractures. Orthopedics 1:365, 1978.

19. Golterman AFL: Diagnosis and treatment of tibiofibular diastasis. Arch Chir Neerl 16:185, 1964.

20. Grath G: Widening of the ankle mortise. A clinical and experimental study. Acta Chir Scand (Suppl) 263:1, 1960.

21. Gristina AG, Rovere GD, Moses TE, Nicastro JF, Poehling GG: Injuries of the ankle syndesmosis: Base slider's ankle fracture. Orthop Rev 8:75, 1979.

22. Heikel H: Open or closed reduction of ankle joint injuries? Acta Orthop Scand 36:338, 1965.

23. Jergesen F: Open reduction of fractures and dislocations of the ankle. Am J Surg 98:136, 1959.

24. Kleiger B: Treatment of oblique fractures of the fibula. J Bone Joint Surg 43:969, 1961.

25. Klossner O: Late results of operative and non-operative treatment of severe ankle fractures. A clinical study. Acta Chir Scand (Suppl) 293:1, 1962.

26. Lauge-Hansen N: Fractures of the ankle. II. Combined experimental-surgical and experimental-roentgenologic investigations. Arch Surg 60:957, 1950.

27. Lauge-Hansen N: Fractures of the ankle. IV. Clinical use of the genetic roentgen diagnosis and genetic reduction. AMA Arch Surg 64:488, 1952.

28. Lauge-Hansen N: Fractures of the ankle. III. Genetic roentgenologic diagnosis of fractures of the ankle. Am J Roentgenol 71:456, 1954.

29. Lee HG, Horan TB: Internal fixation in injuries of the ankle. Surg Gynecol Obstet 76:593, 1943.

30. Lindsjo U: Operative treatment of ankle fractures. Acta Orthop Scand (Suppl) 189:1, 1981.

31. Malka JS, Taillard W: Results of non-operative and operative treatment of fractures of the ankle. Clin Orthop Rel Res 67:159, 1969.

32. Mast JW, Teipner WA: A reproducible approach to the internal fixation of adult ankle fractures: Rationale, technique and early results. Orthop Clin North Am 11:661, 1980.

33. McLaughlin HL: Trauma. Philadelphia, Saunders, 1960.

34. McLaughlin HL, Ryder CT Jr: Open reduction and internal fixation for fractures of the tibia and ankle. Surg Clin North Am 29:1523, 1949.

35. Meyer TL Jr, Kumler KW: A.S.I.F. technique and ankle fractures. Clin Orthop Rel Res 150:211, 1980.

36. Mitchell WG, Shaftan GW, Sclafani S: Mandatory open reduction: Its role in displaced ankle fractures. J Trauma 19:602, 1979.

37. Monk CJE: Injuries of the tibiofibular ligaments. J Bone Joint Surg 51B:330, 1969.

38. Müller ME, Allgöwer M, Schneider R, Willenegger H: Manual of Internal Fixation, 2nd ed. Translated by J. Schatzker. New York, Springer-Verlag, 1979.

39. Mullins JFP, Sallis JG: Recurrent sprain of the ankle joint with diastasis. J Bone Joint Surg 40B:270, 1958.

40. Pankovich AM: Maisonneuve fracture of the fibula. J Bone Joint Surg 58A:337, 1976.

41. Pankovich AM: Fractures of the fibula proximal to the distal tibiofibular syndesmosis. J Bone Joint Surg 60A:221, 1978.

42. Pankovich AM: Fractures of the fibula at the distal tibiofibular syndesmosis. Clin Orthop Rel Res 143:138, 1979.

43. Pankovich AM: Adult ankle fractures. JCE Orthop 7:17, 1979.

44. Quigley TB: Analysis and treatment of ankle injuries produced by rotatory, abduction and adduction forces. Instructional Course Lectures, Am Acad Orthop Surg 19:172, 1970.

45. Rütt A: Surgery of the Lower Leg and Foot. Translated by G. Stiasny. Philadelphia, Saunders, 1980.

46. Smith MGH: Inferior tibiofibular diastasis treated by cross screwing. J Bone Joint Surg 45B:737, 1963.

47. Solonen KA, Lauttamus L: Treatment of malleolar fractures. Acta Orthop Scand 36:321, 1965.

48. Solonen KA, Lauttamus L: Operative treatment of ankle fractures. Acta Orthop Scand 39:223, 1968.

49. Staples OS: Injuries to the medial ligaments of the ankle. J Bone Joint Surg 42A:1287, 1960.

50. Staples OS: Ligamentous injuries of the ankle joint. Clin Orthop 42:21, 1965.

51. Vasli S: Operative treatment of ankle fractures. Acta Chir Scand (Suppl) 226:1, 1957.

52. Wade PA, Lance EM: The operative treatment of fracture-dislocation of the ankle joint. Clin Orthop Rel Res 42:37, 1965.

53. Walsh WM, Hughston JC: Unstable ankle fractures in athletes. Am J Sports Med 4:173, 1976.

54. Watson-Jones R: Fractures and Other Joint Injuries, 4th ed. Baltimore, Williams & Wilkins, 1955.

55. Yablon IG, Heller FG, Shouse L: The key role of the lateral malleolus in displaced fractures of the ankle. J Bone Joint Surg 59A:169, 1977.

56. Yablon IG, Wasilewski S: Management of unstable ankle fracture. In Bateman JE, Trott AW (eds): The Foot and Ankle. New York, Thieme-Stratton, 1980.

57. Yde J: The Lauge-Hansen classification of malleolar fractures. Acta Orthop Scand 51:181, 1980.

Chapter 12   Pronation-Abduction Injuries

WILLIAM C. HAMILTON

In pronation-abduction injuries, the starting position of the foot is that of pronation (dorsiflexion, abduction, eversion). The pathologic talar motion is that of abduction (lateral rotation of the talus about its longitudinal axis) (Fig. 12.1).

The stages of pronation-abduction injuries are as follows [8]:

I. Rupture of the deltoid ligament or avulsion fracture of the medial malleolus (Fig. 12.2A,B).
II. Rupture or avulsion of the anterior (AITFL) and posterior (PITFL/ITTFL) inferior tibiofibular ligaments (Fig. 12.2C,D).

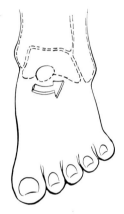

Fig. 12.1. Pronation-abduction mechanism.

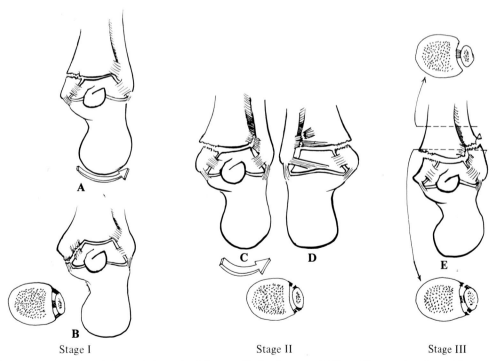

Stage I   Stage II   Stage III

Fig. 12.2. Pronation-abduction injury. **A** Stage I with medial malleolus fracture, **B** Stage I with deltoid ligament rupture, **C** Stage II anterior view with medial malleolar fracture, **D** Stage II posterior view with medial malleolar fracture, **E** Stage III anterior view with medial malleolar fracture.

III. Bending fracture of the distal fibula, 0.5–1 cm above the tibial plafond (Fig. 12.2E).

Mechanism

As already mentioned in reference to pronation-external rotation injuries, a starting position of pronation implies that the deltoid ligament is taut. Lauge-Hansen [8,10] observed that when an abduction force was applied to the talus with the foot in this position, tension was generated initially within the deltoid ligament, resulting in deltoid rupture or medial malleolus avulsion fracture (stage I) (Fig. 12.2A,B). The injury at this stage was identical to that encountered with stage I pronation-external rotation injuries (Fig. 11.2A,B). With continued abduction force, the talus pushed the distal fibula laterally, producing simultaneous rupture or avulsion of the anterior and posterior inferior tibiofibular ligaments (stage II) (Fig. 12.2C,D). If the force were discontinued at this point, the fibula frequently recoiled to its normal position, obscuring the extent of tibiofibular injury.

If the force were continued beyond stage II, Lauge-Hansen observed fracture of the fibula 0.5–1 cm proximal to the tibial plafond at the level where the tibiofibular ligament injury ceased. This resembled a "bending" fracture; it was relatively transverse or short oblique in orientation and frequently was characterized by mild lateral triangular comminution (Fig. 12.2E). The proximal fibular fragment remained in normal relationship to the distal tibia since the interosseous membrane and most of the interosseous ligament remained intact.

Clinical Significance

The pronation-abduction mechanism explains 5–21% of ankle fractures depending on the series [1,2,9–11,14,19]. As already discussed, stage I pronation-abduction injury is identical to stage I pronation-external rotation injury.

Stage II pronation-abduction injury differs from stage II pronation-external rotation injury in that the anterior and posterior inferior tibiofibular ligaments are ruptured or avulsed with the abduction mechanism (Fig. 12.2C,D), whereas the anterior inferior tibiofibular ligament, interosseous ligament, and part of the interosseous membrane are damaged in stage II of the pronation-external rotation injury (Fig. 11.2C). Clinically, however, the pronation-abduction and pronation-external rotation injuries are indistinguishable at stage II; both are characterized by medial injury (deltoid ligament rupture or medial malleolus fracture) and tibiofibular ligament injury (Fig. 12.3).

Stage III pronation-abduction injury is indicated by the typical transverse "bending" fracture of the distal fibula (Fig. 12.4). This is usually located at or just above the tibial plafond (Figs. 12.4 and 12.5), but can occur proximal to the syndesmosis (Fig. 12.6). Frequently the lateral cortex is comminuted (Fig. 12.4). The pronation-abduction fracture of the fibula can usually be differentiated from the typical pronation-external rotation fracture of the fibula since it generally has a transverse or short oblique configuration; even when this fracture has a short oblique configuration in the anteroposterior radiograph, it will usually appear transverse on the lateral view [4]. It is important to distinguish as best as possible between pronation-external rotation and pronation-abduction fractures Stage III since they have different implications in terms of associated ligament damage.

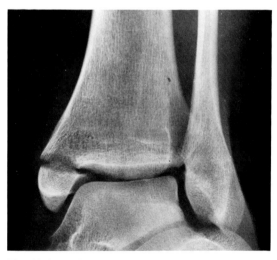

Fig. 12.3. "Isolated" fracture of the medial malleolus associated with tenderness over the syndesmosis. This could represent a stage II pronation-external rotation or stage II pronation-abduction injury.

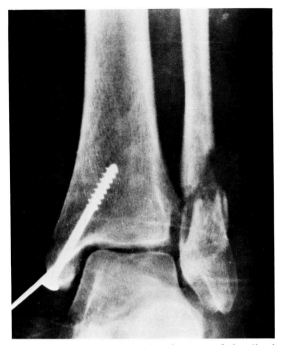

Fig. 12.4. Pronation-abduction fracture of the distal fibula with typical comminution of the lateral cortex.

In pronation-abduction injuries, the fibular fracture generally occurs at the upper limit of the tibiofibular ligamentous injury. The location of the fibular fracture then indicates to what extent the syndesmosis is disrupted. Based on the location of the fibular fracture, three types of pronation-abduction injuries are possible [6, 12,16,18].

Pronation-Abduction Fibular Fracture at the Level of the Tibial Plafond

When a pronation-abduction fracture of the fibula occurs at or just above the tibial plafond, one can usually assume the interosseous membrane and most of the interosseous ligament are intact; therefore the syndesmosis injury is not complete (Fig. 12.5). Because of the intact interosseous ligament, the proximal fibula maintains its normal relationship to the tibia [8], and satisfactory reduction of the fibular fracture automatically protects the anterior and posterior inferior tibiofibular ligaments until healing is complete.

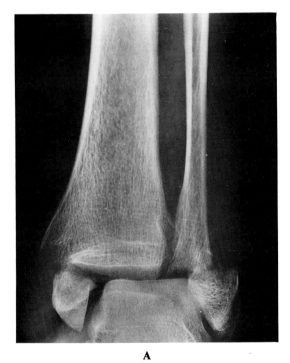

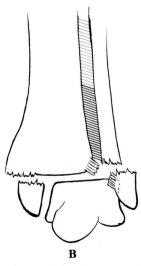

A   B

Fig. 12.5. A PA III with fibular fracture at the level of the tibial plafond. **B** Anterior and posterior inferior tibiofibular ligaments are ruptured but the interosseous ligament is undisturbed; therefore, a complete ligamentous diastasis does not exist.

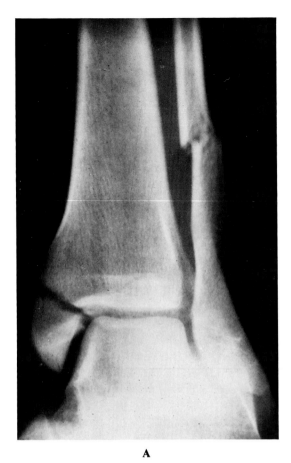

A

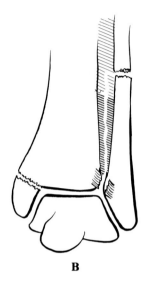

B

Fig. 12.6. A PA III with fibular fracture occurring above the interosseous ligament. **B** One can presume that the interosseous ligament as well as the anterior and posterior inferior tibiofibular ligaments have ruptured; therefore, even after fibular stabilization, a complete tibiofibular ligamentous diastasis will persist.

Pronation-Abduction Fibular Fracture Occurring 6 cm or More Above the Tibial Plafond

When a pronation-abduction fracture of the fibula, however, is situated 6 cm or more above the tibial plafond, the interosseous ligament and part of the interosseous membrane have also been torn; therefore a total ligamentous diastasis exists (Fig. 12.6) [6]. This corresponds to what Bonnin referred to as "diastasis by abduction" [3]. Even if the fibular fracture can be satisfactorily stabilized, the relationship between the fibula and tibia is only maintained by the interosseous membrane, and considerable tibiofibular mobility may persist. Unless the tibiofibular ligament injury consists of bone avulsions that lend themselves to screw fixation, this situation will frequently require temporary stabilization of the syndesmosis with a tibiofibular transfixion screw.

Pronation-Abduction Fibular Fracture in the Intermediate Zone

In the case of pronation-abduction fracture of the fibula occurring in the intermediate area, i.e., the segment 6 cm immediately proximal to the tibial plafond, it is impossible to predict in any given case whether the interosseous ligament has been violated because of individual variation in the length and strength of this structure (Fig. 12.7). This will usually be evident at the time of surgery; but if any question exists, tibiofibular mobility should be assessed with a towel clip after fibular fixation has been completed [15].

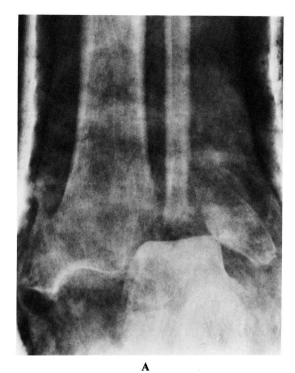

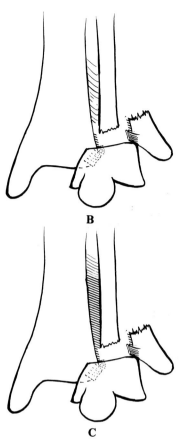

Fig. 12.7. A PA III with fibular fracture occurring in the intermediate area. Lowest fibers of the interosseous ligament as well as the anterior and posterior inferior tibiofibular ligaments have ruptured. Whether the proximal fibula is firmly bound in appropriate relationship to the tibia is determined by the original length of the interosseous ligament. **B** With a short interosseous ligament, a complete tibiofibular ligamentous diastasis exists. **C** With a long interosseous ligament, the proximal fibula remains firmly fixed to the tibia and a complete ligamentous diastasis does not exist.

Thus, pronation-abduction injuries characterized by fracture of the fibula located in this intermediate zone may or may not require temporary tibiofibular fixation (Fig. 12.7B,C).

Combination Abduction-External Rotation Injury

Lauge-Hansen [8] also observed that if the foot was simultaneously externally rotated and abducted, the inferior fibers of the interosseous membrane and interosseous ligament as well as the anterior and posterior tibiofibular ligaments failed, causing the fracture of the fibula to occur somewhat more proximally—at the level where the tibiofibular ligament injury ceased. This combination injury was pathologically similar to the stage IV pronation-external rotation injury, since in the end stage it was characterized by complete ligamentous diastasis.

Golterman [5] believed that in certain instances of abduction violence, the weaker anterior inferior tibiofibular ligament failed, but the stronger posterior inferior tibiofibular ligaments were able to resist rupture, and transform abduction of the talus into external rotation (Fig. 12.8). He postulated that the strong posterior ligaments converted many pronation-abduction injuries into pronation-external rotation injuries. This would certainly be compatible with Lauge-Hansen's cadaver observations concerning the combination injury.

According to Lauge-Hansen [8], the fibular fracture produced by this combination injury be-

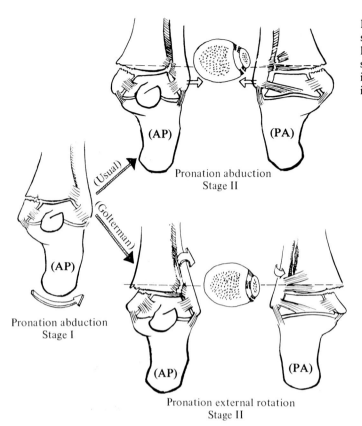

Fig. 12.8. Golterman postulated that the strong posterior inferior tibiofibular ligaments frequently resisted abduction stress, converting pronation-abduction injuries into pronation-external rotation injuries.

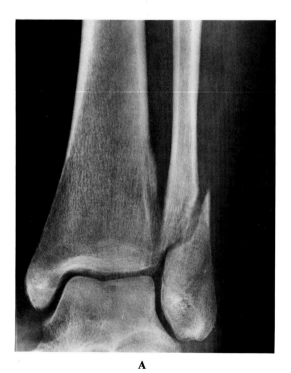

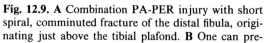

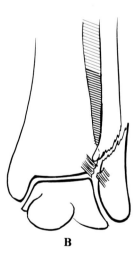

Fig. 12.9. A Combination PA-PER injury with short spiral, comminuted fracture of the distal fibula, originating just above the tibial plafond. **B** One can presume that most of the interosseous ligament is undisturbed.

gins a variable distance above the tibial plafond. The fracture configuration represents a combination of abduction (bending, transverse) and external rotation (spiral, oblique) forces, and generally has a short oblique orientation. As with pronation-abduction injuries, three types of combination (PA-PER) injury are theoretically possible, depending on the location of the fibular fracture.

If the fibular fracture originates near the tibial plafond, most of the interosseous ligament is above the fracture and remains intact (Fig. 12.9). The lateral injury resembles that caused by the supination-external rotation mechanism in that the interosseous ligament is undisturbed and the posterior inferior tibiofibular ligaments are not damaged until late in the sequence of injuries. Unlike supination-external rotation injuries, however, the fibular fracture begins above the syndesmosis rather than at the tibial plafond, and the medial injury occurs in stage I rather than stage IV. The important point to realize is that preservation of the interosseous ligament means a complete ligamentous diastasis has not occurred; therefore fibular fixation will usually

stabilize the lateral ankle and tibiofibular screw fixation is rarely necessary.

If the fibular fracture originates high in the supramalleolar region (i.e., 6 cm or more above the tibial plafond), the injury is identical to a pronation-external rotation injury (Fig. 12.10), and should be treated as such (Chapter 11). Theoretically, the spiral oblique fibular fracture associated with the combination injury should be shorter than the fracture caused exclusively by external rotation forces:

For combination injuries characterized by fibular fracture in the "intermediate zone," the segment 6 cm immediately proximal to the tibial plafond (Fig. 12.11), the status of the interosseous ligament cannot be determined preoperatively. One can assume that it is ruptured as far proximal as the fracture site, but whether this injury involves all or most of the ligament depends on the size (length) of the ligament in the individual patient (Fig. 12.11B,C). As with pronation-abduction injuries in this intermediate zone, the functional status of the interosseous ligament should be determined by stressing the syndesmosis after the fibular fracture has been stabilized.

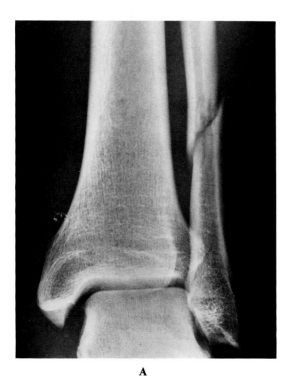

A

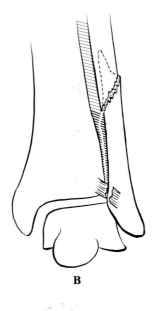

B

Fig. 12.10. A Combination PA-PER injury with short spiral fracture of the fibula occurring 6 cm above the tibial plafond. **B** One should expect that the interosse-ous ligament has been torn. This is analogous to a PER injury—stage III, if the posterior inferior tibio-fibular ligaments are intact; stage IV, if they are torn.

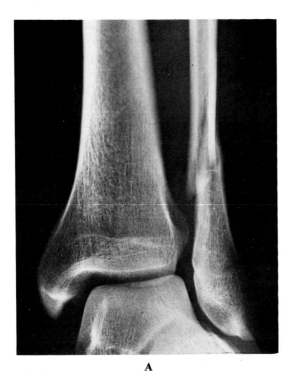

A

Fig. 12.11. A Combination PA-PER injury with fibular fracture in the intermediate zone. Interosseous ligament is ruptured as far proximally as the fracture site. Whether this injury involves all **(B)** or part **(C)** of this ligament cannot be determined preoperatively.

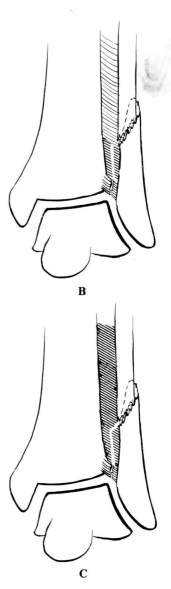

B

C

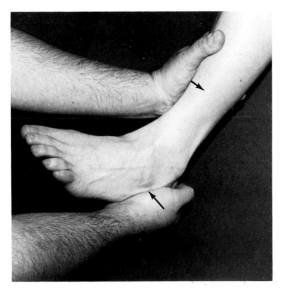

Fig. 12.12. Pronation-abduction injuries: closed reduction technique of Lauge-Hansen.

In summary, there is a clear-cut theoretical distinction between pronation-external rotation and pronation-abduction injuries that can be applied clinically to typical injuries of both types. Some fractures, however, possess features of both injuries, and presumably are caused by a combination mechanism (Figs. 12.9–12.11). Although certain inferences can be drawn from the location of the fibular fracture in pronation-abduction as well as in combination injuries, individual variation in the length of the interosseous ligament will not always permit detection of complete ligamentous diastasis preoperatively. In many instances, this can only be determined by intraoperative testing of syndesmosis stability after fibular stabilization has been achieved.

Pronation-Abduction Injuries: Closed Reduction Technique (Lauge-Hansen) [7,9]

With counterpressure applied to the distal leg, the hindfoot is moved ventrally and medially (Fig. 12.12). The heel should be adducted as the plaster hardens.

Since this injury is caused by abduction rather than rotational violence, a short leg cast will often provide sufficient immobilization [2]. If there is extensive swelling or if the "bending" fracture is atypical, suggesting that rotational forces were partially responsible, it is safer to extend the cast to above the knee.

Pronation-Abduction Injuries: Fixation Techniques

Bending Fracture of the Distal Fibula

The orientation of the fracture line and the associated comminution frequently necessitate use of a small buttress plate to provide fixation (Fig. 12.13) [13]. Occasionally, if the fracture is located distally and is not characterized by significant comminution, a figure-of-eight tension band (Chapter 8), intramedullary device (Chapter 10), or axial screw (Chapter 10) can be employed satisfactorily.

Spiral Fracture of the Distal Fibula

Spiral fractures of the distal fibula usually occur as a result of combination (PA-PER) injuries. These fractures are too short to be satisfactorily fixed with interfragmentary screws alone; therefore a neutralization plate is required (Fig. 12.14).

Fracture of the Medial Malleolus

Since this is an avulsion fracture, it can be stabilized by the same techniques outlined in Chapter 10 for external rotation injuries of the medial malleolus, i.e., lag screw fixation, figure-of-eight tension band, or hook plate.

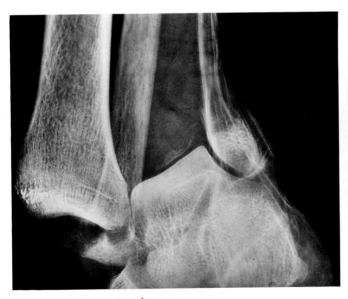
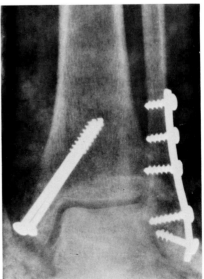

A   **B**

Fig. 12.13. A Pronation-abduction injury occurring at the level of the tibial plafond. **B** Since the interosseous ligament is intact, fibular stabilization satisfactorily restored stability to the ankle mortise.

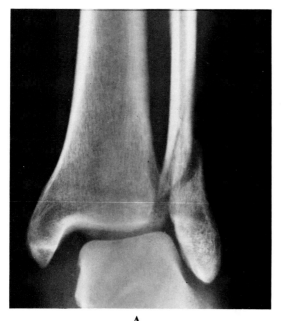

A

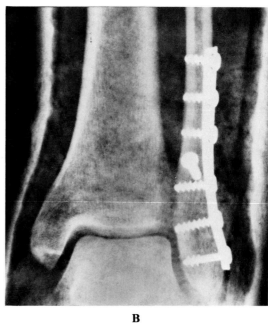

B

Fig. 12.14. A Combination PA-PER injury. **B** Open reduction and fixation of fibular fracture using an interfragmentary screw and neutralization plate restored stability to the ankle joint; after fibular fixation was completed, integrity of the syndesmosis was tested under direct vision and found to be satisfactory.

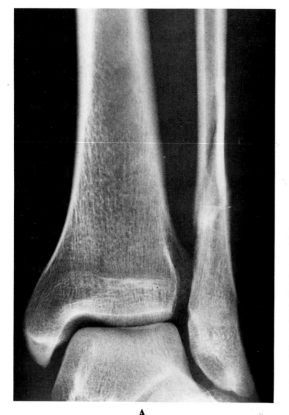

A

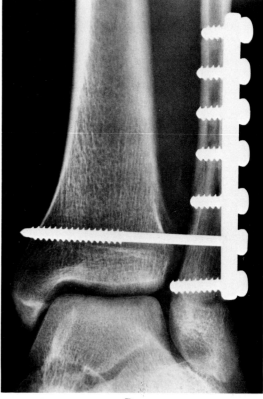

B

Fig. 12.15. A Combination PA-PER injury. **B** Following fibular stabilization, instability of the tibiofibular syndesmosis was demonstrated and a tibiofibular positioning screw was inserted with the syndesmosis held in the reduced position.

Syndesmosis Injury

Syndesmosis injury when complete should be treated as described for pronation-external rotation injuries (Chapter 11). Temporary tibiofibular screw fixation will be required when significant tibiofibular instability persists after fibular stabilization; i.e., in pronation-abduction and combination PA-PER injuries where the fibular fracture occurs a sufficient distance above the syndesmosis to be associated with interosseous ligament rupture (Fig. 12.15). When the fibular fracture occurs near the syndesmosis and all or most of the interosseous ligament is intact, stabilization of the fibula will automatically restore stability to the syndesmosis; therefore, tibiofibular screw fixation is not necessary (Figs. 12.13–12.14).

References

1. Bistrom O: Conservative treatment of severe ankle fractures. A clinical and follow-up study. Acta Chir Scand (Suppl) 168:1, 1952.
2. Bohler L: The Treatment of Fractures, 5th ed. New York, Grune & Stratton, 1956.
3. Bonnin JG: Injuries to the Ankle. New York, Grune & Stratton, 1950.
4. Dabezies E, D'Ambrosia RD, Shoji H: Classification and treatment of ankle fractures. Orthopedics 1:365, 1978.
5. Golterman AFL: Diagnosis and treatment of tibiofibular diastasis. Arch Chir Neerl 16:185, 1964.
6. Henderson MS: Fractures of the ankle. Wisc Med J 31:684, 1932.
7. Kristensen TB: Fractures of the ankle. VI. Follow-up studies. AMA Arch Surg 73:112, 1956.
8. Lauge-Hansen N: Fractures of the ankle. II. Combined experimental-surgical and experimental-roentgenologic investigations. Arch Surg 60:957, 1950.
9. Lauge-Hansen N: Fractures of the ankle. IV. Clinical use of the genetic roentgen diagnosis and genetic reduction. AMA Arch Surg 64:488, 1952.
10. Lauge-Hansen N: Fractures of the ankle. III. Genetic roentgenologic diagnosis of fractures of the ankle. Am J Roentgenol 71:456, 1954.
11. Lindsjo U: Operative treatment of ankle fractures. Acta Orthop Scand (Suppl) 189:1, 1981.
12. Magnusson R: Ligament injuries of the ankle joint. Acta Orthop Scand 36:317, 1965.
13. Mast JW, Teipner WA: A reproducible approach to the internal fixation of adult ankle fractures: rationale, technique and early results. Orthop Clin North Am 11:661, 1980.
14. Mitchell WG, Shaftan GW, Sclafani S: Mandatory open reduction: Its role in displaced ankle fractures. J Trauma 19:602, 1979.
15. Pankovich AM: Fractures of the fibula proximal to the distal tibiofibular syndesmosis. J Bone Joint Surg 60A:221, 1978.
16. Pankovich AM: Adult ankle fractures. JCE Orthop 7:17, 1979.
17. Pankovich AM: Fractures of the fibula at the distal tibiofibular syndesmosis. Clin Orthop Rel Res 143:138, 1979.
18. Platt H: Introduction to a discussion on fractures in the neighborhood of the ankle-joint. Lancet 1:33, 1926.
19. Solonen KO, Lauttamus L: Operative treatment of ankle fractures. Acta Orthop Scand 39:223, 1968.

Chapter 13 Fractures of the Posterior and Anterior Tibial Margins

William C. Hamilton

Fractures of the Posterior Tibial Margin

Fracture of the dorsal aspect of the distal tibia can occur in association with any of the described fracture mechanisms [20] and possibly, in rare instances, as an isolated phenomenon (Fig. 13.7) [44]. Generally, these fractures occur in association with external rotation or abduction injuries and involve the lateral aspect of the dorsal tibia (Fig. 13.1A). Much less commonly, dorsal fractures are encountered with stage II supination-adduction injuries when the talus has subluxated medially; in this situation, the fracture tends to involve the medial aspect of the dorsal tibia (Fig.

13.1B), and occasionally the fragment remains attached to the fractured medial malleolus (Fig. 13.2).

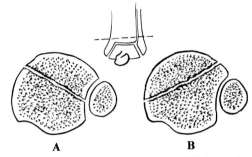

Fig. 13.1. Fractures of the posterior tibial margin. A Dorsolateral fragment. B Dorsomedial fragment, extending into medial malleolus.

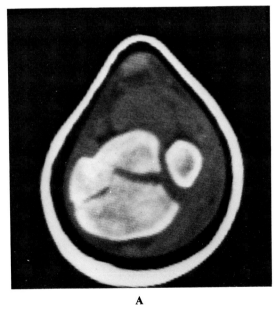

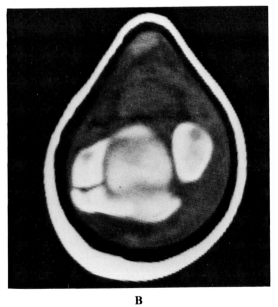

Fig. 13.2. A, B Axial tomography demonstrating distinct dorsolateral and dorsomedial fractures of the tibial margin. Dorsomedial fragment is continuous with the posterior colliculus of the medial malleolus.(B)

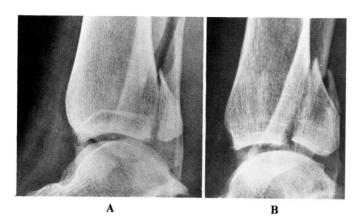

A   B

Fig. 13.3. Fractures of the posterior tibia. **A** Extraarticular/nonsupporting fracture. **B** Articular fracture.

Small fragments that do not involve much or any of the articular surface (extraarticular [11], nonsupporting [17]) generally have no particular clinical significance [48], except to suggest ligament avulsion and thereby facilitate staging of the injury according to the Lauge-Hansen scheme (Fig. 13.3A) [22]. Hall [18] has also suggested that, since the posterior tibial margin fragment remains firmly attached to the distal fibula, its proximal migration provides an index of the degree of fibular shortening. Large fragments that involve the articular surface of the distal tibia are more serious and have important implications in terms of joint stability and congruity (Fig. 13.3B).

The commonly observed small dorso*lateral* fractures result from avulsion (via the posterior inferior tibiofibular ligaments) or from direct pressure exerted by the talus and/or lateral malleolus as they subluxate posterolaterally [4,22], as with external rotation or abduction injuries [9,33]. Less commonly, small dorso*medial* lesions are caused by avulsion (via the tibial periosteum) or by direct pressure exerted on the tibia by the posteromedially subluxating talus, as occurs with supination-adduction injuries. If compression injury is sustained in association with these avulsion/pressure forces, larger lesions involving a significant amount of the articular surface will result [14,22].

Although some authors have tried to separate fractures of the posterior tibial tubercle (posterior inferior tibiofibular ligament origin) from fractures of the posterior tibial margin or lip (inferior transverse tibiofibular ligament origin) (Fig. 13.4), this distinction can sometimes be very hard

to make on the basis of ordinary X-ray examinations [8,22,30]. Also, the clinical significance of this distinction has never been documented. Regardless of whether the fracture involves the posterior tibial tubercle and/or the posterior tibial margin/lip, small fragments do not contribute to instability or incongruity. Moreover, small fragments remain intimately related to the distal fibula via the posterior inferior tibiofibular ligament, and they generally will assume near normal position when the fibular fracture has been satisfactorily reduced by closed or open means (Fig. 10.29) [12,13,17,32,37,43,45,46,50].

In this text, therefore, the terms posterior tibial lip, posterior tibial tubercle, posterior tibial margin, and posterior malleolus will be used synonymously. Lesions will be distinguished by the presence or absence of articular surface involvement (articular/nonarticular) (Fig. 13.3) and by location (posterolateral/posteromedial) (Fig. 13.1).

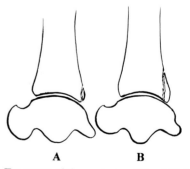

A   B

Fig. 13.4. Fractures of the posterior tibia. A Tubercle. B Margin or lip.

Isolated Fractures of the Posterior Tibial Margin

Although fractures of the posterior tibial margin usually occur in association with other malleolar fractures or ligament injuries [20], there are occasional situations when such a lesion appears to exist as an entirely isolated phenomenon [44]. Frank [15] reported this injury in 2.5% of 194 malleolar fractures; and Hendelberg [4] encountered five such injuries among 223 ankle fractures (2.2%). Recently, Yde [51] found isolated posterior tibial lip fractures on four occasions in a study of 488 patients (0.8%); and Lindsjo [27] encountered this lesion in six of 611 patients (1%).

Palmer [42] believed that isolated posterior tibial lip fractures resulted from excessive plantarflexion of the foot causing an anterior capsular tear and subsequent fracture of the posterior tibial margin. Lucas-Championniere [28,44] as well as Cox and Laxson [11] postulated that this injury was due to compression violence. Magnusson [30] and Bonnin [2] thought that isolated posterior tibial marginal fracture could be caused by stumbling or kicking against a solid block with resultant straight posterior subluxation of the plantarflexed talus.

Lauge-Hansen [24] did not encounter any instances of isolated posterior tibial lip fracture in his experimental or clinical studies, and he concluded that the injury did not exist. He believed that so-called "isolated" fractures of the posterior tibial lip represented stage II pronation-abduction injuries in which the medial injury consisted of ligament rupture and the syndesmosis injury was overlooked (Fig. 13.5). Kristensen [23] similarly found no instances of isolated posterior tibial lip fracture in his review of 500 ankle fractures. He concluded that these apparently "isolated" injuries were, in fact, pronation-external rotation stage IV lesions where the deltoid and tibiofibular ligament damage as well as the fracture of the proximal fibula had been overlooked (Fig. 13.6).

Brostrom [4] studied 18 patients with apparently isolated posterior tibial margin fractures. The proximal fibula as well as the ankle were examined clinically as well as by X ray; arthrography of the ankle was performed in all patients.

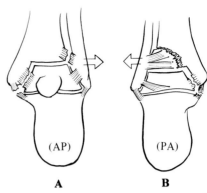

(AP)   (PA)

A   B

Fig. 13.5. Pronation-abduction injury stage II with posterior tibial margin fracture and medial injury characterized by deltoid ligament rupture. A Anterior and B posterior views. If tibia and fibula recoil to normal position, the posterior tibial margin fracture may appear to be "isolated."

No instance of proximal fibular fracture was encountered. Each patient, however, demonstrated tenderness over the anterior syndesmosis and 15 of the 18 patients were found, by arthrography, to have capsular defects corresponding to tears of the anterior inferior tibiofibular ligament. The three patients without arthrographic extravasation had sustained their injury 3, 4, and 7 days previously, and Brostrom believed that the anterior inferior tibiofibular ligament tear might have sealed with clot to obscure this element of the injury. Only one patient of the 18 had any evidence of deltoid ligament injury. Brostrom concluded that "isolated" fracture of the posterior tibial margin was the result of an atypical supination-external rotation injury characterized by rupture of the anterior inferior tibiofibular ligament and avulsion of the posterior tibial margin without fibular fracture or deltoid ligament injury (Fig. 13.7).

McLaughlin [34] believed that isolated posterior tibial margin fracture could occur in association with tibiofibular diastasis when the wide anterior talus was driven into the ankle mortise as a result of tripping or kicking (Fig. 13.8). This explanation although different would correlate with the clinical and arthrographic observations of Brostrom.

On the basis of these findings, it seems safe to presume that "isolated" posterior tibial lip fracture can occur in the absence of malleolar injury but not in the absence of some degree

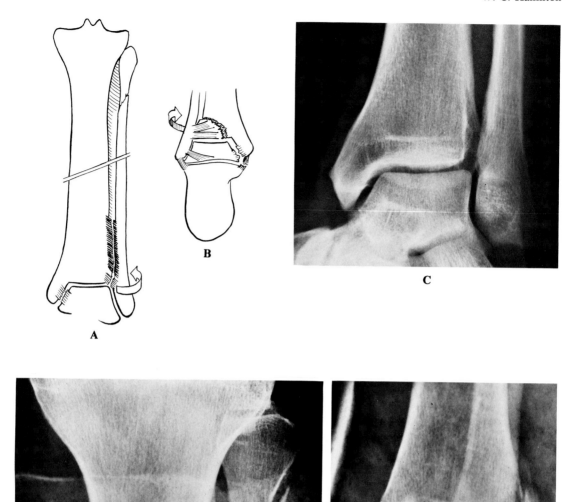

Fig. 13.6. A and **B** Pronation-external rotation injury stage IV with fracture of the posterior tibial margin and proximal fibula; medial injury consists of deltoid ligament rupture. If plain films do not disclose widen-ing of the tibiofibular syndesmosis (**C**) and the proximal fibular fracture (**D**) is overlooked, the injury may masquerade as an "isolated" fracture of the posterior tibial margin (**E**).

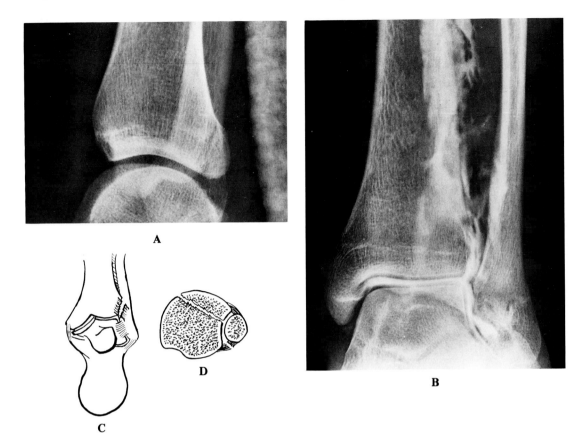

Fig. 13.7. A Apparently "isolated" fracture of the posterior tibial margin. **B** Arthrogram, however, demonstrates leakage of dye through the anterior syndesmosis and proximal extravasation into the tibiofibular interval. Frontal (**C**) and cross-sectional (**D**) schematic interpretation.

of associated soft tissue damage (anterior diastasis–anterior inferior tibiofibular ligament rupture) [4]. Clinically, the demonstration of an "isolated" posterior tibial lip fracture should necessitate a diligent search for associated proximal fibular fracture (pronation-external rotation stage IV injury), deltoid ligament injury (pronation-abduction stage II injury), or anterior diastasis (atypical supination-external rotation injury or straight posterior subluxation of the talus). In this last situation, when the associated injury involves only the anterior inferior tibiofibular ligament, treatment by immobilization in plaster for 3–4 weeks usually results in rapid healing and relief of symptoms [4,10]. When posterior tibial margin fractures occur in association with pronation-external rotation stage IV or pronation-abduction stage II injuries, however, a more aggressive approach is indicated.

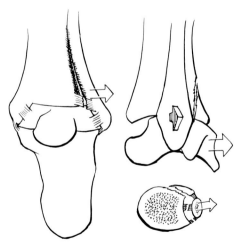

Fig. 13.8. McLaughlin postulated that tripping or kicking could force the wide anterior portion of the talus into the mortise, creating a ligamentous diastasis and an "isolated" fracture of the posterior tibial margin.

Fracture of the Posterior Tibial Margin with Articular Surface Involvement

Like extraarticular (or nonsupporting) fractures of the dorsal tibia, fractures with significant articular surface involvement can occur in association with fracture-dislocations of the ankle or, rarely, as apparent "isolated" injuries [4,44]. The term "trimalleolar" was originally coined to refer to fractures of the medial and lateral malleolus in association with articular fracture of the dorsal tibia and posterior subluxation of the talus [19]. Since then, however, the term has been extended loosely to include injuries characterized by even minor extracapsular fractures of the posterior tibial margin.

It is generally agreed that dorsal fragments involving more than 25–35% [3,5,6,7,8,11,12,20–22,32,33,36,40,41,43,48,52] of the articular surface of the distal tibia (Fig. 13.9A) require specific attempts at reduction and frequently internal fixation to avoid persistent instability and joint incongruity [17]. This is particularly true when the fracture is associated with posterior subluxation of the talus (Fig. 13.9B) [33]. The 25% limit is more appropriate than the 35% figure, since the natural tendency is to underestimate the relative extent of articular surface involvement [33]. Radiographs may also be misleading in this regard since the fracture line is not always perpendicular to the plane of projection of the standard lateral film [27].

Efforts at closed reduction of large posterior tibial lip fragments are frequently unsuccessful [16,19,33,34,41]. McLaughlin has described the dilemma encountered when one tries to treat this injury by closed measures [34] (Fig. 13.10): Because of the relatively lax capsular connection between the talus and the dorsal margin of the tibia, it is frequently necessary to maximally dorsiflex the ankle in order to bring the fragment distally to the appropriate level (Fig. 13.10B). This position, however, will necessarily tighten the calf muscles and bring the talus into contact with the dorsal tibia, and therefore will predispose to recurrent talar subluxation and dorsal redisplacement of the fracture fragment (Fig. 13.10C).

Although traction and percutaneous fixation techniques have been utilized in an attempt to reduce and fix this fracture (Fig. 13.11) [1,41], it is now generally agreed that displaced posterior tibial fractures involving more than 25–35% of the distal tibial articular surface should be treated with formal open reduction and internal fixation, either alone or in combination with surgical treatment of other malleolar and ligamentous injuries. Despite apparently satisfactory reduction and fixation of large posterior tibial fragments, these patients remain at significant risk of developing posttraumatic arthritis, but the incidence is less than is generally incurred by closed treatment of this injury [27,33].

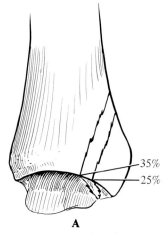

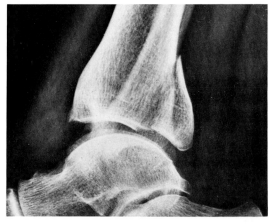

A   B

Fig. 13.9. A Posterior marginal fractures of the tibia involving more than 25–35% of the articular surface require anatomic reduction. **B** This is particularly true when a fracture of this magnitude is associated with dorsal subluxation or dislocation of the talus.

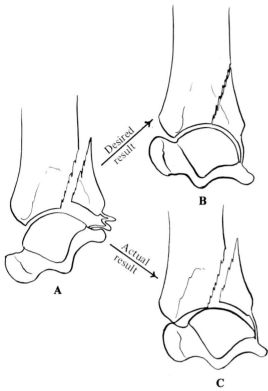

Fig. 13.10. Difficulty is likely to be encountered with attempted closed reduction of large posterior tibial fractures **(A)**. Extreme dorsiflexion of the ankle required to bring large posterior fragments down to the appropriate level **(B)** increases tension within the gastrocnemius-soleus complex and frequently results in recurrent dorsal dislocation of the talus **(C)**.

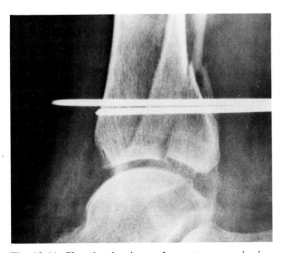

Fig. 13.11. Closed reduction and percutaneous pinning of large posterior tibial marginal fractures is frequently unsuccessful.

Posterior Tibial Fractures with Significant Articular Surface Involvement: Fixation Technique

The classical surgical approach to this lesion has been posterolaterally, as described by Henry (Fig. 13.12) [6,10,49]. This exposure permits direct mobilization of the tibial fragment and fixation by screws inserted posteriorly [38] or anteriorly through a separate incision [26,31,39,47]. In the less common situation, where the fragment arises from the posteromedial corner of the tibia, a posteromedial surgical exposure is preferable [20]. Rarely, both approaches are necessary [20].

Neither of these approaches, however, provides for direct inspection of the distal tibial articular surface because of overhang of the posterior tibial margin. Radiographic control is helpful but, even so, it is quite easy to fix the fragment in less than anatomic position (Fig. 13.13) [43]. To facilitate reduction and fixation of this fracture, medial or lateral transmalleolar approaches with malleolar osteotomy have been recommended [16]. Since this injury is frequently associated with a medial and/or lateral malleolar fracture, these fractures can frequently be utilized as osteotomies to permit distal reflection of one or both malleoli with minimal additional tissue violation (Fig. 13.14) [12,35,43,47]. This permits direct medial and/or lateral visualization of the articular surface of the distal tibia and facilitates precise reduction of posterior tibial fragments.

Once reduced, the fracture should be stabilized temporarily with two Kirschner wires, as one or, preferably, two screws (malleolar, cancellous, or lagged cortical) are inserted to provide compression across the fracture site. The screws can be inserted from the back or from the front through a separate small incision [31,32,35]. When inserted from the front, the screws should be angled laterally or medially, depending on whether the fragment originates from the lateral or medial side of the posterior tibia (Fig. 13.15) [12]. Care should be taken to be sure that no threads of the screw cross the fracture site, as this will jeopardize compression [32]; sometimes it is necessary to alter the screws to fulfill this requirement.

Miller [37] has recommended use of a dorsal buttress plate to stabilize this fracture. This

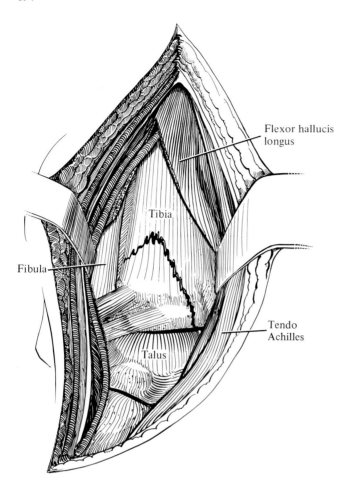

Fibula

Tibia

Flexor hallucis
longus

Talus

Tendo
Achilles

Fig. 13.12. Posterolateral approach to the dorsal aspect of the distal tibia (after Henry).

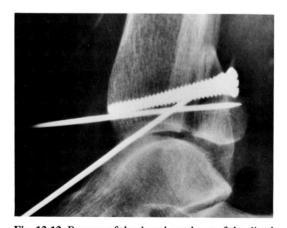

Fig. 13.13. Because of the dorsal overhang of the distal tibia, open reduction of posterior tibial fragments via a posterolateral or posteromedial approach does not permit accurate visualization of the articular surface and it is easy to fix the fragment in less than anatomic position.

should rarely be necessary, however, if the fragment is large; if the fragment is small, then reduction is usually not necessary.

Fractures of the Anterior Tibial Margin

Small fractures, involving little if any of the articular surface, of the anterior tibial margin are occasionally seen (Fig. 13.16). They are caused by anterior capsular avulsion and occur in association with lateral ankle sprains where the injuring force includes a significant element of plantarflexion, in addition to internal rotation and adduction. Clinically, these injuries are characterized by an inordinate amount of anterior and anterolateral soft tissue swelling and tenderness.

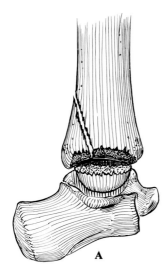

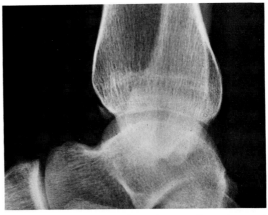

Fig. 13.16. Capsular avulsion fracture from the anterior aspect of the distal tibia.

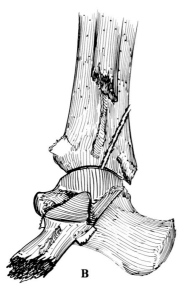

Fig. 13.14. Reflection of the medial (**A**) and/or lateral (**B**) malleolus will provide optimal visualization of the entire distal tibial articular surface.

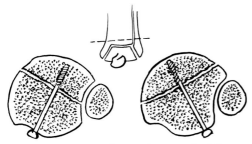

Fig. 13.15. Fixation of posterior marginal fractures. If screws are inserted from anterior, they need to be angled medially or laterally, depending on the origin of the fragment.

They are treated similarly to other lateral ankle sprains; recovery is usually complete but convalescence is frequently prolonged.

Large anterior tibial lip fractures involving the articular surface rarely, if ever, occur as an isolated phenomenon. They are usually seen in association with pilon or pronation-dorsiflexion injuries [25] or in association with fractures of the neck of the talus [2,29]. Treatment is discussed in Chapter 14.

References

1. Bohler L: The Treatment of Fractures, 5th ed. New York, Grune & Stratton, 1956.
2. Bonnin JG: Injuries to the Ankle. New York, Grune & Stratton, 1950.
3. Braunstein PW, Wade PA: Treatment of unstable fractures of the ankle. Ann Surg 149:217, 1959.
4. Brostrom L, Liljedahl SO, Lindvall N: Isolated fractures of the posterior tibial tubercle aetiologic and clinical features. Acta Chir Scand 128:51, 1964.
5. Burgess E: Fractures of the ankle. J Bone Joint Surg 26:721, 1944.
6. Burwell HN, Charnley AD: Treatment of displaced fractures at the ankle by rigid internal fixation and early joint movement. J Bone Joint Surg 47B:634, 1965.
7. Cave EF: Complications of the operative treatment of fractures of the ankle. Clin Orthop Rel Res 42:13, 1965.
8. Cedell A-A: Supination-outward rotation injuries of the ankle. Acta Orthop Scand (Suppl) 110:1, 1967.
9. Cotton FJ: A new type of ankle fracture. JAMA 64:318, 1915.

10. Cox FJ: Fractures of the ankle involving the lower articular surface of the tibia. Clin Orthop 42:51, 1965.
11. Cox FJ, Laxson WW: Fractures about the ankle joint. Am J Surg 83:674, 1952.
12. Dabezies E, D'Ambrosia RD, Shoji H: Classification and treatment of ankle fractures. Orthopaedics 1:365, 1978.
13. Denham RA: Internal fixation for unstable ankle fractures. J Bone Joint Surg 46B:206, 1964.
14. DeSouza DL, Foerster TP: Traumatic lesions of the ankle joint. The supination-external rotation mechanism. Clin Orthop Rel Res 100:219, 1974.
15. Frank S: Isolerede brud i Nedre Skinnebenskant (Marginale brud). Nord Med 9:643, 1941.
16. Gatellier J: The juxtoretroperoneal route in the operative treatment of fractures of the malleolus with posterior marginal fragment. Surg Gynecol Obstet 52:67, 1931.
17. Golterman AFL: Diagnosis and treatment of tibiofibular diastasis. Arch Chir Neerl 16:185, 1964.
18. Hall H: A simplified workable classification of ankle fractures. In Bateman JE, Trott AW (eds): The Foot and Ankle. New York, Thieme-Stratton, 1980.
19. Henderson MS: Fractures of the ankle. Wisc Med J 31:684, 1932.
20. Jergeson F: Open reduction of fractures and dislocations of the ankle. Am J Surg 98:136, 1959.
21. Key JA, Conwell HE: Injuries in the Region of the Ankle. The Management of Fractures, Dislocations and Sprains, 6th ed. St. Louis, Mosby, 1956.
22. Kleiger B: Mechanisms of ankle injury. Orthop Clin North Am 5:127, 1974.
23. Kristensen TB: Treatment of malleolar fractures according to Lauge-Hansen's method. Preliminary results. Acta Chir Scand 97:362, 1949.
24. Lauge-Hansen N: Fractures of the ankle. II. Combined experimental-surgical and experimental-roentgenologic investigations. Arch Surg 60:957, 1950.
25. Lauge-Hansen N: Fractures of the ankle. V. Pronation-dorsiflexion fracture. AMA Arch Surg 67:813, 1953.
26. Lee HG, Horan TB: Internal fixation in injuries of the ankle. Surg Gynecol Obstet 76:593, 1943.
27. Lindsjo U: Operative treatment of ankle fractures. Acta Orthop Scand (Suppl) 189:1, 1981.
28. Lucas-Championniere J: Precis du Traitement des Fracture. Paris, Steinheil, 1910.
29. MacKinnon AP: Fracture of the lower articular surface of the tibia in fracture dislocation of the ankle. J Bone Joint Surg 10:352, 1928.
30. Magnusson R: On the late results in non-operated cases of malleolar fractures. I. Fractures by external rotation. Acta Chir Scand (Suppl) 84:1, 1944.
31. Malka JS, Taillard W: Results of non-operative and operative treatment of fractures of the ankle. Clin Orthop Rel Res 67:159, 1969.
32. Mast JW, Teipner WA: A reproducible approach to the internal fixation of adult ankle fractures: Rationale, technique and early results. Orthop Clin North Am 11:661, 1980.
33. McDaniel WJ, Wilson FC: Trimalleolar fractures of the ankle. An end result study. Clin Orthop Rel Res 122:37, 1977.
34. McLaughlin HL: Trauma. Philadelphia, Saunders, 1960.
35. McLaughlin HL, Ryder CT Jr: Open reduction and internal fixation for fractures of the tibia and ankle. Surg Clin North Am 29:1523, 1949.
36. Meyer TL Jr, Kumler KW: A.S.I.F. technique and ankle fractures. Clin Orthop Rel Res 150:211, 1980.
37. Miller AJ: Posterior malleolar fractures. J Bone Joint Surg 56B:508, 1974.
38. Monk CJE: Injuries of the tibiofibular ligaments. J Bone Joint Surg 51:330, 1969.
39. Müller ME, Allgöwer M, Schneider R, Willenegger H: Manual of Internal Fixation, 2nd ed. Translated by J. Schatzker. New York, Springer-Verlag, 1979.
40. Neufeld AJ: Ankle joint fractures and their treatment. Clin Orthop 42:91, 1965.
41. Nyström G: A contribution to the treatment of fractures of the posterior border of the tibia by malleolar fractures. Acta Radiol 25:672, 1944.
42. Palmer I: Fotledens Skador. En Översikt. Nord Med 12:3167, 1941.
43. Patrick J: A direct approach to trimalleolar fractures. J Bone Joint Surg 47B:236, 1965.
44. Platt H: Introduction to a discussion on fractures in the neighborhood of the ankle-joint. Lancet 1:33, 1926.
45. Solonen KA, Lauttamus L: Treatment of malleolar fractures. Acta Orthop Scand 36:321, 1965.
46. Solonen KA, Lauttamus L: Operative treatment of ankle fractures. Acta Orthop Scand 39:223, 1968.
47. Staples OS: Ligamentous injuries of the ankle joint. Clin Orthop 42:21, 1965.
48. Stören G: Conservative treatment of ankle fractures: Follow-up of 99 fractures treated conservatively. Acta Chir Scand 128:45, 1964.
49. Wade PA, Lance EM: The operative treatment of fracture-dislocation of the ankle joint. Clin Orthop Rel Res 42:37, 1965.
50. Walsh WM, Hughston JC: Unstable ankle fractures in athletes. Am J Sports Med 4:173, 1976.
51. Yde J: The Lauge-Hansen classification of malleolar fractures. Acta Orthop Scand 51:181, 1980.
52. Yde J, Kristensen KD: Ankle fractures: supination-eversion fractures of stage IV. Acta Orthop Scand 51:981, 1980.

Chapter 14 Comminuted Fractures of the Tibial Plafond

WILLIAM C. HAMILTON

Axial compression caused by gravity and/or muscular forces has a role in the production of virtually all ankle injuries. In some situations, however, such as falls from a height, axial compression forces predominate. The resultant "impact" [23] or "compression" [15] injuries are characterized by more articular surface disruption than injuries caused primarily by rotational forces. The immediate effects are more devastating and the ultimate result is less favorable [16,24]. Fortunately, these injuries are relatively uncommon [14,23,24,33,40].

The morphology of axial compression or impact fractures is quite variable, depending on the position of the foot at the moment of injury and the nature of the applied forces (Fig. 14.1) [17,26,33]. Generally, compression force directed posteriorly with the foot in plantarflexion results in separation of a large posterior tibial fragment [1,18,25]. On the other hand, compression force concentrated anteriorly, as with the foot in dorsiflexion, generates a large anterior tibial fragment [1,18,25]. Force directed vertically with the foot in neutral position may shatter the entire articular surface of the tibia or talus [19,32]. The position of the foot, however, may change during production of the injury, and angular and rotational forces may be superimposed, resulting in fracture patterns that sometimes defy all attempts at explanation [24].

The pronation-dorsiflexion mechanism of Lauge-Hansen explains some but not all of these complex injuries.

Pronation-Dorsiflexion Injuries

In pronation-dorsiflexion injuries, the starting position of the foot is that of pronation (dorsiflexion, abduction, eversion) [21]. The pathologic talar motion is that of extreme dorsiflexion and axial compression.

The stages of pronation-dorsiflexion injuries are as follows (Fig. 14.2) [21]:

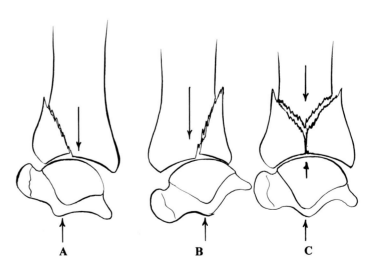

Fig. 14.1. Axial compression injuries: configuration of the fracture will be determined, at least in part, by the tibiotalar relationship at impact.

A   B   C

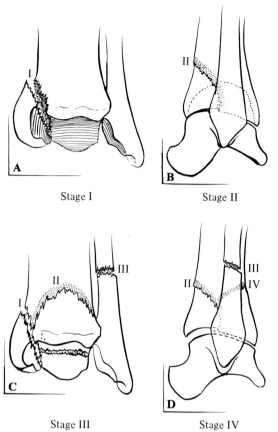

Fig. 14.2. Pronation-dorsiflexion injury. **A** Stage I, **B** Stage II, **C** Stage III , **D** Stage IV.

I   Fracture of the medial malleolus.
II   Large anterior tibial lip fracture (with significant involvement of the articular surface).
III Fracture of the supramalleolar part of the fibula.
IV   Fracture of the posterior tibia, frequently level with the proximal margin of the anterior tibial fracture.

Unlike his other categories, Lauge-Hansen did not produce this injury in cadaver specimens. His observations were based on the study of radiographs and a single injury subjected to postmortem dissection. His conclusions were as follows:

1. The starting position, pronation, implies that the ankle is dorsiflexed. Dorsiflexion beyond this point, combined with axial loading, wedges the wide distal and inferior portions

of the talus into the malleolar fork. This produces a fracture at the base of the medial malleolus (stage I) (Fig. 14.2A). This degree of talar dorsiflexion far exceeds the physiologic range and would seem to require rupture of the dorsal tibiotalar capsule, which in fact was observed by Lauge-Hansen in the one specimen that he dissected. He also observed that the medial malleolar fracture did not quite reach the cortex posteriorly, suggesting that the malleolus had been wedged medially and opened anteriorly by the wide distal and inferior dimension of the trochlea tali (Fig. 14.2A).

2. With the loss of medial and posterior restraints, the talus is permitted to dorsiflex even further and to subluxate anteriorly and proximally, splitting off the anterior articular surface of the tibia with which it is in contact (stage II) (Figs. 14.2B and 14.12). If, because of medial disruption, the talus is permitted to simultaneously externally rotate during or immediately prior to this stage, the anterior tibial lip fracture may be based anterolaterally, rather than straight anteriorly.

3. With continued force, the distal fibula fails above the malleolar region (stage III) (Fig. 14.2C) and frequently the posterior tibia fractures transversely at a level corresponding to the proximal extent of the anterior tibial lip fragment (stage IV) (Figs. 14.2D and 14.3).

A completely satisfactory explanation for the stage III and stage IV lesions was not offered by Lauge-Hansen. Since the fibular fracture, however, has been observed in the absence of the posterior tibial fracture, this sequence of injury is presumably correct. Lauge-Hansen observed this fracture infrequently and he did not (or could not) reproduce this injury in cadaver specimens. Therefore, this particular mechanism does not have as sound a scientific basis as the other four types of injury that he described.

Pilon Fractures

European fracture surgeons have coined the term "pilon fracture" to describe comminuted, intraarticular injuries of the distal tibia and fibula,

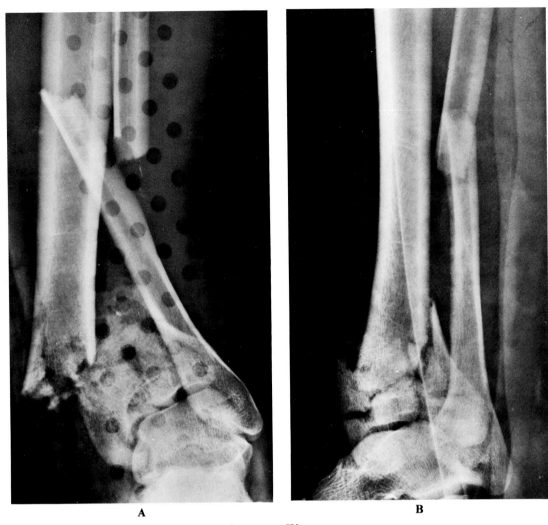

A
B

Fig. 14.3. A and **B** Pronation-dorsiflexion injury, stage IV.

usually occurring as a result of high velocity accidents [13,34]. Generally (75% of cases) the fibula is fractured at or above the ankle joint. In some instances (25%) the fibula is intact, in which case some degree of tibiofibular diastasis usually occurs. Rüedi and Allgöwer have classified pilon fractures into three types, based on the degree of displacement and comminution (Fig. 14.4) [32,34]. This injury in its milder form (type I) corresponds well to the pronation-dorsiflexion injury described by Lauge-Hansen. Even in its more severe form (type III) characterized by extensive displacement and comminution (the "explosion" fracture of some authors) [9], it bears some resemblance to Lauge-Hansen's pronation-dorsiflexion injury.

The term "pronation-dorsiflexion" does not thoroughly explain or include all the different lesions encountered in clinical practice. The term "pilon fracture" has recently acquired rather specific connotation, and with the Rüedi-Allgöwer classification scheme it represents a better designation for these comminuted, intraarticular injuries.

Pilon fractures represent difficult therapeutic problems for several reasons. The articular surface of the tibia and sometimes the talus are injured to a degree that makes anatomic restitution very difficult [4,24]. They are usually associated with severe local soft tissue damage and frequently occur in patients with multiple injuries [24]. Even in those instances where anatomic re-

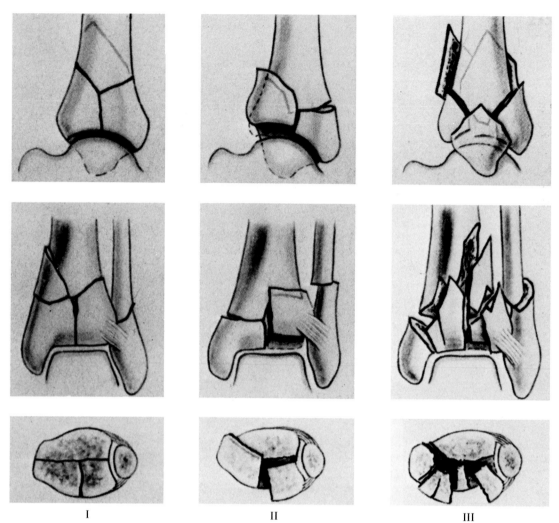

Fig. 14.4. Classification of pilon fractures. Reprinted with permission from Rüedi T, Allgöwer M: The operative treatment of intra-articular fractures of the lower end of the tibia. Clin Orthop Rel Res 138:106, 1979. Lippincott/Harper & Row.

duction can be achieved, ultimate function may be impaired because of irreparable damage to articular cartilage and/or periarticular soft tissues [3,9,16,19,20]. Nevertheless, every effort within reason should be made to restore stability, congruity, and mobility to the ankle joint.

Treatment

The complexity of the pilon fracture becomes obvious when one reviews the various techniques that have been employed to treat it. Virtually every modality or combination of modalities—including closed treatment, skeletal traction, skeletal fixation, open reduction, and primary ar-

throdesis—has been advocated for this fracture [24].

Comminuted fractures of the tibial plafond are potentially devastating injuries. Treatment cannot be standardized but must be individualized based on the nature of the fracture, circumstances of the patient and experience of the treating physician. Optimal restoration of function requires that the surgeon be well-versed in the full spectrum of treatment modalities available.

Closed Reduction and External Immobilization

Because of the degree of soft tissue disruption as well as bone comminution and impaction, pilon fractures do not generally lend themselves well to treatment by closed means [4]. Even Lauge-Hansen, one of the staunchest proponents of closed treatment, conceded that it was difficult to obtain good anatomic and functional results with pronation-dorsiflexion injuries by closed measures [20,21].

Less severe injuries, characterized by anterior tibial lip fracture with preservation of a substantial portion of the posterior tibial articular surface, can occasionally be reduced by plantarflexing the foot as direct pressure is applied to the displaced anterior fragment [17,21,26]. Not uncommonly, however, one encounters a dilemma similar to that described by McLaughlin [26] in reference to large posterior tibial margin fractures: efforts to tighten the anterior capsule by plantarflexing the ankle result in anterior dislocation of the talus and perpetuation of the deformity (Fig. 14.5) [9]. With many pilon injuries,

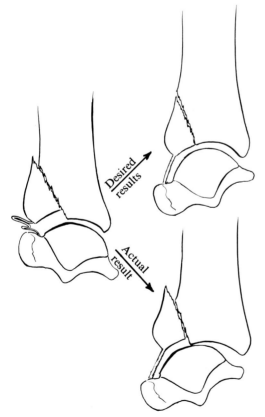

Fig. 14.5. Pronation-dorsiflexion injuries are difficult to reduce by closed means, even when limited to stage II. Sufficient plantarflexion to pull the anterior fragment down to the level of the tibial plafond will frequently cause the talus to redislocate anteriorly.

the entire articular surface is involved and this technique should not even be attempted.

Skeletal Traction–Skeletal Fixation

Various forms of skeletal traction and/or fixation with plaster or frames have also been recommended for pilon injuries [1,9,10,11,17,26,30,36]. These methods rely on tension generated across the ankle and subtalar joints to reduce and maintain the fracture fragments. Although the medial fragment can usually be brought out to length by traction through the deltoid ligament, it is not usually possible to exert sufficient force through the relatively lax anterior and posterior capsules to disengage and reduce the impacted anterior and posterior articular fragments (Fig. 14.6) [21]. In those cases where shortening and impaction are not marked, and some combination of manipulation and longitudinal traction succeeds in aligning the fracture fragments, position can generally be maintained by skeletal traction or external skeletal fixation (Fig. 14.7). Skeletal traction combined with early motion to mold the fragments into position is also indicated for "explosion"-type pilon fractures characterized by such extensive comminution that reduction by any means is impossible (Fig. 14.8) [1,6,7,10, 27,31,39]. Although prognosis should be guarded under these circumstances, some patients will regain a surprising degree of relatively painless function. If nothing else, maintenance of approximate alignment will facilitate reconstructive surgery if it becomes necessary at a later date.

Limited Open Reduction Combined with External Skeletal Fixation

Burgess [4] and later Scheck [36] recommended skeletal fixation in combination with limited open reduction of "key" articular fragments. This approach provides for restoration of the joint surface and removal of intraarticular fragments, as well as maintenance of limb length and alignment, while inflicting only a minimum of surgical trauma [4,24,36]. This technique is especially well suited for comminuted fractures where the articular surface can be reassembled but the metaphyseal defect defies operative reduction and stable internal fixation.

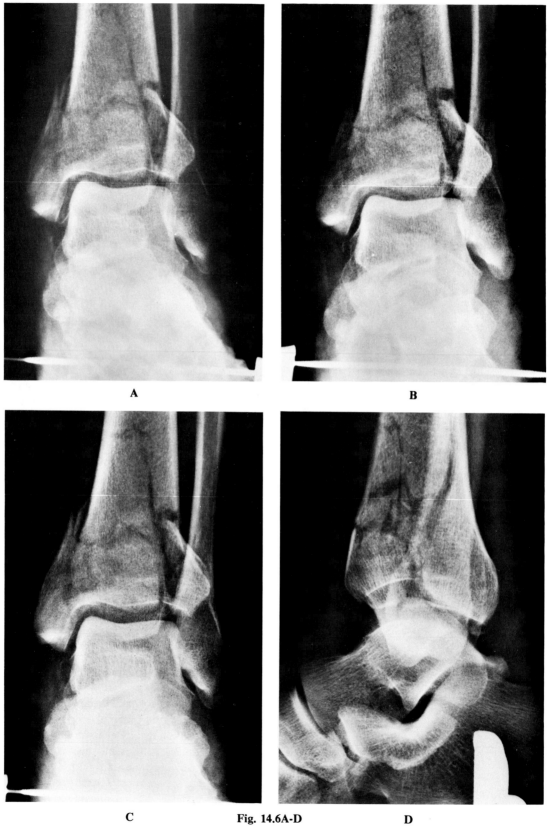

A   B

C   **Fig. 14.6A-D**   D

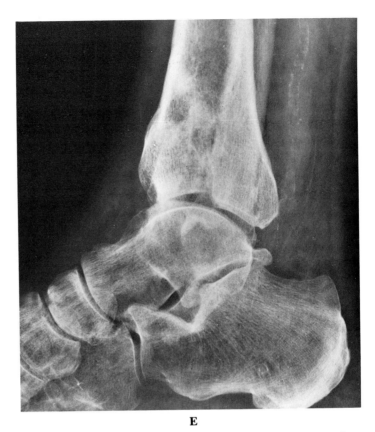

E

Fig. 14.6. Comminuted fracture of the distal tibia. **A–D** Increasing skeletal traction serves to distract the tibiotalar joint with little or no change in the position of the fracture fragments. **E** Anterior tibial fragment healed with residual step-off in the articular surface; follow-up film demonstrates persistent anterior subluxation of the talus.

Technique (Scheck) [36]

Under general or spinal anesthesia, 3/16-in. Steinmann pins are inserted through the os calcis and the proximal tibia and attached to a reduction frame [36]. Traction is slowly applied across the fracture site as an attempt is made to directly manipulate the fragments into position. Radiographs are obtained and, if a "key" fragment remains displaced, the skin between the pins is prepared and isolated from the frame using plastic drapes. Through a limited, carefully placed incision, the major "key" fragment is approached and, with a minimum of soft tissue damage, reduced and stabilized with one or more screws. Distraction is maintained for approximately 6 weeks by incorporation of the tibial and calcaneal pins into a toe-to-groin plaster (Fig. 14.9).

One of the problems reported by Scheck [36] was late angular deformity due to comminution and bone loss. This can be avoided to a large degree by cancellous bone grafting of the metaphyseal defect and/or a longer period of immobilization.

Limited Internal Fixation Combined with External Immobilization

Along similar lines, Leach [22] has recommended fibular stabilization with a Rush or Steinmann pin (Fig. 14.10) as a minimally invasive method of maintaining limb length and conferring some degree of stability to comminuted fractures of the distal tibia. If the attachments of the stout inferior tibiofibular ligaments are intact, restoration of fibular length will often effect approximate reduction of large anterior and/or posterior tibial fragments, without further jeopardizing their blood supply by even a limited surgical exposure.

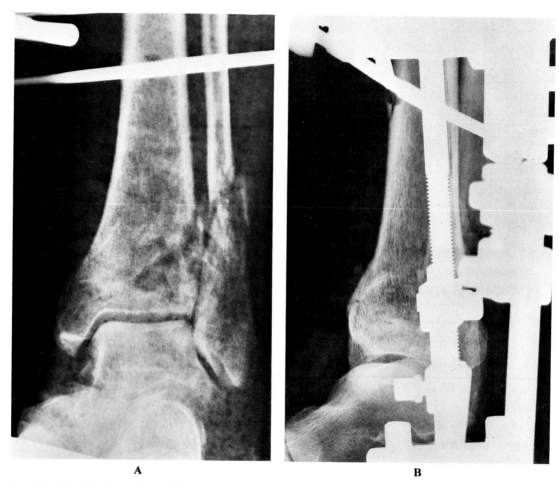

A   B

Fig. 14.7. A and **B** Pilon fracture (pronation-dorsiflexion injury, stage III) treated by closed reduction; position satisfactorily *maintained* by use of a Hoffman external fixator.

Fig. 14.8. A Severely comminuted pilon fracture in an elderly patient. **B** and **C** Treated with skeletal traction and early active motion. **D** Despite a poor radio- graphic result, the patient regained an excellent degree ▷ of relatively painless function.

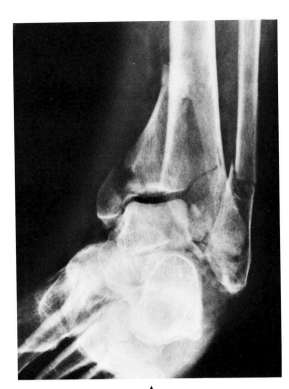

A

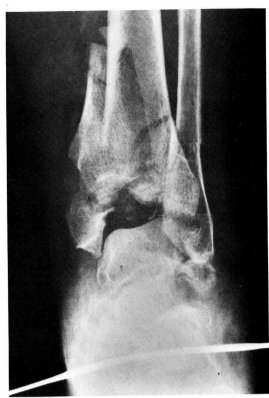

B

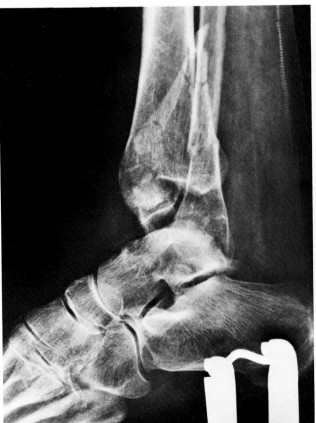

C

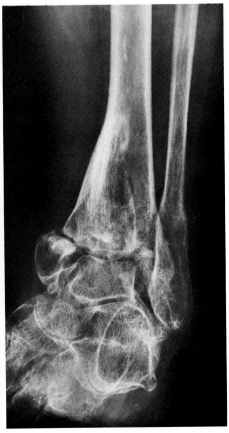

D

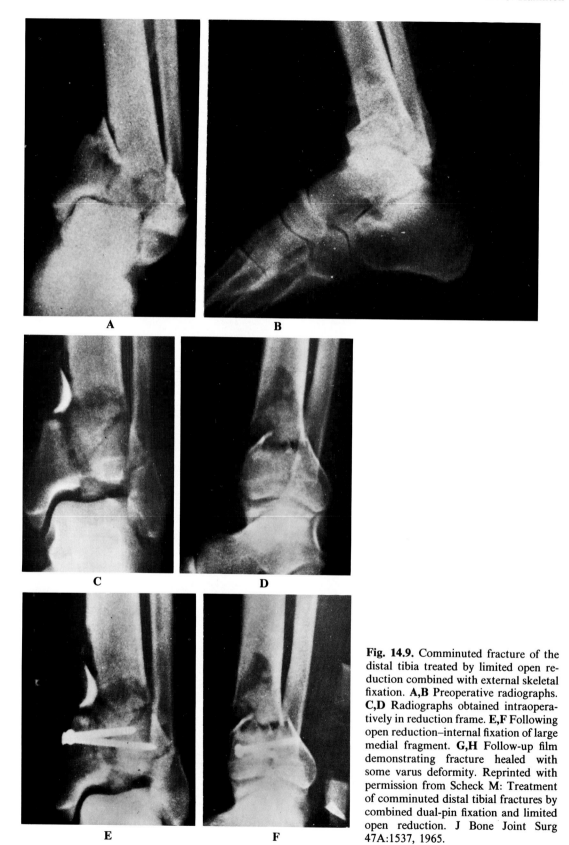

Fig. 14.9. Comminuted fracture of the distal tibia treated by limited open reduction combined with external skeletal fixation. **A,B** Preoperative radiographs. **C,D** Radiographs obtained intraoperatively in reduction frame. **E,F** Following open reduction–internal fixation of large medial fragment. **G,H** Follow-up film demonstrating fracture healed with some varus deformity. Reprinted with permission from Scheck M: Treatment of comminuted distal tibial fractures by combined dual-pin fixation and limited open reduction. J Bone Joint Surg 47A:1537, 1965.

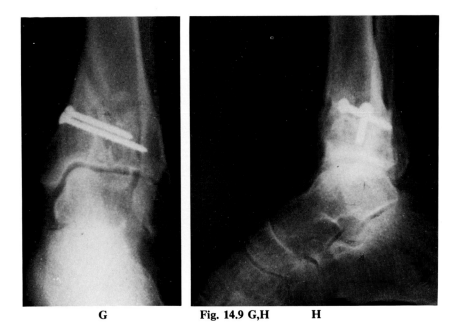

G   **Fig. 14.9 G,H**   **H**

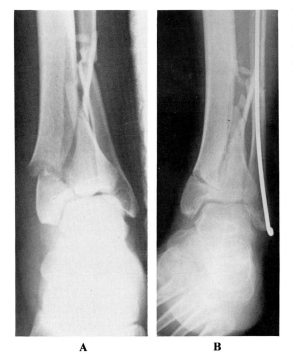

A   **B**

Fig. 14.10. A and **B** Comminuted fracture of the distal tibia and fibula treated by fibular fixation and external immobilization in plaster. Reprinted with permission from Leach RE: A means of stabilizing comminuted distal tibial fractures. J Trauma 4:723, 1964. The Williams & Wilkins Co., Baltimore.

This technique is especially applicable when extensive comminution or damage to the anterior or medial soft tissues precludes formal open reduction. With extensive soft tissue disruption, however, fibular fixation may have very little if any beneficial effect on tibial fracture position (Fig. 14.11).

Complete Open Reduction and Internal Fixation

By far, the most promising results with pilon injuries have been obtained by complete internal fixation and early motion [5,10,13,30,32,33, 34,38]. Rüedi and Allgöwer [32,34] have recommended aggressive surgical treatment of these injuries as follows:

1. Reduction and fixation of the fibula at normal length.
2. Restoration of the tibial articular surface.
3. Cancellous bone grafting of any metaphyseal defect.
4. Stabilization of the medial aspect of the distal tibia with a buttress plate to prevent late varus deformity.

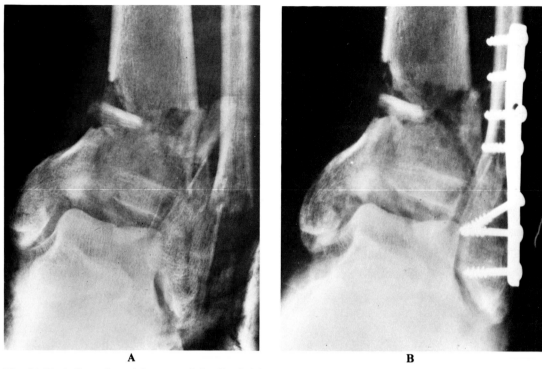

| A | B |

Fig. 14.11. A Comminuted fracture of the distal tibia and fibula. **B** Fibular stabilization had negligible effect on the distal tibial fracture.

5. Early active motion but prolonged avoidance of weight bearing.

These authors reported very good or good results in 85% of patients treated by this scheme [32,34]. They conceded, however, that results might be affected by the age of the patient, the nature of the injury, and the experience of the operating surgeon. This latter variable is probably even more important than they have suggested. Under the best circumstances, satisfactory open reduction and internal fixation of pilon fractures represents a demanding technical challenge that may consume up to 6 hours [33]. In order to justify subjecting a severely traumatized limb to a procedure of this magnitude, the surgeon must be experienced and reasonably confident that he can safely effect anatomic reduction and complete internal fixation [10,13,30], since unsatisfactory reduction or unstable fixation almost always leads to painful joint degeneration [34]. Otherwise, one of the less invasive approaches is preferred.

Technique (Ruedi and Allgöwer) [33,34]

The procedure is performed under tourniquet control. If plain radiographs or tomograms suggest that reduction of the articular fragments will produce a significant metaphyseal defect, cancellous bone graft is obtained from the greater trochanter or other site prior to tourniquet inflation.

Provided the fibular fracture is amenable to fixation (60% of cases), this component of the injury is fixed initially using a plate or intramedullary device. This will restore length to the limb and effect approximate reduction of the distal tibial fragments.

Next the distal tibia and ankle are exposed utilizing anteromedial and anterolateral skin incisions, preserving as wide a skin bridge as possible (minimum 7 cm). The articular fragments are carefully elevated from their impacted position, assembled with smooth Kirschner wires, and fixed to each other with screws. The resultant metaphyseal defect is packed with cancellous graft and then the medial or anterior aspect of

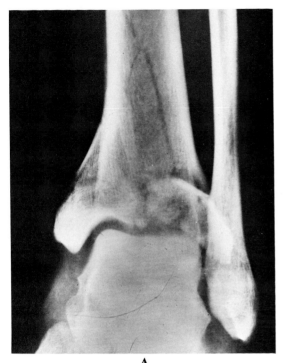

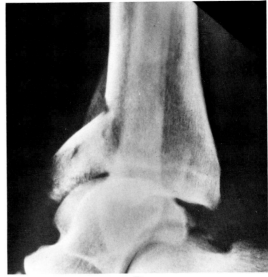

B

A

Fig. 14.12. A and **B** Pilon fracture. **C** Treated with open reduction and internal fixation using interfragmentary screws and a medial buttress plate. Metaphyseal defect was packed with autogenous cancellous bone graft.

the distal tibia is buttressed by application of a T-shaped or cloverleaf plate (Fig. 14.12) [28]. After wound closure, a U-shaped splint that allows active and passive dorsiflexion of the ankle is applied. Provided wound healing is satisfactory, patients are allowed to ambulate on the sixth postoperative day, but are kept non–weight bearing for 8–10 weeks, and then partial weight bearing is allowed until a total of 14–20 weeks has elapsed since surgery.

Primary Arthrodesis

Since fusion of the ankle is often required for painful joint degeneration following comminuted fractures of the distal tibia, some authors have recommended it as primary treatment when satisfactory reduction cannot be obtained by closed or open means [26,35,37]. However, this ignores the fact that some patients will regain a considerable degree of painless motion despite rather

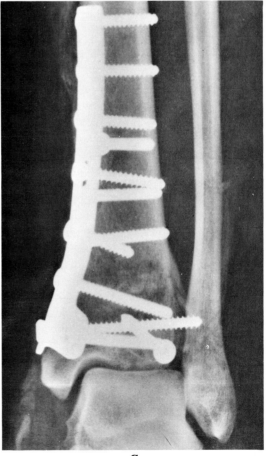

C

marked deformity [29]. Also, primary arthrodesis is technically difficult and potentially dangerous in the presence of comminution and soft tissue disruption [2,9,12]. Therefore, most authors presently believe that primary arthrodesis is rarely, if ever, indicated for the treatment of these injuries [9,30,39].

Impaction of the Lateral Weight-Bearing Surface of the Tibia

Coonrad [8] called attention to impaction of the lateral weight-bearing surface of the tibia as an important cause of unsatisfactory results following injury to the ankle. He was able to demonstrate this lesion in 12 of 25 patients who eventually required arthrodesis because of unsatisfactory results following ankle injuries. Coonrad described two types of injuries.

The first type corresponds to the posterior (actually posterolateral) fracture of the tibial margin commonly observed in association with external rotation and abduction injuries. Since the fracture line runs in an oblique direction, the full extent of the articular surface involvement is frequently underestimated, and the fragment, therefore, may be left in an unreduced position with resultant instability and incongruity (Fig. 14.13B). The joint usually undergoes progressive degenerative change with articular cartilage attrition most marked on the lateral side (Fig. 14.13A).

The other type of lateral impaction injury described by Coonrad is characterized by subchondral compression of the lateral tibial plafond. This can occur in association with stable as well as unstable ankle injuries. The lesion is frequently occult and easy to overlook at the time of initial treatment (Fig. 14.14A). Eventually, despite an otherwise satisfactory reduction, degenerative changes develop (Fig. 14.14B). Initially, the degenerative changes are confined to the lateral tibiotalar joint and are associated with valgus deformity, but eventually the entire joint becomes involved. Coonrad suggested that early diagnosis with open wedge osteotomy and bone grafting might improve the outcome from this injury; to date, however, this has not been proved. McLaughlin [26] has also alluded to this injury

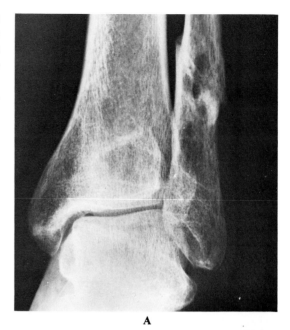

A

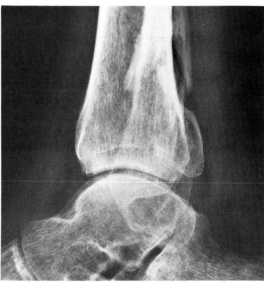

B

Fig. 14.13. Pronation-external rotation injury associated with a large displaced articular fragment from the posterolateral aspect of the tibia. Fragment healed in a proximal position (**B**) with resultant degenerative changes in the lateral tibiofibular joint (**A**).

and Cox [9] has described a similar clinical situation caused by occult subchondral fracture which is frequently overlooked until degenerative changes ensue.

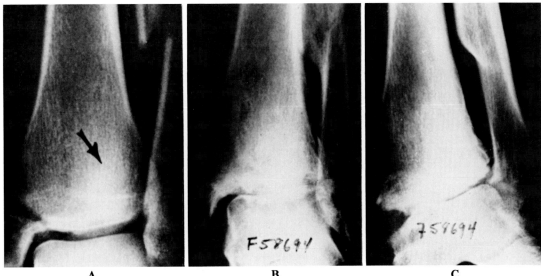

Fig. 14.14. A Subchondral compression fracture of the lateral tibial plafond occurring in association with fractures of the medial malleolus and distal fibula. **B** and **C** Fifteen months following injury, there is extensive arthrosis of the tibiotalar joint. Reprinted with permission from Coonrad RW: Fracture-dislocations of the ankle joint with impaction injury of the lateral weight-bearing surface of the tibia. J Bone Joint Surg 52A:1337, 1970.

References

1. Bohler L: The Treatment of Fractures, 5th ed. New York, Grune & Stratton, 1956.
2. Bonnin JG: Injuries to the Ankle. New York, Grune & Stratton, 1950.
3. Brodie IAOD, Denham RA: The treatment of unstable ankle fractures. J Bone Joint Surg 56B:256, 1974.
4. Burgess E: Fractures of the ankle. J Bone Joint Surg 26:721, 1944.
5. Burwell HN, Charnley AD: Treatment of displaced fractures at the ankle by rigid internal fixation and early joint movement. J Bone Joint Surg 47B:634, 1965.
6. Cave EF (ed): Ankle injuries. In: Fractures and Other Injuries. Chicago, Year Book Medical, 1958.
7. Chapman MW: The use of immediate internal fixation in open fractures. Orthop Clin North Am 11:579, 1980.
8. Coonrad RW: Fracture-dislocations of the ankle joint with impaction injury of the lateral weight-bearing surface of the tibia. J Bone Joint Surg 52A:1337, 1970.
9. Cox FJ: Fractures of the ankle involving the lower articular surface of the tibia. Clin Orthop 42:51, 1965.
10. Cox FJ, Laxson WW: Fractures about the ankle joint. Am J Surg 83:674, 1952.
11. Dabezies E, D'Ambrosia RD, Shoji H: Classification and treatment of ankle fractures. Orthopedics 1:365, 1978.
12. DePalma AF: The Management of Fractures and Dislocations, 2nd ed. Philadelphia, Saunders, 1970.
13. Ferguson AB Jr, Mears DC: Pilon fracture. The challenge for internal fixation. Orthop Consult 1:1, 1980.
14. Gaston SR, McLaughlin HL: Complex fracture of the lateral malleolus. J Trauma 1:69, 1961.
15. Jergesen F: Open reduction of fractures and dislocations of the ankle. Am J Surg 98:136, 1959.
16. Joy G, Patzakis MJ, Harvey JP Jr: Precise evaluation of the reduction of severe ankle fractures. Technique and correlation with end results. J Bone Joint Surg 56A:979, 1974.
17. Key JA, Conwell HE: Injuries in the region of the ankle. In: The Management of Fractures, Dislocations and Sprains, 6th ed. St. Louis, Mosby, 1956.
18. Kleiger B: The mechanism of ankle injuries. J Bone Joint Surg 38A:59, 1956.
19. Kleiger B: Mechanisms of ankle injury. Orthop Clin North Am 5:127, 1974.
20. Kristensen TB: Treatment of malleolar fractures according to Lauge-Hansen's method. Preliminary results. Acta Chir Scand 97:362, 1949.
21. Lauge-Hansen N: Fractures of the ankle. V. Pronation-dorsiflexion fracture. AMA Arch Surg 67:813, 1953.
22. Leach RE: A means of stabilizing comminuted distal tibial fractures. J Trauma 4:722, 1964.
23. Lindsjo U: Operative treatment of ankle fractures. Acta Orthop Scand (Suppl) 189:1, 1981.
24. Maale G, Seligson D: Fractures through the dis-

tal weight-bearing surface of the tibia. Orthopedics 3:517, 1980.

25. MacKinnon AP: Fracture of the lower articular surface of the tibia in fracture dislocation of the ankle. J Bone Joint Surg 10:352, 1928.

26. McLaughlin HL: Trauma. Philadelphia, Saunders, 1960.

27. Mitchell CL, Fleming JL: Fractures and fracture-dislocations of the ankle. Postgrad Med 26:773, 1959.

28. Müller ME, Allgöwer M, Schneider R, Willenegger H: Manual of Internal Fixation, 2nd ed. Translated by J. Schatzker. New York, Springer-Verlag, 1979.

29. Neufeld AJ: Ankle joint fractures and their treatment. Clin Orthop 42:91, 1965.

30. Pankovich AM: Adult ankle fractures. JCE Orthop 7:17, 1979.

31. Perkins G: Injuries around the ankle. In: Fractures and Dislocations. London, Athlone Press, 1958.

32. Rüedi TP: Fractures of the lower end of the tibia into the ankle joint. Results 9 years after open reduction and internal fixation. Injury 5:130, 1973.

33. Rüedi TP, Allgöwer M: Fractures of the lower end of the tibia into the ankle-joint. Injury 1:92, 1969.

34. Rüedi TP, Allgöwer M: The operative treatment of intraarticular fractures of the lower end of the tibia. Clin Orthop Rel Res 138:105, 1979.

35. Rütt A: Surgery of the Lower Leg and Foot. Translated by G. Stiasny. Philadelphia, Saunders, 1980.

36. Scheck M: Treatment of comminuted distal tibial fractures by combined dual-pin fixation and limited open reduction. J Bone Joint Surg 47A:1537, 1965.

37. Solonen KA, Lauttamus L: Treatment of malleolar fractures. Acta Orthop Scand 36:321, 1965.

38. Spiegel PG: Distal tibial intraarticular fractures. Clin Orthop Rel Res 138:17, 1979.

39. Williams CW, Langston J, Sanders A: Comminuted fractures of the distal tibia into the ankle joint. J Bone Joint Surg 49A:192, 1967.

40. Yde J: The Lauge-Hansen classification of malleolar fractures. Acta Orthop Scand 51:181, 1980.

Chapter 15 Malleolar Injuries: Aftercare, Prognosis, and Complications

WILLIAM C. HAMILTON AND ROBERT P. GOOD

Aftercare and Rehabilitation

> If things have gone well, no physical therapy is necessary and movement is restored by function. If things have not gone well, physical therapy will rarely remedy the fault.
>
> Key and Conwell [43]

Although formal rehabilitation efforts may be unnecessary for most patients, certain simple measures will minimize complications and facilitate complete recovery. The entire patient and injured limb must be rehabilitated before recovery can be called complete. Toward this end, patients should be encouraged to remain active from the very beginning and exercise body parts not encumbered by immobilization. As soon as immobilization is discontinued or immediately following surgery, if external immobilization is not employed, active effort to regain ankle (plantarflexion-dorsiflexion) as well as subtalar (inversion-eversion) motion should be instituted [18].

When plaster is first removed, following open or closed treatment, most patients will experience a tendency to dependent edema. This results from the trauma of injury and/or surgery and is frequently perpetuated by muscular atrophy and gait disturbance, secondary to discomfort, stiffness, or habit. Swelling can cause pain and impede recovery. When swelling persists, it is frequently disturbing to the patient who by this point thinks he should have recovered. Some form of support (e.g., gel cast, elastic anklet, or surgical stocking) is helpful at this stage to minimize this complication [18,20,85], as well as to impart a sense of ankle security without frustrating efforts to regain motion. Patients should also be advised to elevate their leg whenever they are not ambulating or doing something purposeful. Older patients or patients with associated vascular disease frequently will require support and

intermittent limb elevation for an extended period of time [7].

Patients initially ambulate with crutches or a cane and are encouraged to bear increasing amounts of weight on their injured extremity (provided fracture healing is secure and the nature of the injury does not require further protection of the articular surface). Even during this stage, however, every effort should be made to restore normal heel-toe gait, with appropriate contraction of the gastrocnemius-soleus muscle group during toe rise.

As weight bearing becomes more comfortable and motion approaches normal, walking aids can gradually be withdrawn [18]. Recovery of more active individuals and athletes can be facilitated at this stage by adding resistance exercises to increase strength and endurance, as well as proprioceptive exercises using a tilting board, as described by Freeman et al. [32]. Although drills are permissible much earlier, return to competitive athletics should be discouraged until motion, strength, and coordination of the individual as well as the limb return to normal.

Patients, especially older individuals, should be made to understand that it may be several months before full recovery is realized, so that they are not discouraged by persistent mild discomfort, stiffness, or weakness.

Malleolar Injuries: Prognosis

As with any injury, prognosis following ankle trauma is determined by many factors—psychologic and social, as well as physical. It is generally agreed that the most important factor within the surgeon's control is the exactness of reduction [14,17,30,39,43,49,50]. The manner in which this is accomplished appears to be much less critical than the actual quality of the ultimate anatomic result.

Although many factors are beyond the physician's control, their role needs to be considered since they will frequently influence the selection of treatment and they must be studied carefully in any attempt to compare the effectiveness of different treatment modalities. As the reader will note, there is unfortunately little consensus to date regarding the importance of these variables. Elucidation of the true role of each of these factors must await the results of long-term prospective studies, using standardized definitions and evaluation criteria.

Age

Lewis and Graham [52] believed that older patients were predisposed to degenerative arthritis following fractures because of "impaired restorative powers," and because they generally demonstrated a higher incidence of severe injuries with articular surface involvement. Burwell and Charnley [17] found that older patients were more likely to sustain supination-external rotation injuries—a type of fracture that they thought implied a less favorable prognosis. Walheim [102] and Klossner [47] documented a higher incidence of radiographic arthrosis with advanced age, but they did not relate these changes to subjective symptoms specifically for the older age group. Magnusson [56] noted that radiographic arthrosis was more common in older patients with external rotation injuries, but the incidence of subjective symptoms was not increased.

Kristensen [50] Klossner [47], and Wheelhouse and Rosenthal [105] could not demonstrate any relationship between age and result, provided satisfactory reduction was achieved and maintained. Wilson and Skilbred [107] observed that older patients, with incomplete reduction, were more prone to develop arthrosis but complained of surprisingly few symptoms. Similarly, Joy et al. [41] did not find any statistically significant relationship between age and the clinical result. Sarkisian and Cody [86] found that patients over age 70 actually demonstrated good results, despite often inadequate reduction; they concluded that this was due to the limited demands older patients placed on their ankles.

Sex

Lewis and Graham [52] noted that two-thirds of the 18 patients with post-traumatic arthritis of the ankle they studied were women, and concluded that the patient's sex had a definite role in determining outcome following ankle fracture. However, Magnusson [56,57], Klossner [47], Wheelhouse and Rosenthal [105], and Joy et al. [41] were unable to demonstrate any relationship between the patient's sex and the ultimate result. Lindsjo [53], in a series of patients treated operatively, observed that women of all ages faired less well than men, with the highest incidence of poor results occurring in the 45- to 64-year-old group; he attributed this to postmenopausal osteoporosis that impaired fracture fixation.

Obesity

Lewis and Graham [52] also believed that the patient's weight was instrumental in determining the result following injury. This relationship was subsequently denied by Kristensen [50], as well as by Joy et al. [41].

Type of Fracture

Generally those fractures, regardless of mechanism, which are associated with significant injury to the articular surface of the tibia or talus carry a less favorable prognosis than those without such injury [10,25,30,37,47,52,53,55,65,67,72, 86,89,100,102,103,107]. Included in this group are large displaced posterior tibial lip fractures [23,25,29,61,98,105], lateral impaction fractures of the distal tibia [24], and diffuse comminution of the talar or tibial articular surfaces [25,53, 105]. Articular fractures of the posterior tibial margin, even if satisfactorily reduced, carry a substantial risk of arthritis [53].

Also, it is generally accepted that regardless of type, unstable injuries characterized by disruption of multiple structures carry a less favorable prognosis than do stable unimalleolar fractures [12]. So-called "trimalleolar" fractures generally have a graver prognosis, especially when associated with posterior dislocation of the talus. This probably reflects significant articular cartilage damage as well as instability [24,36,47,58,98, 100].

Kristensen [49] encountered no poor results in patients with supination-adduction fractures treated nonoperatively. Similarly, Eventov et al. [31] noted that supination injuries, whether treated by open or closed means, resulted in a better outcome than fractures of other types. Phillips and Spiegel [79] concluded that Weber type A fractures (which correspond to supination-adduction injuries of Lauge-Hansen) generally did well with either open or closed treatment. Lindsjo [53], on the other hand, found that the highest incidence of unsatisfactory clinical results in his operative series was associated with Weber type A injuries and concluded that many of these fractures were on the "border" of impact (axial loading) fractures.

Burwell and Charnley [17] concluded that supination-external rotation injuries were more prone than other fractures to produce traumatic arthritis. Yet other authors have identified advanced stage pronation-external rotation injuries (PER III and PER IV) as more likely to impair the ultimate result [14,41,59,86]. Perkins [77] believed that external rotation fractures were more "pleasant" than abduction injuries. However, he did not distinguish between external rotation injuries occurring in supination and those occurring in pronation and he probably included many pronation-external rotation injuries in his group of abduction fractures.

Kristensen [49] found the greatest incidence of poor clinical results in patients with pronation-abduction injuries. Burns [16] also noted that most of the problems encountered with ankle fractures were due to abduction violence.

Klossner [47] stated that the type of injury was only of minor importance provided satisfactory reduction was achieved and maintained. Finally, Wheelhouse and Rosenthal [105] concluded that the type of fracture had no particular influence on the final result.

Diastasis

Some degree of diastasis or distal tibiofibular disruption can be encountered with virtually any mechanism of ankle injury, but total ligamentous diastasis is generally only seen with pronation-external rotation and certain pronation-abduction injuries. Persistent widening of the tibiofibular syndesmosis due to ligamentous diastasis

has been recognized as a common cause of unsatisfactory results following ankle injury [3,16, 22,24,30,36,52,57,103]. Mild distortion of distal tibiofibular relationship, secondary to fibular malrotation and/or shortening in association with anterior (or intraosseous) diastasis, is also thought to produce ill effects [17,34,53,68,87], but as yet this has not been well documented.

Initial Degree of Displacement

In studying this variable, there is considerable inherent error because the initial radiographs frequently will not reveal the full degree of displacement that occurred during production of the injury [41]. In general, stable nondisplaced fractures carry a more favorable prognosis than unstable displaced injuries [12]. This difference could be related to the extent of bone, cartilage, and soft tissue damage or to the degree of difficulty likely to be encountered in securing and maintaining satisfactory reduction of the unstable fractures [57].

Cedell [20], in a series of 132 operatively treated supination-external rotation injuries, observed that the best clinical results occurred in stage II injuries and the worst results in stage IV injuries. Even so, 94.7% of the stage II and 83.6% of the stage IV injuries experienced good results. Joy et al. [41] found that the degree of initial talar displacement affected the final clinical result and simultaneously demonstrated a positive correlation between the adequacy of reduction and the final result; they did not, however, specifically analyze their data to determine whether the effect of initial displacement could be nullified by exact anatomic repositioning. Similarly, Wheelhouse and Rosenthal [105] observed that the magnitude of initial talar displacement (> 5 mm) and the completeness of reduction both affected the final clinical result. Unfortunately, they also did not offer an opinion as to whether the prognosis was impaired by the greater degree of displacement or by difficulties encountered in securing and maintaining satisfactory reduction of the more unstable injuries.

Neither Kristensen [50] nor Klossner [47] could demonstrate any difference in end results between those patients with satisfactory fracture position on admission and those patients in whom satisfactory position was not achieved until after reduction; this suggested that the degree of initial displacement was not especially significant, provided satisfactory reduction was maintained. Burwell and Charnley [17] provided the best synthesis when they concluded that the degree of initial displacement was more important than the type of fracture, but less important than the adequacy of reduction, in affecting the final clinical outcome.

Fractures characterized by significant displacement imply a greater degree of soft tissue and bone violation, are likely to be associated with articular surface damage, and frequently are difficult to reduce and maintain in satisfactory position. The extent of bone, soft tissue, and articular damage are beyond the control of the treating physician and undoubtedly will have some influence on the ultimate result. The accuracy of reduction, however, is within the physician's control; if this is satisfactory, it appears to nullify, at least in part, the effect of initial displacement and instability on the clinical outcome [17,21, 39,47,49,52,53].

Malleolar Injuries: Complications

Although the emphasis should be placed on prevention of complications, they are to some degree unavoidable with either open or closed treatment. This section deals with diagnosis and treatment of complications encountered with malleolar fractures. Complications associated with lateral ligamentous rupture, fractures and dislocations of the talus, and epiphyseal injuries are discussed in the specific chapters concerned with these entities.

Infection

Although sepsis has been reported in association with closed fractures [61], it is for the most part a complication of open fractures and fractures treated by operative means. Deep sepsis complicating ankle fractures is relatively uncommon (Table 15.1). It requires prompt diagnosis with early drainage, aggressive debridement, and appropriate parenteral antibiotics. Metallic implants should not be removed if they continue to provide fixation [2,64,82,94]. If they are non-

functional, they should be removed and the fracture should be stabilized by another means. Deep sepsis is a serious event that frequently compromises the outcome and occasionally culminates in arthrodesis or amputation.

Superficial infection, on the other hand, is more common. It usually responds to local wound care and antibiotics without compromising the ultimate result. The incidence of superficial infection is difficult to ascertain, since it frequently cannot be distinguished from incisional skin necrosis with marginal inflammation and the two may frequently coexist (Table 15.1).

Skin Necrosis

Vasli [101] as well as Boettcher et al. [53] reported extremely high incidences of marginal necrosis; other authors, however, have found the incidence of incisional necrosis to be much lower (Table 15.1) [14,20,47,53,60,67,110]. Marginal skin necrosis can be minimized by appropriately designed surgical approaches, straight rather than curved incisions, careful handling of skin edges, and wound closure without excessive or concentrated tension. In some instances, however, skin loss is secondary to irreversible damage incurred at the moment of injury or immediately afterward, especially if the ankle has been permitted to remain too long in a dislocated position. This occurs most frequently in association with high velocity injuries, especially in older patients with preexisting vascular disease [20]. A favorite site for this complication is medially where the skin is stretched over the medial malleolus or jagged surface of the tibia with displaced external rotation or abduction injuries [20,46]. With local wound care, minor degrees of incisional necrosis usually heal by secondary intention without compromising the ultimate result. Rarely are plastic procedures required to provide satisfactory coverage.

Deep Vein Thrombosis

Deep vein thrombosis is a potential complication with both open and closed treatment [14,17, 20,84,110]. On the one hand, open treatment subjects the limb to additional trauma that may predispose to thrombosis. On the other hand, effec-

Table 15.1. Incidence of Infection and Marginal Skin Necrosis Reported in the Literature.

Source	Infection (Total) (%)	Infection (Superficial) (%)	Infection (Deep) (%)	Marginal Skin Necrosis (%)
Vasli [101] 1957	2.2	NA	2.2	19.5
Klossner [47] 1962	8	5.2	0.5	2.3
Burwell and Charnley [17] 1965	6.6	5.9	0.7	NA
Cedell [20] 1967	2.6	2.2	0.4	2.2
Boettcher et al. [53] 1970	NA	NA	NA	18
Weber [53] 1972	0.6	NA	NA	NA
Brodie and Denham [14] 1974	2.6	2.3	0.3	0.7
Muller [53] 1975	0.5	NA	0.5	4
Mitchell et al. [67] 1979	1	NA	NA	1
Mast and Teipner [60] 1980	0	NA	NA	0
Yde and Kristensen [110] 1980	0	NA	NA	1.6
Lindsjo [53] 1981	2.3	NA	NA	2.9

NA, not available.

tive internal fixation will usually permit more rapid mobilization of the patient and the limb, so as to reduce the likelihood of thrombotic phenomena [53]. Despite a voluminous amount of literature concerning deep vein thrombosis in general, there are little data concerned specifically with ankle injuries to support either method of treatment in this regard. Prophylactic anticoagulation should be seriously considered, especially in high risk patients undergoing closed or open treatment of lower extremity injuries. The development of deep vein thrombosis can be insidious and prompt diagnosis requires a high index of clinical suspicion. Any unexplained discomfort or edema should suggest this possibility and prompt further investigation.

Reflex Sympathetic Dystrophy (Sudeck's Atrophy, Mimocausalgia)

Reflex sympathetic dystrophy has been reported to occur once in every 2000 injuries [48]. This estimate is probably low, however, since many milder forms resolve spontaneously [9]. Although the upper extremity is most commonly involved, the condition can affect the lower ex-

tremity as well [26,40,48]. Reflex sympathetic dystrophy can follow even the most trivial injury [99], and is not related to the adequacy of treatment [1]. Emotionally labile and psychoneurotic patients, as well as those with low pain thresholds or in quest of monetary gains, are particularly susceptible [42,75,99]. The etiology is unknown but probably is related to dysfunction of the central and/or sympathetic nervous systems [1, 42,48,75,99,108].

The syndrome is heralded by pain seemingly out of proportion to the extent of injury. This frequently has a burning quality [108], but may be described as dull, aching or throbbing [9]. Physical findings include diffuse tenderness and swelling, as well as vasomotor or trophic disturbances, depending on the stage of the disease process [75,106]. Within 4 to 8 weeks of onset, radiographs will demonstrate pronounced osteoporosis [42]. While all the signs and symptoms may be present, the patient will frequently manifest one out of proportion to the others [1,9].

If recognized early, active motion and restoration of function with or without formal physical therapy will often reverse the situation [1,9, 40,42,75,108]. Later, treatment becomes more difficult and usually requires systemic corticosteroids [40,48], sympathetic block (or sympathectomy) [1,9,40,75,99], or some combination of the two [99].

Pseudoarthrosis (Nonunion)

Pseudoarthrosis complicating ankle fractures may involve the medial or, less commonly, the lateral malleolus [90]. It can cause local discomfort and may predispose to painful joint instability, deformity, or incongruity. The incidence of pseudoarthrosis is higher in fractures characterized by marked displacement and/or inadequate reduction [65]. It also occurs more frequently in fractures treated by closed rather than open means [53]; this reflects the increased likelihood of inadequate reduction, interposed soft tissue, and/or poor stabilization with closed treatment. A single instance of nonunion of the posterior malleolus has also been reported by Mendelsohn [65] who considers this to be a "rara avis."

Pseudoarthrosis of the Medial Malleolus

The incidence of pseudoarthrosis involving the medial malleolus has been reported to be 5–18% with closed treatment [6,47,49,57,65,98,101] and less than 1% with operative measures [20,101]. Many causative factors have been implicated; however, interposed soft tissue and persistent diastasis at the fracture site appear to be most significant [6,15,19,47,65]. Although nonunion may occur at any site along the medial malleolus, proximal lesions at or near the level of the tibial plafond are more likely to produce symptoms than are more distal lesions [6,47,62,107]. A pseudoarthrosis need not produce any symptoms [47,71,92,98], however, since the fibrous union that occurs in the absence of bone healing may be quite firm [8,65,91]. Mindell and Rogers [66] have reported two cases that attest to this fact. In each instance, acute ankle injury produced avulsion fracture of the medial malleolus proximal to a preexisting pseudoarthrosis from prior injury.

The relationship between medial malleolar pseudoarthrosis and arthritis is unclear. Cox and Laxson [26] as well as McLaughlin [62] believed that pseudoarthrosis predisposed to instability and traumatic arthritis. Other authors [5,66], however, have been unable to demonstrate any relationship between medial malleolar pseudoarthrosis and the ultimate results following ankle injury. Mendelsohn [65] specified that pseudoarthrosis at this site was consistent with a stable painless ankle provided talotibial alignment was maintained. Sneppen [89,90] did not think a malleolar pseudoarthrosis should necessarily predispose to a poor ultimate result because of the excellent results achievable with bone grafting procedures.

Patients with radiographic evidence of nonunion and local symptoms of 6 months duration should be considered for surgical intervention. Ideally, there should be no tibiotalar malalignment nor evidence of traumatic arthritis. In some instances, however, the latter requirement can be overlooked if the pseudoarthrosis itself seems to be responsible for most of the patient's complaints. Small distal fragments below the level of the tibial plafond do not as a rule produce symptoms. When they do, however, they can be readily treated by simple excision of the fragment and reattachment of the deltoid ligament to the proximal malleolus [27,85,90]. Larger fragments at or near the mortise angle need to be preserved. Various procedures have been described to foster union at this site [5,27,62,90]. Sneppen reported excellent results by combining excision of the pseudoarthrosis and screw fixation of the fragment with autogenous bone grafting [90]. Other authors have questioned the need to excise the pseudoarthrosis except in situations where the fracture position must be improved [37,85]. Sliding tibial bone grafts [27] are technically difficult to perform due to osteoporosis and the small size of the malleolar fragment. Bone pegs [10] can be used, but great care must be taken not to split or comminute the softened malleolar fragment. Simple drilling of the nonunion site seems to be of little value and is not recommended [90].

In those instances where tibiotalar alignment is normal, the author's preference is to use cancellous bone obtained from the distal tibial metaphysis. This is packed into a trough created with a high speed burr on the external surface of the pseudoarthrosis. Screw fixation of a stable pseudoarthrosis is rarely necessary. When tibiotalar or malleolar alignment is not satisfactory, the pseudoarthrosis should be excised and the fragment repositioned and fixed internally (Fig. 15.1).

Presently, there is considerable enthusiasm for the use of electrical stimulation as a means of

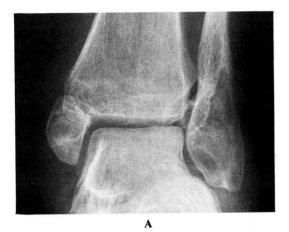

A

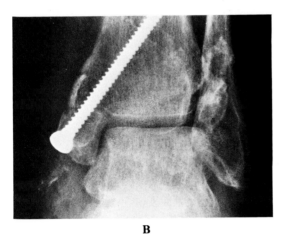

B

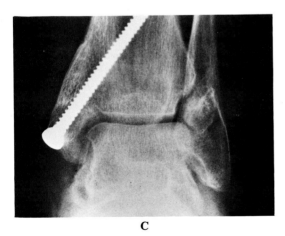

C

Fig. 15.1. A Painful pseudoarthrosis at the base of the medial malleolus. **B** Treated by excision of pseudoarthrosis, repositioning of the medial malleolar fragment, internal fixation with a lagged cortical screw, and bone grafting from the medial aspect of the distal tibia. **C** Follow-up film 4 months after surgery demonstrates healing of malleolar fracture. Note also an asymptomatic anterior tibial tubercle pseudoarthrosis.

treating symptomatic nonunion [13]. Since the occurrence of malleolar nonunion is low, little experience with this specific application has been obtained. The technique offers promise, however, and may eventually prove to be the method of choice for those nonunions in which tibiotalar and malleolar position is normal.

Pseudoarthrosis of the Lateral Malleolus

Lateral malleolar pseudoarthrosis is relatively uncommon [74], occurring in 1% of conservatively treated fractures [47,65,89] and even less frequently in operatively treated injuries [20,91]. When it does occur, it usually (69%) involves the transverse, avulsion-type fractures, especially those supination-adduction injuries characterized by medial fracture and varus displacement of the talus [65,89]. Provided the lateral malleolus is nondisplaced, pseudoarthrosis does not appear to play a significant role in the development of traumatic arthritis [89]. Although the nonunion may cause persistent local discomfort [65], conservatism is indicated since lateral malleolar pseudoarthrosis shows a marked propensity to eventual spontaneous union [89]. Rarely, a lateral malleolar pseudoarthrosis will persist and remain symptomatic enough to warrant surgical intervention [19,90]. Alternatives include internal fixation with bone grafting and electrical stimulation.

Malunion

Malunion of malleolar fractures with residual subluxation of the talus, tibiofibular diastasis, or gross angular/rotational deformity is obviously undesirable and likely to predispose to painful joint dysfunction and traumatic arthritis [44, 68,69,104]. Lesser degrees of malunion, such as are seen with mild fibular shortening or malrotation, are suspected to produce similar effects if allowed to persist over an extended period of time [79,107]. Until the exact margin of tolerance is established for malleolar injuries, the emphasis should be placed on prevention of malunion of any degree, since "joint preserving" reconstructive attempts at this site are difficult and the results, unfortunately, are rarely entirely satisfactory [17,70].

Once a malpositioned fracture is recognized, an attempt should be made to properly realign the fragments. If the malunion is established, consideration should be given to corrective osteotomy [33]. In the presence of tibiotalar arthritis, however, the success rate of realignment osteotomy diminishes greatly [76,88]. With mild to moderate arthritic changes, it is often difficult to choose between realignment malleolar osteotomy and ankle arthrodesis. The time interval since injury is not always a reliable factor in predicting the success or failure of osteotomy or other "joint preserving" reconstructive surgery [38,73,104]. The authors believe that when in doubt, the more conservative procedure (osteotomy) should be performed first; if osteotomy is unsuccessful, arthrodesis can be performed at a later date.

According to Speed and Boyd [93], requirements for successful reconstructive surgery about the ankle include (1) restoration of the proper weight-bearing alignment; (2) restoration of normal tibiotalar relationship; and (3) restoration of satisfactory painless range of motion. If it does not seem likely that these three requirements can be fulfilled, attempts at "joint preserving" reconstructive surgery should be abandoned. Several specific situations involving malleolar malunion deserve discussion.

Fibular Fracture With Widened Mortise and Lateral Shift of the Talus

Relatively mild degrees of fibular shortening and external rotation may be responsible for persistent symptoms and may predispose to eventual traumatic arthritis [104]. Weber has referred to this condition as the "sprung mortise" and has described the characteristic roentgenographic findings demonstrable on the 20° internal rotation view of the ankle [104]: (1) slight widening of the medial clear space; (2) interruption of the dense subchondral bone contour of the syndesmotic edge of the fibula; and (3) interruption of the symmetric relationship between the articular surface of the fibula and lateral facet of the talus (Fig. 15.2). For this deformity, Weber [104] and others [38,73] have advised lengthening-derotation osteotomy of the fibula. It is suggested that the procedure can be performed successfully any time prior to the demonstration of significant traumatic arthritis.

Technique (Weber) [104]

The distal fibula is exposed and the fibular incisura freed of scar tissue, so as to permit eventual reduction of the syndesmosis [104]. A narrow five-hole plate is fixed to the distal end of the

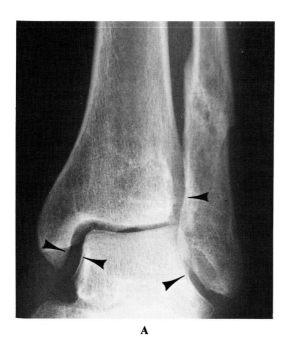

A

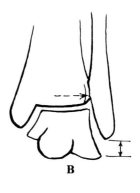

B

Fig. 15.2. "Sprung mortise." A Radiograph. B Schematic. See text for explanation.

fibula, and a special device which allows for distraction and compression is applied to the proximal end of the plate and fixed to the adjacent fibula with a screw. The fibula is then osteotomized transversely. Using the special device, the fibula is simultaneously lengthened and internally rotated approximately 10° until it fits properly between the anterior and posterior tubercles of the distal tibia. A radiograph is obtained to confirm restoration of fibular length and tibiotalar alignment. If normal tibiotalar relationship cannot be readily restored, the medial ankle must be explored for excision of scar tissue or osteotomy of the medial malleolus. A small corticocancellous graft obtained from the medial aspect of the distal tibia is then inserted into the osteotomy site and the osteotomy is compressed using the special device. The plate is then affixed to the proximal fibular fragment with three screws (Fig. 15.3).

Ordinarily, this will correct rotatory deformity as well as shortening. If there is any question about maintaining reduction of the tibiofibular syndesmosis, however, a transfixion screw can be employed to provide temporary tibiofibular fixation. This should be removed at 8 to 12 weeks.

Malunited Trimalleolar Fracture

For trimalleolar fractures characterized by a large posterior tibial lip fragment and posterior dislocation of the talus, attempts at malleolar reconstruction are uniformly unsuccessful [88,93]. Due to soft tissue scarring and osteoporosis of the displaced posterior fragment, it is extremely difficult to correct longstanding deformity of this type. Even if corrected, the result is likely to be impaired by irreversible damage to the articular cartilage. Under these circum-

stances, arthrodesis of the ankle is the procedure of choice.

Supramalleolar Fractures

Residual varus or valgus deformity at the ankle secondary to supramalleolar fracture lends itself well to correction by osteotomy provided tibiotalar relationship is normal [88,93]. Ideally, the osteotomy should be fixed internally so as to permit early resumption of active ankle motion.

Pes Planovalgus

At one time, when strictly conservative treatment of ankle fractures was practiced more widely, pes planovalgus deformity was occasionally encountered as a complication of external rotation and abduction injuries of the ankle [50,53,56–58]. It has never been satisfactorily explained; but it is probably a manifestation of external rotation deformity of the talus, secondary to residual deltoid ligament insufficiency and/or rotational deformity at the fibular fracture site [50,80]. It is rarely mentioned in the recent literature, presumably because increased attention to restoration of fibular anatomy, with both open and closed treatment, has made it an uncommon sequela [53, 101].

Tibiofibular Synostosis

A mild degree of ossification or dystrophic calcification within the interosseous ligament and/or interosseous membrane occurs commonly following injury to these structures. Complete ossification or tibiofibular synostosis, however, is un-

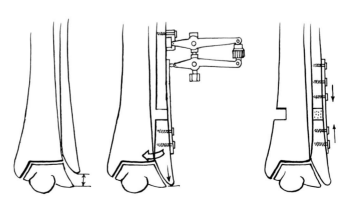

Fig. 15.3. Lengthening-derotation osteotomy of the distal fibula (after Weber). See text.

common. It can complicate injuries treated by closed or operative means [35,63,81].

Complete synostosis which eliminates tibiofibular motion is certain to impair ankle resiliency, and theoretically should predispose to joint dysfunction and degenerative arthritis. Grath [35], however, studied this phenomenon in great detail, and was unable to demonstrate any association between apparent complete synostosis and functional disturbance. Of 14 patients with complete tibiofibular synostosis, ten had neither symptoms nor evidence of functional disability. Grath observed that most tibiofibular widening occurred between plantarflexion and neutral position and very little occurred with weight bearing or with dorsiflexion above neutral. He concluded that a complete synostosis with the foot at or near 90° with respect to the leg need not have any detrimental effect on joint function. Since the introduction of axial tomography, our experience and that of others [54] indicate that many apparent synostoses do not constitute a complete osseous bridge between the two bones, even though they may appear quite dense on plain radiographs (Fig. 15.4). Grath did not have the benefit of axial tomography and it is quite possible that many of his ten asymptomatic patients did not have a truly complete synostosis. However, we have also observed some patients with apparently normal, painless function following longstanding surgical arthrodesis of the tibiofibular joint for persistent diastasis (Fig. 15.5). Why this condition is well tolerated by some patients and not by others is unknown at present.

Little can be done to prevent spontaneous tibiofibular ossification, but to reduce the incidence of this complication following operation on the fibula or tibiofibular interval, surgical trauma to this area should be minimized and tibiofibular fixation should only be employed when absolutely necessary to temporarily stabilize tibiofibular relationship [68].

McMaster and Scranton [63] have reported successful excision of a symptomatic tibiofibular synostosis in seven patients.

Instability

The consequences and treatment of lateral ligamentous insufficiency have been discussed in Chapter 9.

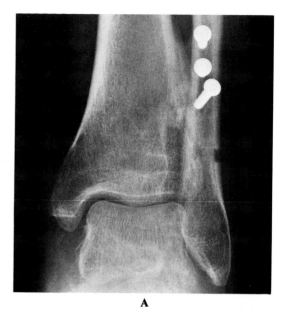

A

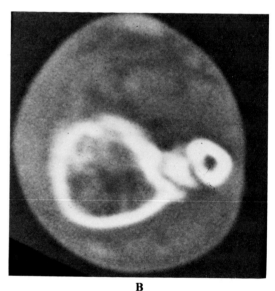

B

Fig. 15.4. A Pronation-external rotation injury, stage IV, treated with interfragmentary screw fixation of the fibular fracture and temporary tibiofibular screw transfixion. Four months following surgery, plain films suggested that a tibiofibular synostosis had developed. **B** Axial tomography, however, demonstrated that the apparent synostosis was incomplete.

Although isolated deltoid ligament rupture theoretically is possible, it is not common [95]. Moreover, medial instability of the ankle cannot persist as an isolated phenomenon [60,78,81, 95,96,109]. Any widening of the medial clear space suggesting deltoid insufficiency must neces-

Traumatic Arthritis

The ankle is rarely involved by primary osteoarthritis [51,97]. When degenerative arthritis affects this joint, it is usually as a result of injury. Premature degenerative arthritis is the most common cause of serious disability following injury of the ankle. It may occur as a result of primary irreversible cartilage damage at the time of injury, or secondarily as a consequence of instability or uncorrected deformity. In either event, signs and symptoms will usually become apparent within 2 to 3 years of injury [53,107]. Certain mechanical disturbances by themselves, however, may cause pain and disability prior to the development of articular cartilage changes, and it is sometimes difficult or impossible to ascertain exactly when degenerative arthritis intervenes.

Magnusson [56–58] and Klossner [47] relied heavily on marginal osteophytes and contour changes of bone as an indication of arthrosis. These changes, however, do not correlate especially well with symptoms [56,98,101,107], and in many instances, probably only reflect posttraumatic bone reaction. One is on much firmer ground if the diagnosis of "arthritis" is reserved for those patients with demonstrable joint space narrowing [20,53], in addition to the peripheral joint changes and appropriate clinical symptoms. Mild cases of traumatic ankle arthritis can often be managed by conservative measures, including analgesics, nonsteroidal antiinflammatory agents, local corticosteroid injection, physical therapy, and customized footwear. Baker [4] has recommended the use of a SACH heel and rocker bottom sole for this condition. If symptoms remain uncontrolled by conservative measures, surgical intervention should be considered. Options are generally limited to joint replacement or arthrodesis.

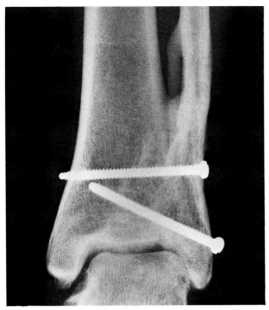

Fig. 15.5. Patient without pain or functional limitation 15 years after distal tibiofibular arthrodesis, performed because of persistent painful diastasis.

sarily be associated with tibiofibular ligamentous diastasis or displaced fracture of the distal fibula [41]. Primary treatment that includes satisfactory reduction of the lateral side of the ankle will indirectly close the medial clear space and oppose the ends of the torn deltoid ligament [11,28, 60,109], unless there is interposed ligament or flexor tendon at this site; in this case, medial exploration will be necessary as well [17,45,95].

When widening of the medial clear space persists after treatment, it implies coexisting malunion of the fibular fracture or disturbance of the distal tibiofibular syndesmosis. The radiographic "clear" space is actually occupied by an interposed structure or becomes filled with scar tissue. Mediolateral instability of the talus is generally not increased, but the talus is forced to articulate in an incongruous fashion with the tibial plafond [102]. The net result is reduction in contact surface of the tibiotalar joint with abnormal concentration of forces rather than true instability. This condition should be prevented if at all possible. Fibular malunion, if recognized early before the advent of significant degenerative changes, can often be improved by osteotomy as already described.

References

1. Abramson DI, Miller DS: Vascular Problems in Musculoskeletal Disorders of the Limbs. New York, Springer-Verlag, 1981.
2. Alho A, Koskinen EVS, Malmberg H: Osteomyelitis in nonoperative and operative fracture treatment. Clin Orthop Rel Res 82:123, 1972.
3. Alldredge RH: Diastasis of the distal tibiofibular joint and associated lesions. JAMA 115: 2136, 1940.

4. Baker PL: SACH heel improves results of ankle fusion. J Bone Joint Surg 52A:1485, 1970.

5. Banks SW: The treatment of nonunion of fractures of the medial malleolus. J Bone Joint Surg 31A:658, 1949.

6. Bistrom O: Conservative treatment of severe ankle fractures. A clinical and follow-up study. Acta Chir Scand (Suppl) 168:1, 1952.

7. Bohler L: The Treatment of Fractures, 5th ed. New York, Grune & Stratton, 1956.

8. Bolin H: The fibula and its relationship to the tibia and talus in injuries of the ankle due to forced external rotation. Acta Radiol 56:439, 1961.

9. Bonica JJ: Causalgia and other reflex sympathetic dystrophies. Postgrad Med 53:143, 1973.

10. Bonnin JG: Late results and complications of ankle injuries. In: Injuries to the Ankle. New York, Grune & Stratton, 1950.

11. Bonnin JG: Injury to the ligaments of the ankle. J Bone Joint Surg 47B:609, 1965.

12. Braunstein PW, Wade PA: Treatment of unstable fractures of the ankle. Ann Surg 149:217, 1959.

13. Brighton CT, Black J, Friedenberg ZB, Esterlai JL, Day LJ, Connolly JF: A multicenter study of the treatment of non-union with constant direct current. J Bone Joint Surg 63A:2, 1981.

14. Brodie IAOD, Denham RA: The treatment of unstable ankle fractures. J Bone Joint Surg 56B:256, 1974.

15. Burgess E: Fractures of the ankle. J Bone Joint Surg 26:721, 1944.

16. Burns BH: Diastasis of the inferior tibio-fibular joint. Proc Roy Soc Med 36:330, 1943.

17. Burwell HN, Charnley AD: Treatment of displaced fractures at the ankle by rigid internal fixation and early joint movement. J Bone Joint Surg 47B:634, 1965.

18. Cave EF, (ed): Ankle injuries. In: Fractures and Other Injuries. Chicago, Year Book Medical, 1958.

19. Cave EF: Complications of the operative treatment of fractures of the ankle. Clin Orthop Rel Res 42:13, 1965.

20. Cedell C-A: Supination-outward rotation injuries of the ankle. Acta Orthop Scand (Suppl) 110:1, 1967.

21. Cedell C-A, Wiberg G: Treatment of eversion-supination fracture of the ankle (second degree). Acta Chir Scand 124:41, 1962.

22. Close R: Some applications of the functional anatomy of the ankle joint. J Bone Joint Surg 38A:761, 1956.

23. Coonrad RW: Fracture-dislocations of the ankle joint with impaction injury of the lateral weight-bearing surface of the tibia. J Bone Joint Surg 52A:1337, 1970.

24. Coonrad RW, Lincoln CR: Unstable ankle injuries. Important factors and errors in evaluation, diagnosis and treatment. J Bone Joint Surg 49A:1013, 1967.

25. Cox FJ: Fractures of the ankle involving the lower articular surface of the tibia. Clin Orthop 42:51, 1965.

26. Cox FJ, Laxson WW: Fractures about the ankle joint. Am J Surg 83:674, 1952.

27. Crenshaw AH: Delayed union and nonunion of fractures. In Edmonson AS, Crenshaw AH (eds): Campbell's Operative Orthopaedics, 6th ed. St. Louis, Mosby, 1980.

28. Denham RA: Internal fixation for unstable ankle fractures. J Bone Joint Surg 46B:206, 1964.

29. Dewar FP, Martin RF: A survey of fractures involving the ankle joint. J Bone Joint Surg 50B:433, 1968.

30. Dewar FP, Martin FR: Ankle fusions following closed ankle fractures. J Bone Joint Surg 54B:768, 1972.

31. Eventov I, Salama R, Goodwin DRA, Weissman SL: An evaluation of surgical and conservative treatment of fractures of the ankle in 200 patients. J Trauma 18:271, 1978.

32. Freeman MAR, Dean MRE, Hanham IWF: The etiology and prevention of functional instability of the foot. J Bone Joint Surg 47B:678, 1965.

33. Gaston SR, McLaughlin HL: Complex fracture of the lateral malleolus. J Trauma 1:69, 1961.

34. Golterman AFL: Diagnosis and treatment of tibiofibular diastasis. Arch Chir Neerl 16:185, 1964.

35. Grath G: Widening of the ankle mortise. A clinical and experimental study. Acta Chir Scand (Suppl) 263:1, 1960.

36. Henderson MS, Stuck WG: Fractures of the ankle: Recent and old. J Bone Joint Surg 15:882, 1933.

37. Hughes J: The medial malleolus in ankle fractures. Orthop Clin North Am 11:649, 1980.

38. Hughes JL: Corrective Osteotomies of the fibula after defectively healed ankle fractures. J Bone Joint Surg 58A:728, 1976.

39. Jergesen F: Open reduction of fractures and dislocations of the ankle. Am J Surg 98:136, 1959.

40. Johnson JB, Cavallaro DC: Post-traumatic reflex sympathetic dystrophy. J Am Podiatry Assoc 67:870, 1977.

41. Joy G, Patzakis MJ, Harvey JP Jr: Precise evaluation of the reduction of severe ankle fractures. Technique and correlation with end results. J Bone Joint Surg 56A:979, 1974.

42. Julsrud ME: A review of reflex sympathetic dystrophy. J Am Podiatry Assoc 70:512, 1980.

43. Key JA, Conwell HE: Injuries in the region of the ankle. In: The Management of Fractures, Dislocations and Sprains, 6th ed. St. Louis, Mosby, 1956.

44. Kimizuka M, Kurosawa H, Fukubayashi T: Load-bearing pattern of the ankle joint. Contact area and pressure distribution. Arch Orthop Trauma Surg 96:45, 1980.

45. Kleiger B: Treatment of oblique fractures of the fibula. J Bone Joint Surg 43:969, 1961.

46. Kleiger B: Mechanisms of ankle injury. Orthop Clin North Am 5:127, 1974.

47. Klossner O: Late results of operative and non-operative treatment of severe ankle fractures. A clinical study. Acta Chir Scand (Suppl) 293:1, 1962.

48. Kozin F, McCarty DJ, Sims J, Genant H: The reflex sympathetic dystrophy syndrome. Am J Med 60:321, 1976.

49. Kristensen TB: Treatment of malleolar fractures according to Lauge-Hansen's method. Preliminary results. Acta Chir Scand 97:362, 1949.

50. Kristensen TB: Fractures of the ankle. VI. Follow-up studies. AMA Arch Surg 73:112, 1956.

51. Laurin CA: The surgical management of degenerative lesions of the foot and ankle. In Cruess RL, Mitchell NS (eds): Surgical Management of Degenerative Arthritis of the Lower Limb. Philadelphia, Lea & Febiger, 1975.

52. Lewis RW, Graham WC: Secondary osteoarthritis following fractures of the ankle. Am J Surg 49:210, 1940.

53. Lindsjo U: Operative treatment of ankle fractures. Acta Orthop Scand (Suppl) 189:1, 1981.

54. Lindsjo U, Hemmingsson A, Sahlstedt B, Danckwardt-Lilliestrom G: Computed tomography of the ankle. Acta Orthop Scand 50:797, 1979.

55. MacKinnon AP: Fracture of the lower articular surface of the tibia in fracture dislocation of the ankle. J Bone Joint Surg 10:352, 1928.

56. Magnusson R: On the late results in non-operated cases of malleolar fractures. I. Fractures by external rotation. Acta Chir Scand (Suppl) 84:1, 1944.

57. Magnusson R: On the late results in non-operated cases of malleolar fractures. II. Fractures by pronation. Acta Chir Scand 92:162, 1945.

58. Magnusson R: On the late results in non-operated cases of malleolar fractures. III. Fractures by supination together with a survey of the late results in non-operatively treated malleolar fractures. Acta Chir Scand 92:259, 1945.

59. Malka JS, Taillard W: Results of non-operative and operative treatment of fractures of the ankle. Clin Orthop Rel Res 67:159, 1969.

60. Mast JW, Teipner WA: A reproducible approach to the internal fixation of adult ankle fractures: Rationale, technique and early results. Orthop Clin North Am 11:661, 1980.

61. McDaniel WJ, Wilson FC: Trimalleolar fractures of the ankle. An end result study. Clin Orthop Rel Res 122:37, 1977.

62. McLaughlin HL: Trauma. Philadelphia, Saunders, 1960.

63. McMaster JH, Scranton PE Jr: Tibiofibular synostosis: A cause of ankle disability. J Bone Joint Surg 57A:1035, 1975.

64. McNeur JC: The management of open skeletal trauma with particular reference to internal fixation. J Bone Joint Surg 52B:54, 1970.

65. Mendelsohn HA: Nonunion of malleolar fractures of ankle. Clin Orthop 42:103, 1965.

66. Mindell ER, Rogers WJ III: Refracture of ununited medial malleolus. Clin Orthop 11:233, 1958.

67. Mitchell WG, Shaftan GW, Sclafani S: Mandatory open reduction: Its role in displaced ankle fractures. J Trauma 19:602, 1979.

68. Müller ME, Allgöwer M, Schneider R, Willenegger H: Manual of Internal Fixation, 2nd ed. Translated by J. Schatzker. New York, Springer-Verlag, 1979.

69. Nahigian SH, Oh I, Zahrawi FB: Wire-loop fixation of the lateral malleolus in ankle fractures. In Bateman JE, Trott AW (eds): The Foot and Ankle. New York, Thieme-Stratton, 1980.

70. Neer CS II: Injuries of the ankle joint. Evaluation. Conn State Med J 17:580, 1953.

71. Neufeld AJ: Ankle joint fractures and their treatment. Clin Orthop 42:91, 1965.

72. Nyström G: A contribution to the treatment of fractures of the posterior border of the tibia by malleolar fractures. Acta Radiol 25:672, 1944.

73. Offierski CM, Hall JH, Harris WR, Graham JD, Schatzker J: Late revision of fibular malunion in ankle fractures. J Bone Joint Surg 63B:460, 1981.

74. Packard AG Jr: Unusual fractures and orthopedic problems. Maryland State Med J 23(10):93, 1974.

75. Pak TJ, Martin GM, Magness JL, Kavanaugh GJ: Reflex sympathetic dystrophy. Minnesota Med 53:507, 1970.

76. Pankovich AM: Adult ankle fractures. JCE Orthop 7:17, 1979.

77. Perkins G: Injuries around the ankle. In: Fractures and Dislocations. London, Athlone Press, 1958.

78. Phillips RS, Balmer GA, Monk CJE: The external rotation fracture of the fibular malleolus. Br J Surg 56:55, 1969.

79. Phillips WA, Spiegel PG: Evaluation of ankle fractures, non-operative vs. operative. Clin Orthop Rel Res 138:17, 1979.

80. Purvis GD: The unstable oblique distal fibular fracture. Clin Orthop Rel Res 92:330, 1973.

81. Quigley TB: Analysis and treatment of ankle injuries produced by rotatory, abduction and adduction forces. Instructional Course Lectures. Am Acad Orthop Surg 19:172, 1970.

82. Rittmann WW, Schibli M, Matter P, Allgöwer M: Open fractures. Clin Orthop Rel Res 138:132, 1979.

83. Rüedi TP, Allgöwer M: Fractures of the lower end of the tibia into the ankle-joint. Injury 1:92, 1969.

84. Rüedi TP, Allgöwer M: The operative treatment of intra-articular fractures of the lower end of the tibia. Clin Orthop Rel Res 138:105, 1979.

85. Rütt A: The talocrural joint. In Stiasny G (ed): Surgery of the Lower Leg and Foot. Philadel-

phia, Saunders, 1980.

86. Sarkisian JS, Cody GW: Closed treatment of ankle fractures: A new criterion for evaluation. A review of 250 cases. J Trauma 16:323, 1976.

87. Sisk TD: In Edmonson AP, Crenshaw AH (eds): Campbell's Operative Orthopaedics, 6th ed. St. Louis, Mosby, 1980.

88. Smith H: Malunited fractures. In Edmonson AP, Crenshaw AH (eds): Campbell's Operative Orthopaedics, 6th ed. St. Louis, Mosby, 1980.

89. Sneppen O: Pseudoarthrosis of lateral malleolus. Acta Orthop Scand 42:187, 1971.

90. Sneppen O: Treatment of pseudoarthrosis involving the malleolus. A postoperative follow-up of 34 cases. Acta Orthop Scand 42:201, 1971.

91. Solonen KA, Lauttamus L: Treatment of malleolar fractures. Acta Orthop Scand 36:321, 1965.

92. Solonen KA, Lauttamus L: Operative treatment of ankle fractures. Acta Orthop Scand 39:223, 1968.

93. Speed JS, Boyd HB: Operative reconstruction of malunited fractures about the ankle joint. J Bone Joint Surg 27:270, 1936.

94. Spiegel PG: Early internal fixation in open fractures. Clin Orthop Rel Res 138:20, 1979.

95. Staples OS: Injuries to the medial ligaments of the ankle. J Bone Joint Surg 42A:1287, 1960.

96. Staples OS: Ligamentous injuries of the ankle joint. Clin Orthop 42:21, 1965.

97. Stauffer RN: Total ankle joint replacement as an alternative to arthrodesis. Geriatrics 31:79, 1976.

98. Stören G: Conservative treatment of ankle fractures: Follow-up of 99 fractures treated conservatively. Acta Chir Scand 128:45, 1964.

99. Thompson JE: The diagnosis and management of post-traumatic pain syndromes (causalgia). Aust NZ J Surg 49:299, 1979.

100. Trethowan WH: Fractures in the neighborhood of the ankle-joint. II. The operative treatment of ankle fractures. Lancet 1:90, 1926.

101. Vasli S: Operative treatment of ankle fractures. Acta Chir Scand (Suppl) 226:1, 1957.

102. Walheim T: Intra-articular malleolar fractures. A survey. Acta Chir Scand 79:166, 1937.

103. Watson-Jones R: Fractures and Other Joint Injuries, 4th ed. Baltimore, Williams & Wilkins, 1955.

104. Weber BG: Lengthening osteotomy of the fibula to correct a widened mortise of the ankle after fracture. Int Orthop 4:289, 1981.

105. Wheelhouse WW, Rosenthal RE: Unstable ankle fractures: Comparison of closed versus open treatment. South Med J 73:45, 1980.

106. Williams WR: Reflex sympathetic dystrophy. Rheumat Rehabil 16:119, 1977.

107. Wilson FC Jr, Skilbred LA: Long-term results in the treatment of displaced bimalleolar fractures. J Bone Joint Surg 48A:1065, 1966.

108. Wilson RL: Management of pain following peripheral nerve injuries. Orthop Clin North Am 12:343, 1981.

109. Yablon IG, Heller FG, Shouse L: The key role of the lateral malleolus in displaced fractures of the ankle. J Bone Joint Surg 59A:169, 1977.

110. Yde J, Kristensen KD: Ankle fractures: Supination-eversion fractures of stage IV. Acta Orthop Scand 51:981, 1980.

Chapter 16 Injuries of the Talus

S. Terry Canale and James H. Beaty

Anatomy

The most distal bone of the ankle is the talus, consisting of a body, dome, neck, and head (Fig. 1.5). Coltart [13] has referred to it as the "universal joint of the foot" because of its mechanical importance. Besides articulating with the distal tibia and fibula to form the ankle joint, the talus articulates with the os calcis and navicular to form the talocalcaneal and talonavicular joints, respectively.

Ligament attachments to the talus are numerous to provide stability at the ankle, subtalar, and talonavicular joints. At the ankle level, insertions include the deep deltoid ligament from the tibia (Fig. 16.1B) and the talofibular ligaments (anterior and posterior) from the fibula (Fig. 16.1B,C). The interosseous talocalcaneal ligament forms the chief bond between the talus and the os calcis (Fig. 16.1B). It is supplemented by the anterior, posterior, medial, and lateral talocalcaneal ligaments (Fig. 16.1A,C). The strong dorsal talonavicular ligament provides most of the stability of the talonavicular joint (Fig. 16.1C) [19].

Anatomically, the talus has two unique characteristics. First, most of its surface is articular so that deformity or incongruity is poorly tolerated. Second, it has a retrograde blood supply derived from three main sources: through the neck of the talus, through the foramina in the sinus tarsi and tarsal canal, and through the foramina in the medial surface of the body (Fig. 16.2) [22,26,35]. Because of this retrograde blood supply, fractures of the neck of the talus account for a much higher incidence of avascular necrosis of the body of the talus than do fractures of the body itself [10,22].

Fractures of the Neck of the Talus

Fractures of the neck of the talus have received considerable attention in the literature because of their potentially disabling effects, especially when associated with avascular necrosis of the body [3,5,6,10,11,13,17,21,22,25,26,30,31,33,35, 37,43,45]. Anderson, [1] and Shands [41] noted that these fractures occur secondary to major trauma, usually as a result of dorsiflexion injury (aviator's astragalus). Talar neck fractures have been classified by Hawkins [22] into three types (Fig. 16.3). The type of fracture indicates the degree to which the blood supply of the talus has been disturbed. The incidence of avascular necrosis increases with the severity of the fracture type.

Type I   Talar neck fracture with minimal displacement; only one source of blood supply (that entering through the neck) is possibly disrupted.

Type II   Talar neck fracture associated with subtalar subluxation or dislocation; at least two of the three sources of blood supply are jeopardized (that entering through the neck and that entering through the tarsal canal) (Fig. 16.4).

Type III   Talar neck fracture associated with dislocation of the body of the talus from the ankle joint; all three sources of blood supply are disrupted (Fig. 16.5).

We have also observed and described a type IV injury, characterized by fracture of the talar neck in association with subluxation/dislocation of the body of the talus from the ankle or subtalar joint as well as subluxation/dislocation of the head of the talus from the talonavicular joint (Figs. 16.6 and 16.7) [10].

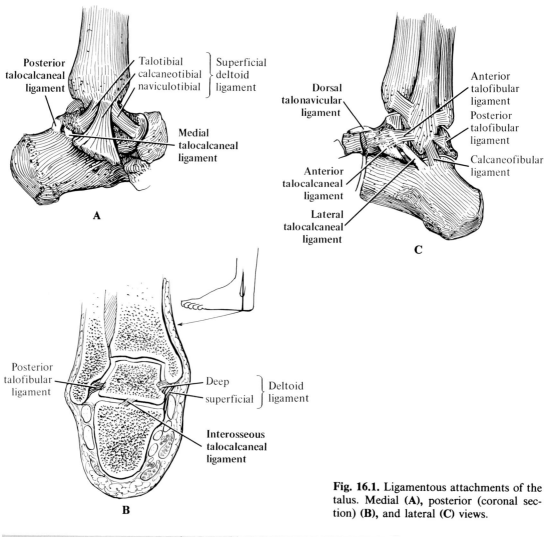

Fig. 16.1. Ligamentous attachments of the talus. Medial **(A)**, posterior (coronal section) **(B)**, and lateral **(C)** views.

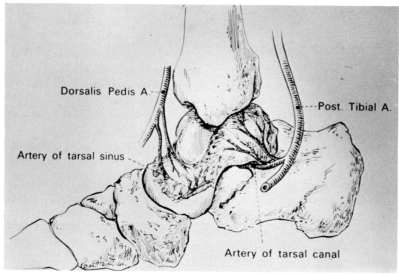

Fig. 16.2. Sources of blood supply to the talus. Reprinted with permission from Buckingham WW Jr: Subtalar dislocation of the foot. J Trauma 13:753, 1973. The Williams & Wilkins Co., Baltimore.

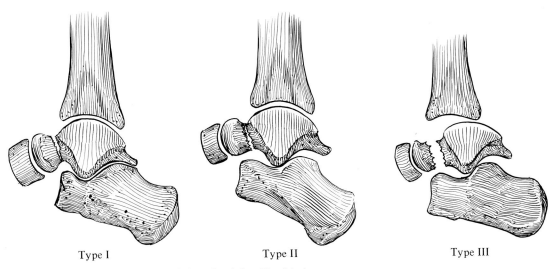

Type I   Type II   Type III

Fig. 16.3. Fractures of the neck of the talus (after Hawkins).

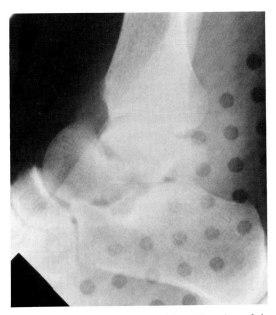

Fig. 16.4. Talar neck fracture with subluxation of the subtalar joint (type II).

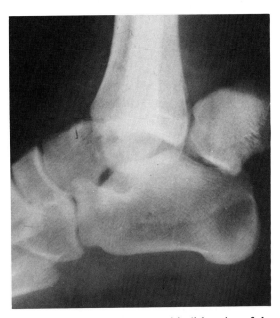

Fig. 16.5. Talar neck fracture with dislocation of the body of the talus from the ankle and subtalar joints (type III). Reprinted with permission from Canale ST, Kelly FB Jr: Fractures of the neck of the talus. Long-term evaluation of 71 cases. J Bone Joint Surg 60A:143, 1978.

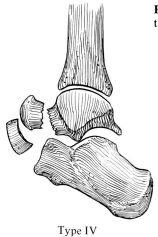

Fig. 16.6. Type IV fracture of the talar neck, characterized by disruption of the subtalar and talonavicular joints.

Type IV

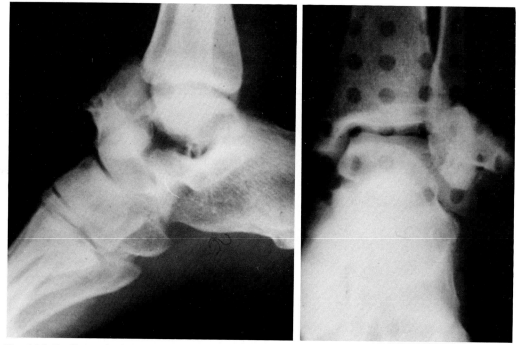

Fig. 16.7. Radiograph of a type IV fracture of the talar neck: talonavicular joint is dislocated.

At the Campbell Clinic, we have reviewed the long-term results of 71 patients with fractures of the neck of the talus [10]. The distribution of the 71 injuries was as follows: type I, 15 (21%); type II, 30 (42%); type III, 23 (32%); and type IV, 3 (4%). Fifty-four of the 71 fractures were closed and 17 (24%) of the injuries were open. There were ten associated medial malleolus fractures and one associated lateral malleolus fracture.

Treatment

We continue to subscribe to the treatment recommendations of Boyd and Knight [6]: mild to moderately displaced fractures are treated by closed reduction, followed by immobilization in non–weight-bearing plaster. A reduction characterized by less than 5 mm of displacement and less than 5° of malalignment is considered adequate. If satisfactory reduction cannot be obtained by

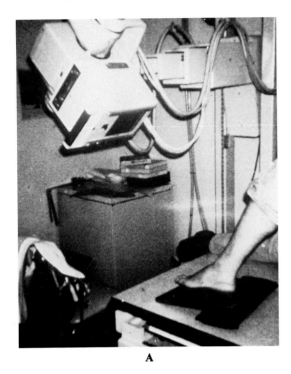

A

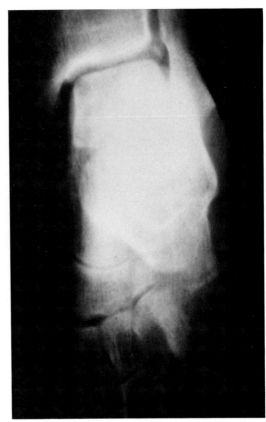

B

Fig. 16.8. A Roentgenographic projection to determine adequacy of reduction of talar neck fractures. **B** Radiograph obtained with this technique demonstrating excellent alignment of talar head, neck, and body.

closed measures, open reduction with internal fixation is performed. Because of the difficulty in obtaining and maintaining adequate closed reduction in highly displaced type II, III, and IV fractures, open reduction is frequently necessary for these injuries. Open fractures are treated by wound debridement and irrigation; internal fixation is used only if necessary to secure fracture position. These wounds generally are left open.

For optimal radiographic visualization of the talus to ensure adequate reduction, we employ a modification of the "oblique dorsiplantarflexion" view (Chapter 4) in addition to routine anteroposterior and lateral projections [10]. This radiograph is made with the cassette directly under the foot. The ankle is placed in maximum equinus (this usually being the proper position following reduction of fractures of the talar neck). Positioning can be facilitated by flexing the hip and knee. The foot is then pronated 15° and the tube is directed cephalad at a 75° angle from the horizontal (Fig. 16.8A). This technique readily permits detection of any offset or varus deformity of the head and neck of the talus (Fig. 16.8B).

When operative intervention is required, we prefer to approach the talus through an anteromedial, rather than anterolateral, incision, since the malalignment is medial in most instances [16]. We routinely use a cancellous screw to maintain reduction (Fig. 16.9). Occasionally, in type III fractures with displacement of the talar neck and body, the displaced fragment may be trapped behind the medial malleolus and, on rare occasions, osteotomy of the medial malleolus is required (Fig. 16.10). Occasionally, the displacement is so significant that repositioning of the talar body into proper articular alignment is exceptionally difficult; the surgeon can easily be misled because of the many articulations of the talus.

Complications

In our experience, type I fractures generally do well following closed reduction and immobili-

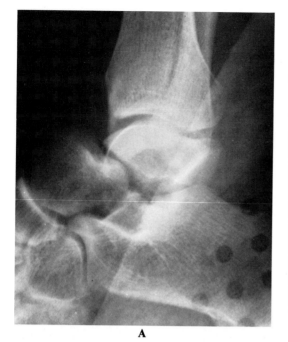

A

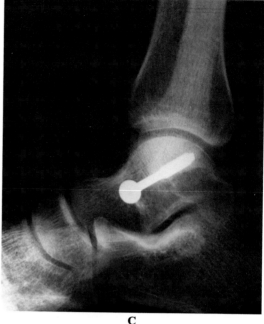

C

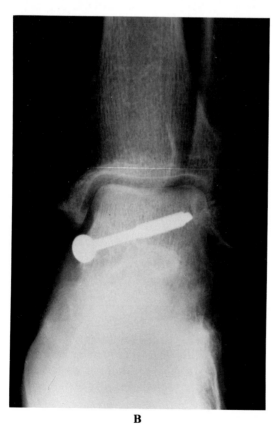

B

Fig. 16.9. Type II talar neck fracture. **A** Preoperative radiograph. **B** and **C** Following open reduction and cancellous screw fixation using an anteromedial surgical approach.

zation in non–weight-bearing plaster. Type II, III, and IV injuries, however, regardless of treatment, are complicated in a high percentage of cases by avascular necrosis, malunion, infection, and/or degenerative arthritis of the ankle or subtalar joint.

Avascular Necrosis

In our series, avascular necrosis of the talar body occurred in 37 of 71 fractures (52%). The incidence was lowest (13%) in type I fractures. The development of avascular necrosis in minimally or nondisplaced fractures is uncommon because only one source of blood supply is involved. In type II fractures, however, two or possibly three sources of blood supply to the talus may be jeopardized and avascular necrosis is much more common. This complication occurred in 50% of the type II fractures in our series. Like other investigators [3,6,22,25,26,31,37], we were unable to identify which type II fractures would eventually develop avascular necrosis. The occurrence of this complication did not appear, however, to be increased in open injuries, and the incidence did not correlate with either open or closed methods of treatment. In type III fractures, all three sources of blood supply are likely to be compromised and avascular necrosis can be expected in a high percentage of cases. We

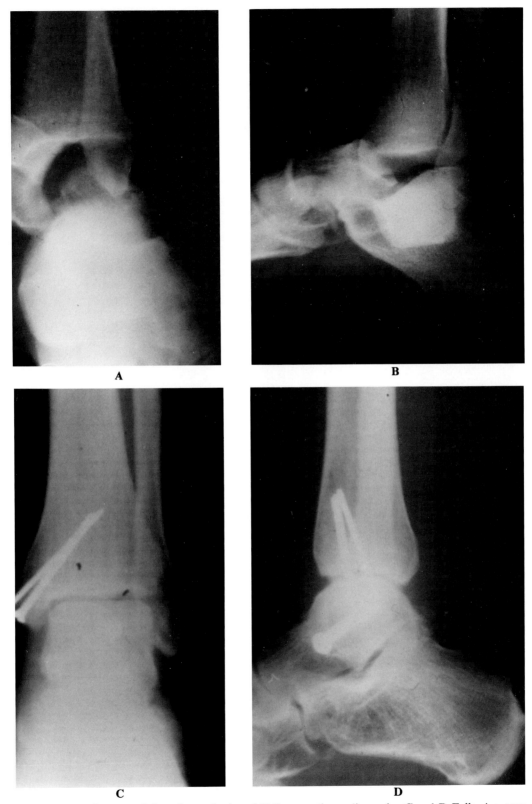

Fig. 16.10. Type III fracture of the talar neck. **A** and **B** Preoperative radiographs. **C** and **D** Following open reduction and screw fixation, facilitated by medial malleolar osteotomy.

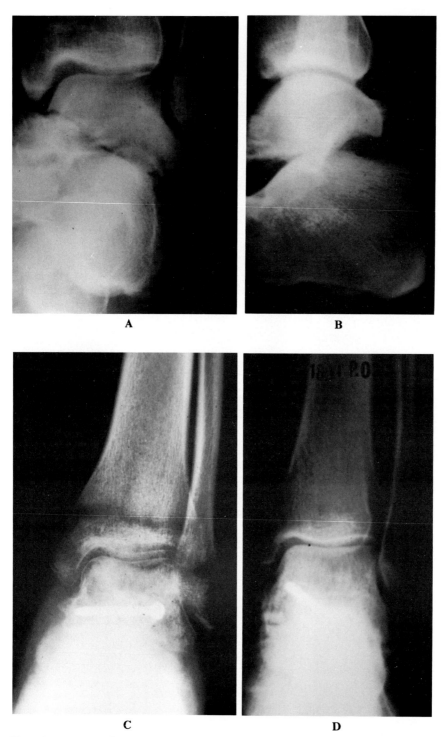

Fig. 16.11. Type II fracture of the talar neck. **A** and **B** Preoperative radiographs. **C** Four months following open reduction and internal fixation. A subchondral radiolucency (Hawkins sign) had developed indicating viability of the body of the talus. **D** Eighteen years later, the patient had no symptoms and no roentgenographic evidence of avascular necrosis. Reprinted with permission from Canale ST, Kelly FB Jr: Fractures of the neck of the talus. Long-term evaluation of 71 cases. J Bone Joint Surg 60A:143, 1978.

observed this complication in 84% of our type III injuries. Other authors have reported a 75 to 100% incidence [6,13,22,25,26,33,37]. Similarly, in type IV fractures, all primary sources of blood supply are likely to be disrupted and avascular necrosis can be anticipated in a large percentage of cases [10].

Hawkins [22] described a subchondral radiolucency visible in the body of the talus, best seen on anteroposterior radiographs 6–8 weeks after fracture. He thought this was caused by disuse osteopenia or vascular congestion and postulated that it implied maintenance of blood supply to the body of the talus. In order to verify this observation, we retrospectively examined serial radiographs available for 49 of our patients. The Hawkins radiolucency was noted in 23 patients within 12 weeks after injury; only one of these patients developed avascular necrosis (Fig. 16.11). The other 26 patients did not demonstrate a subchondral radiolucency, and in 20 instances avascular necrosis eventually developed (Fig. 16.12). The six patients who failed to demonstrate the subchondral radiolucency and yet did not develop avascular necrosis had all been treated with relatively short periods of immobilization which may explain the absence of osteopenia and subchondral radiolucency, despite preservation of talar blood supply. Our experience, then, paralleled that of Hawkins, in that the presence of a radiolucent zone in the subchondral area of the talus suggested that the body of the talus would not undergo an avascular process; but the absence of this sign did not necessarily imply that avascular necrosis would develop [10].

Because of the variable incidence and uncertain pathogenesis of avascular necrosis of the talus, many forms of treatment have been advocated for this complication, [3,5,6,31,33]. Talectomy was favored for a time, but subsequently lost popularity [32,33]. Blair [3] suggested removing the body of the talus and fusing the remaining head and neck of the talus to the tibia. Mindell et al [33] reviewed 40 cases and concluded that avascular necrosis should be treated conservatively with protection from weight bearing until the necrotic area has been sufficiently replaced by viable bone.

In our series, 23 patients with established avascular necrosis were treated nonoperatively. Nine patients were kept non–weight bearing for an average of 8 months. Partial weight bearing in a patellar tendon brace or short leg brace with limited ankle motion was allowed in six patients. No specific treatment was employed in the remaining eight patients. Table 16.1 reveals that those patients treated by non–weight bearing had more excellent and good results. However, partial weight bearing in a patellar tendon brace appeared to offer a suitable substitute, and was superior to no treatment at all or to unrestricted weight bearing. None of these 23 patients with an average follow-up of 15 years required surgery or developed degenerative joint disease secondary to avascular necrosis. Occasionally, avascular necrosis will develop in a child. Three of our patients with avascular necrosis were under 12 years of age. All were kept non–weight bearing for an average of 5 months. Two of the three developed cystic changes in the talus, but at long-term follow-up all three were considered to have good results (Fig. 16.13).

Many authors have recommended definitive procedures at the time of injury in an attempt to prevent avascular necrosis in type III fractures. These procedures include primary subtalar fusion [22,26,31]. Blair fusion [3], talocalcaneal fusion [32,33,40], and talectomy [8]. Three patients in our series underwent primary subtalar arthrodesis in an attempt to accelerate revascularization of the talus by creeping substitution. Two of these patients experienced poor results with severe degenerative changes in the ankle joint. For this reason, we no longer perform subtalar arthrodesis as a primary procedure to promote talar revascularization. We prefer to restrict

Table 16.1. Results of Nonoperative Treatment of Avascular Necrosis.

	Excellent	Good	Fair	Poor
Non–weight bearing [9]	4	4	1	0
Brace [6]	0	2	3	1
No treatment [8][a]	0	2	1	5

[a] Non–weight bearing for less than 3 months.
From ref. 10.

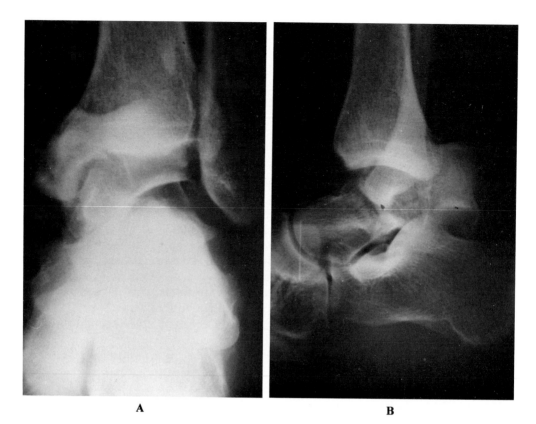

A   B

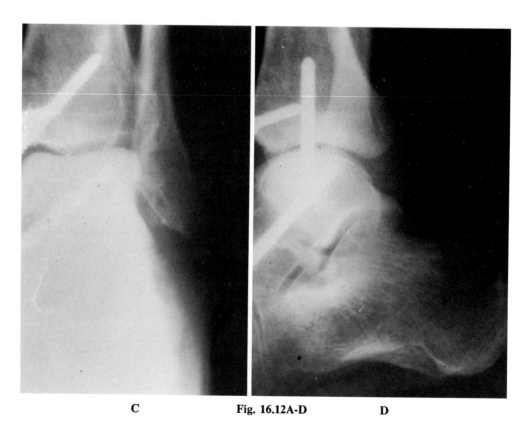

C   Fig. 16.12A-D   D

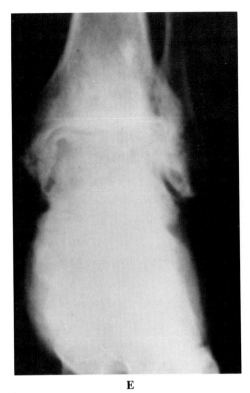

E

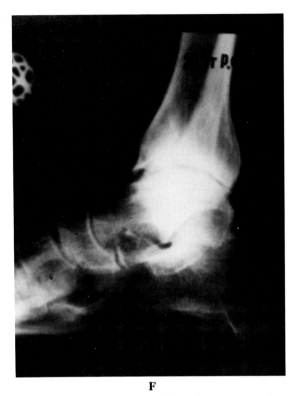

F

Fig. 16.12. Type II fracture of the talar neck. **A** and **B** Preoperative radiographs, **C** and **D** Six months following open reduction and internal fixation with a cancellous screw (via medial malleolar osteotomy). There was no evidence of subchondral radiolucency, suggesting that the body of the talus was avascular. **E** and **F** Twenty years after injury, there was evidence of severe avascular necrosis. The patient fortunately remained asymptomatic.

our initial surgery to open reduction and internal fixation, since one cannot usually predict with any degree of certainty which type II and type III fractures will develop avascular necrosis. Furthermore, many patients with avascular necrosis will obtain satisfactory results following conservative treatment.

Also, when persistent pain associated with avascular necrosis necessitated a secondary procedure, talectomy alone was frequently unsatisfactory in our experience. Instead, we would presently recommend tibiotalar fusion if there is only moderate avascular necrosis of the talus, or tibiocalcaneal fusion is there is extensive involvement (Fig. 16.14).

Recently, we have employed radionuclide bone scanning to examine both tali in patients with suspected or established avascular necrosis. We have not used this as a diagnostic tool because a positive scan after injury could indicate either fracture healing or early revascularization. In-stead, we are using the scan for evaluation for 2 to 3 years following the onset of avascular necrosis, to determine if there is any pattern which could signify "creeping substitution" and healing of the lesion. We hope that this test ultimately will be useful to indicate how long non–weight bearing or bracing should be continued. The bone scan has also helped to determine how much of the talus is involved in the avascular process and has indicated in many instances that the entire body, rather than just the dome, of the talus is involved. This may explain why degenerative changes in the subtalar joint are sometimes observed in association with avascular necrosis of the body of the talus [10].

Malunion

Malunion of a talar neck fracture is usually characterized by angulation in either dorsal or varus position. Malunion was encountered in 18 of our

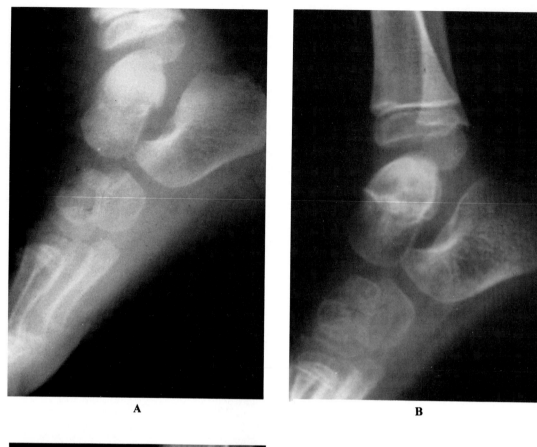

A   B

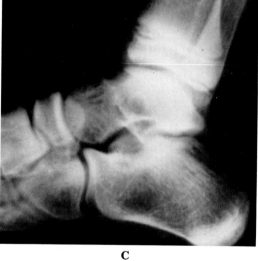

C

Fig. 16.13. A Fracture of the talar neck in a 6-year-old child. B Satisfactory fracture healing, but there is evidence of avascular necrosis with cystic changes in the body of the talus. C Nine years following injury, the patient was asymptomatic and there was no roentgenographic evidence of avascular necrosis.

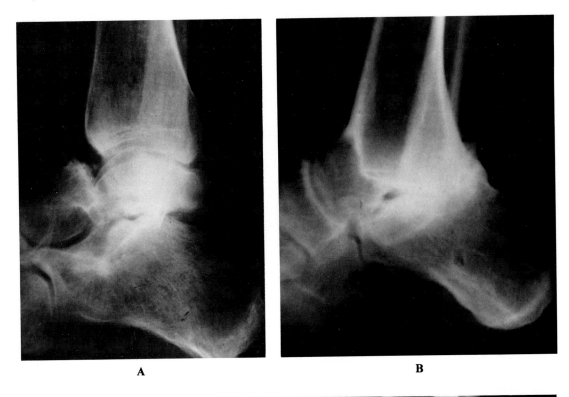

A   B

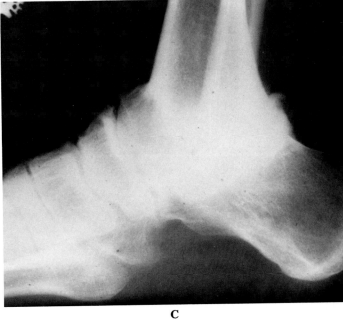

Fig. 16.14. A Type II fracture of the talar neck, complicated by malunion and avascular necrosis of the entire body of the talus. **B** Nine years following Blair tibiotalar fusion, there was a painful false articulation between the tibia and the calcaneus. **C** Symptoms were relieved following tibiocalcaneal fusion.

C

71 patients (25%). The majority occurred in type II fractures. Eleven of these 18 patients had been treated by closed reduction and plaster immobilization.

Four of our patients demonstrated dorsal malunion with pain and restricted dorsiflexion of the ankle. Three of these were converted to satisfactory results following dorsal beak resection of the talar neck. Varus malunion is frequently associated with a prominent fibula (Fig. 16.15). This appears to be a rotational deformity, secondary to varus position of the foot, with the fibula displaced anterior to its normal position. Most patients with this deformity bear an excessive amount of weight on the lateral side of the foot, and in some instances painful degenerative changes develop in the subtalar joint (Fig. 16.16). Five of our 11 patients with varus malunion eventually required triple arthrodesis for severe subtalar degenerative changes. Good results were subsequently obtained in three of these patients.

Traumatic Arthritis of the Ankle and Subtalar Joint

The most common cause of degenerative arthritis of the ankle following fracture of the talar neck is avascular necrosis of the body of the talus [6,10,13,22,25,26,33,37]. Our series, however, did

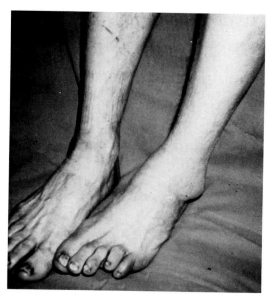

Fig. 16.15. Clinical appearance of a varus malunion of the talar neck. Note the prominent fibula and tendency to bear weight on the lateral aspect of the foot.

include two patients with traumatic arthritis of the ankle secondary to poor reduction of the talar neck fracture and talar body within the ankle mortise. Both patients had associated malleolar fractures. A third patient had an associated fracture of the talar dome and developed mild arthritic changes in the ankle, presumably on this basis.

Degenerative changes in the subtalar joint were observed in 50% of our patients. One-third of these demonstrated malunion. Subtalar arthritis in the remaining patients was thought to be related to disruption of the subtalar joint or, possibly, to avascular necrosis of the inferior aspect of the body of the talus.

Arthrodesis for severe degenerative arthritis of the ankle joint, whether secondary to avascular necrosis or malunion/incongruity, is a satisfactory salvage procedure. Evaluation of the subtalar joint, however, is mandatory. If pain and degenerative changes are present within the subtalar joint, as well as the ankle, an ankle fusion will only serve to accentuate stress on the subtalar articulation. Similarly, triple arthrodesis is a satisfactory salvage procedure for degenerative arthritis localized to the subtalar joint (Fig. 16.17), but a degenerated ankle will be overstressed if the underlying subtalar joint alone is fused (Fig. 16.18). If both the ankle and subtalar joints are involved, we recommend tibiocalcaneal fusion. Some of our worst results occurred following talectomy alone, and we cannot recommend this procedure.

Infection

Open fractures of the talar neck, and rarely closed injuries treated by open reduction, can be complicated by osteomyelitis of the talus with chronic pain and drainage. We observed this complication in five instances. Four of these followed open injuries. All had been treated by early debridement. The wounds had been left open in two cases and internal fixation had not been employed. The fifth infection developed in a closed type III fracture treated by open reduction and internal fixation with primary subtalar fusion.

In our experience, drainage usually persisted following simple soft tissue and bone debridement procedures. Four of our five patients eventually underwent arthrodesis; in each case, fusion was obtained and drainage ceased. One patient

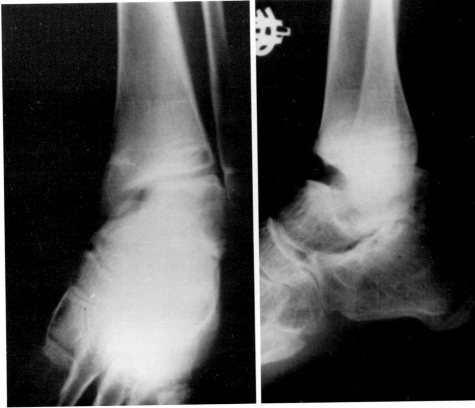

Fig. 16.16. Varus malunion of the talar neck with narrowing, incongruity, and degenerative changes of the subtalar joint.

was treated by talectomy alone without fusion; he experienced persistent disabling pain and was considered a poor result. Because of this, we recommend that chronic infection be treated by excision of all infected material—including part or all of the talus if necessary—followed by ankle, subtalar, or tibiocalcaneal arthrodesis.

Fractures of the Body of the Talus

Fractures of the body account for 10–20% of talar fractures [13,18,25,37]. These injuries can be categorized as nondisplaced, displaced, or comminuted (Fig. 16.19).

Nondisplaced Fractures

Nondisplaced fractures should be treated by immobilization in a short leg, non–weight-bearing cast for 4–8 weeks. Mindell et al. [33] reported a 20% incidence of avascular necrosis in nondisplaced fractures. This is contrary, however, to the experience of Kenwright and Taylor [25], as well as Pennall [37], who observed no instances of avascular necrosis complicating nondisplaced fractures of the body.

Displaced Fractures

Fractures of the body of the talus with displacement ordinarily will require open reduction with internal fixation (Fig. 16.20). The two most important factors affecting prognosis are the amount of initial displacement and the accuracy of reduction. Closed reduction may be attempted, but is almost invariably unsuccessful. Open reduction is best performed through an anteromedial incision. Osteotomy of the medial malleolus may be required to effect truly anatomic restoration. Following fixation of the talar fracture with

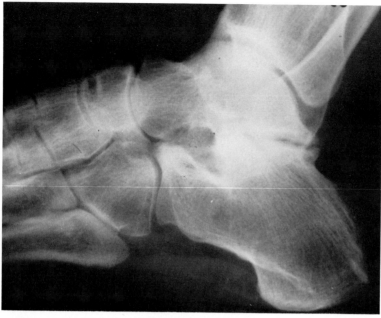

A

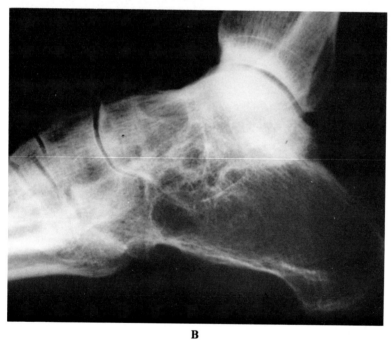

B

Fig. 16.17. A Roentgenogram obtained 3 years after talar neck fracture demonstrating subtalar arthritis. The patient complained of chronic pain. **B** Nine years following triple arthrodesis, the patient was entirely asymptomatic.

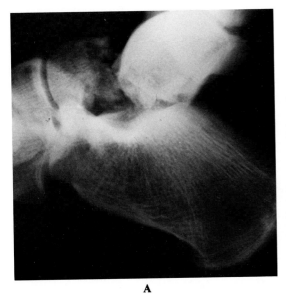

A

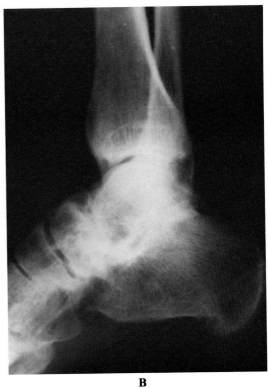

Fig. 16.18. A Type II fracture of the talar neck. **B** Triple arthrodesis was performed 1 year following injury because of painful subtalar arthritis. **C** and **D** Twenty-three years later, the patient had persistent pain and radiographs demonstrated a solid triple arthrodesis with narrowing of the ankle joint.

B

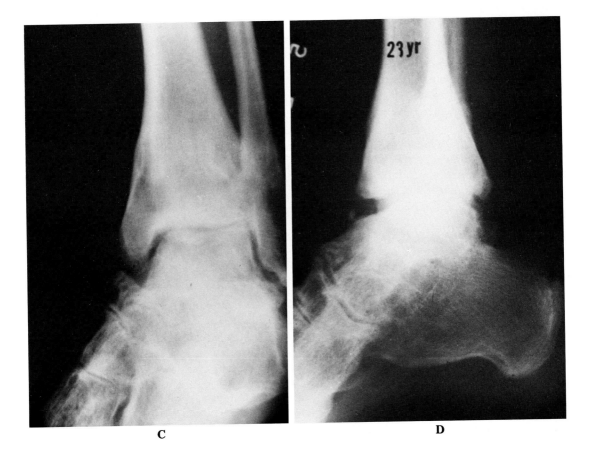

C   D

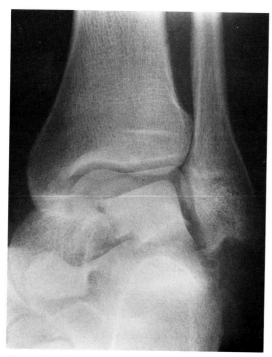

Fig. 16.19. Comminuted fracture of the body of the talus (courtesy of Dr. John Chandler).

Comminuted Fractures

For comminuted fractures of the body of the talus with gross displacement, there is little hope of producing a functionally normal ankle. These fractures are difficult to treat and have been characterized by poor long-term results in most series. Initial treatment should consist of compression dressing, splinting, and elevation. Soft tissue edema and skin conditions are usually improved within 3 to 6 weeks following injury, allowing operative intervention at the discretion of the surgeon. The results of talectomy alone are generally poor and frequently characterized by persistent pain, instability, and lack of endurance. Coltart [13] advocated fusion of the tibia to the calcaneus after talectomy in irreparable fractures of the body of the talus. Pennall [37] suggested early tibiocalcaneal fusion 3 to 4 weeks after injury for grossly comminuted fragments of the body of the talus. Blair [3] recommended excision of the comminuted fragments of the body of the talus combined with a sliding graft from the anterior surface of the tibia to the remaining head and neck of the talus. With this procedure, the position of the foot is unchanged and a more normal relationship between the foot and ankle is maintained. Also, the shortening usually encountered with tibiocalcaneal fusion can be avoided if significant collapse of the talus has not already occurred. If there is already significant loss or collapse of the talar body, then there is little to recommend a Blair fusion over conventional tibiocalcaneal arthrodesis. Postoperative care for tibiocalcaneal or Blair fusion involves 12–16 weeks of cast immobilization, a long leg cast followed by a short leg cast, until the fusion is solid [16].

Steinmann pins or cancellous lag screws, the medial malleolus osteotomy can be secured with one or two malleolar screws. Postoperatively, the foot should be immobilized in neutral or slight equinus position in a well-molded short leg cast. If, after 6 to 8 weeks, radiographs show evidence of early union, a walking cast is applied and weight bearing is permitted. If no healing can be demonstrated by this time, non–weight bearing is continued for an additional 6 to 8 weeks [16].

Complications of displaced fractures of the body of the talus include avascular necrosis of the talus and posttraumatic arthritis of the ankle and/or subtalar joint. Avascular necrosis has been reported to occur in 50% of patients when the body of the talus remains in the ankle mortise, compared to an incidence approaching 100% when the body of the talus is dislocated from the ankle and subtalar joints [10,22]. Treatment of avascular necrosis is outlined above. If disabling posttraumatic arthritis develops, arthrodesis of the appropriate joint is recommended (ankle fusion or triple arthrodesis) (Fig. 16.21).

Isolated Subtalar Dislocations

Subtalar dislocation occurs when there is combined dislocation of the talonavicular and talocalcaneal joints, usually with preservation of tibiotalar joint relationship. The injury has also been termed "subastragalar dislocation" [42] and "peritalar dislocation" [20].

Shands [41] surveyed the literature in 1928 and found 139 cases of subtalar dislocation. Smith [42] reviewed 535 consecutive dislocations

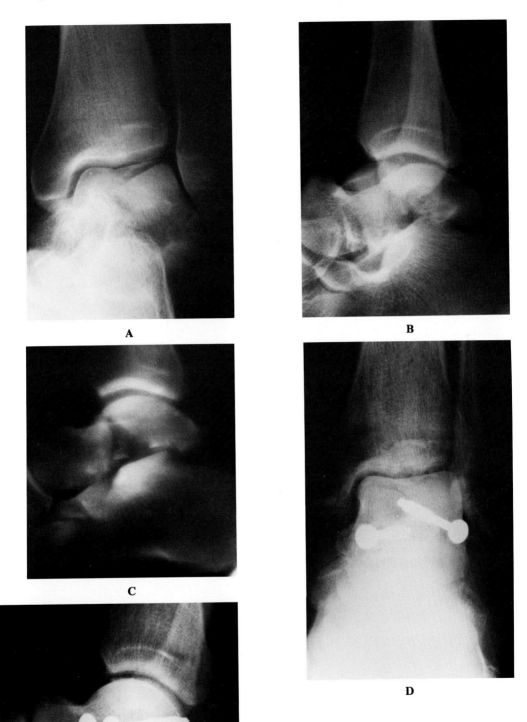

A

B

C

D

E

Fig. 16.20. A and **B** Anteroposterior and lateral radiographs demonstrating a comminuted, displaced fracture of the body of the talus. **C** Conventional tomograms illustrating the degree of comminution. **D** and **E** Radiographs obtained several months following open reduction–internal fixation, demonstrating satisfactory position and healing but suggestive of early avascular necrosis.

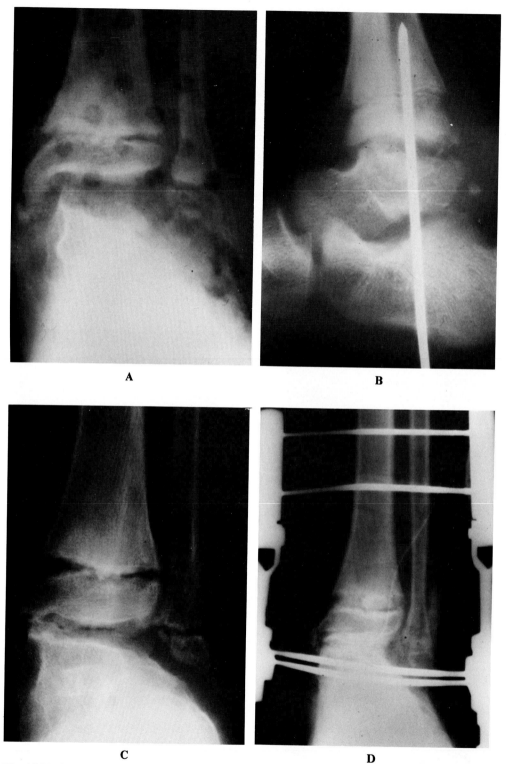

A

B

C

D

Fig. 16.21. A and **B** Anteroposterior and lateral radiographs of a severe open fracture of the body of the talus, occurring in a child. The wound was debrided and the ankle was stabilized using a vertical pin. **C** Six months following injury, there was evidence of avascular necrosis and severe traumatic arthritis. **D** Anteroposterior radiograph following ankle fusion utilizing a Calandruccio compression clamp and autogenous bone graft from the iliac crest.

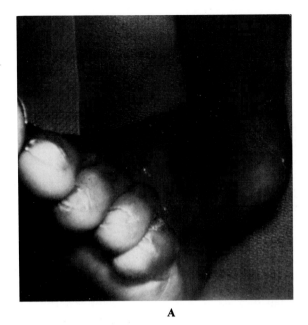

A

B

Fig. 16.22. Clinical appearance of medial (**A**) and lateral (**B**) subtalar dislocation (courtesy of Dr. John Chandler).

of all types and observed that subtalar dislocation occurred with an incidence of 1.3%. He noted no particular age preference but observed a six-fold greater incidence in males than females. Severe trauma was usually required to produce this injury.

Buckingham [7] classified subtalar dislocations as medial or lateral, according to the position of the foot in relation to the talus following injury. Medial dislocation is more common than lateral dislocation with reported incidences of 56% [42] and 85% [28]. Anterior and posterior dislocations have been reported but are generally considered to be rare phenomena.

Mechanism of Injury

The mechanism of injury for medial subtalar dislocation combines plantarflexion, adduction, and supination of the foot. Buckingham postulated that the sustentaculum tali acts as a fulcrum for the posterior aspect of the body of the talus. Dislocation of the talonavicular joint occurs in association with a rotatory subluxation of the talocalcaneal joint. With further force, the talocalcaneal joint then dislocates, completing the injury. Anatomically, the head of the talus appears between the extensor hallucis longus and the extensor digitorum longus tendons, resting on either the navicular or the cuboid bone [7].

Lateral subtalar dislocation is produced by abduction and pronation of the hindfoot. The anterior calcaneal process serves as a fulcrum for the anterolateral aspect of the talus, forcing the head of the talus medially through the talonavicular joint capsule.

Physical Findings

Subtalar dislocations may be open or closed, depending on the severity of the trauma. On physical examination, pain is severe with any attempted motion of the ankle or subtalar joints. Swelling of the foot and ankle is usually significant. The prominent head of the talus may distort the overlying skin and promote local ischemia if the deformity is not promptly corrected. Clinically, the head of the talus is prominent on the dorsolateral aspect of the foot with medial dislocations (Fig. 16.22A) and on the medial side (Fig. 16.22B) with lateral subtalar dislocations [7].

Radiographic Diagnosis

Anteroposterior, lateral, and oblique radiographs of the foot and ankle are required to determine the relationship of the talus to the remaining tarsal bones, as well as to delineate associated fractures. Frontal views of the ankle demonstrate a normal ankle mortise with the body of the talus intact.

With medial subtalar dislocation, the anteroposterior view of the foot reveals disruption of the talonavicular joint, with the navicular seen medial to the head of the talus, and the calcaneus displaced medially. On the lateral projection, the head of the talus is inferior to the navicular and the calcaneus lies parallel to or behind the talus (Fig. 16.23).

In lateral subtalar dislocation, the anteroposterior projection is also the most informative view. The navicular is seen to be displaced lateral to the head of the talus and the calcaneus is dislocated laterally. In the lateral roentgenogram, the talocalcaneal joint appears to be obliterated and the talonavicular joint is disrupted with the navicular appearing to rest on the neck of the talus.

Treatment

Treatment should be accomplished immediately, whether by closed or open means. In our experience, gentle reduction can usually be accomplished in the emergency room with or without intravenous sedation. Any difficulty usually signifies an obstacle that will require open reduction. Forceful reduction using intravenous sedation is not recommended for fear of further damaging the articular surfaces. If in doubt, closed reduction under general or regional anesthesia is preferred. An open dislocation should be irrigated, debrided, and reduced in the operating room under general or regional anesthesia [16].

Closed reduction is best accomplished by exaggerating the existing deformity and then reversing the forces which produced the dislocation [42]. The surgeon should grasp the foot and calcaneus while an assistant applies countertraction at the thigh with the knee flexed. Traction should be applied to the foot and calcaneus as direct pressure is exerted on the head of the talus. With medial dislocations, the foot should first be adducted and plantarflexed. Then traction and ab-

duction are applied to the plantarflexed foot with pressure on the head of the talus to reduce the talonavicular joint. The calcaneus will usually reduce simultaneously beneath the talus. With lateral dislocations, the deformity is exaggerated by abducting the foot in plantarflexion with traction applied. Following this, adduction of the hindfoot with direct pressure on the head of the talus is utilized to achieve reduction. Postreduction immobilization is recommended for 3–6 weeks. Weight bearing can be allowed in uncomplicated cases. McKeever [31] believed that early mobilization would prevent stiffness of the subtalar joint, but this has not been recommended by other authors [12,16].

If closed reduction under general anesthesia is unsuccessful, open reduction is indicated. Leitner [28], in a review of the literature in 1954, found that 8% of medial dislocations and 15% of lateral dislocations required open reduction. Many obstacles to closed reduction have been described [7,20,28,36,42,44]. Smith [42] noted that the toe extensor tendons, the anterior and posterior tibial tendons, and/or the talonavicular capsule–ligament complex may become looped over the head and neck of the talus, preventing closed reduction. Instances of medial subtalar dislocation with "buttonholing" of the talar head through the extensor retinaculum have been reported by both Leitner [28] and Haliburton [20]. Leitner [28] believed that closed reduction could be accomplished even in this situation by alternating dorsiflexion and plantarflexion of the foot during reduction maneuver. Other less common causes of irreducible medial subtalar dislocation include impaction fracture of the head of the talus into the lateral aspect of the navicular, entrapment by the peroneal tendons, and buttonholing of the talus through the extensor digitorum brevis muscle [28,44]. Closed reduction of lateral subtalar dislocations has reportedly been blocked by the posterior tibial tendon or osteochondral separations of the talus and navicular which become interlocked [7,28,36].

If open reduction of subtalar dislocation is required, the incision should be placed laterally over the sinus tarsi in order to avoid skin necrosis which is frequently encountered with the medial approach. Usually the entire anterolateral approach (Chapter 2) is required. After the subtalar and midtarsal joints are exposed, the head and neck of the talus should be freed of all structures

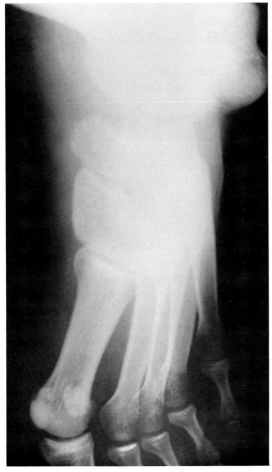

A

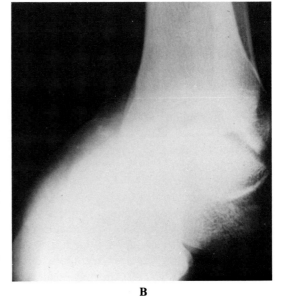

B

Fig. 16.23. Radiographic appearance of medial subtalar dislocation. **A** Navicular displaced medial to the head of the talus. **B** Calcaneus and hindfoot displaced medially. **C** Head of the talus inferior to the navicular and mid-foot.

that prevent reduction. By inserting a bone skid or periosteal elevator into the subtalar joint, and by applying traction to the subtalar and talonavicular joints, the dislocation can usually be reduced. When the dislocation is medial, an assistant simultaneously abducts and everts the foot, and when it is lateral, he adducts and inverts the foot. Occasionally, more extensive dissection is necessary to identify and release other soft tissues that impede reduction. Postoperatively, a short leg cast is applied and bivalved if necessary to allow for swelling. At 3 weeks, this cast is removed and a walking boot is applied and worn for 8 weeks. During this time, weight bearing is gradually resumed [16].

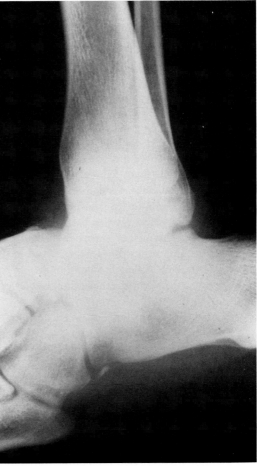

C

The long-term results of isolated subtalar dislocations are generally good, even in those instances where open reduction is required. The major complications reported include avascular necrosis, subtalar and midtarsal stiffness, and late posttraumatic arthritis. The incidence of avascular necrosis ranges from 0 to 20% [7,25,33,37]. Treatment is similar to that described for avascular necrosis complicating fractures of the neck of the talus. Pennall [37] reported 15 cases of subtalar dislocation, nine of which had associated marginal fractures and developed varying degrees of posttraumatic arthritis. Only one case, however, required triple arthrodesis for pain relief. The six patients without associated fractures did well at long-term follow-up. Although it would appear that marginal fractures predispose to late posttraumatic arthritis, Christensen et al. [12] reported that six of 13 cases of late subtalar arthritis were not associated with fracture. The injury in these patients may have been more severe, since four of the six patients had sustained open injuries. Christensen also hypothesized that excessive immobilization (beyond 8 weeks) might play a role in the development of posttraumatic arthritis.

Osteochondral Lesions of the Talus

Since the small osteochondral lesion of the talus was first observed, there has been considerable controversy as to whether this represents a true transchondral fracture or a lesion caused by another process, such as avascular necrosis. This distinction has important therapeutic implications. If the lesion is indeed a fracture, then healing can be expected following immobilization in proper position. If, on the other hand, the lesion is due to an avascular process, then the possibility of healing with either closed or open treatment is remote.

The term "osteochondritis dissecans" was first used by König [27] in 1888 to describe loose bodies within the knee joint. He theorized that these were caused by spontaneous necrosis of bone. Kappis [23] noted a similar lesion in the ankle in 1922 and was the first to refer to osteochondritis dissecans at this site. In 1932, Rendu [38] described an intraarticular fracture of the talus similar to the lesion of osteochondritis dissecans. Roden [39] and others [15,29,46] collected 55 lesions of the talus and concluded that most of the lateral lesions were secondary to trauma, rarely healed spontaneously, and caused more symptoms than lesions occurring elsewhere in the ankle. They observed that arthritis developed if early operative treatment was not accomplished. On the other hand, a large percentage of the medial lesions they encountered were not associated with trauma, had fewer symptoms, frequently healed spontaneously, and seemed to develop little or no arthrosis when treated by conservative means. They recommended excision of medial lesions only if there was a loose body causing mechanical symptoms.

Following an exhaustive study, Berndt and Harty [2] concluded that both medial and lateral lesions of osteochondritis dissecans were largely secondary to trauma and, in fact, were transchondral or osteochondral fractures. In their series, 43% of lesions were located in the lateral portion, usually the middle third, of the talus; 57% occurred in the medial talus, usually the posterior third. In experiments with cadaver limbs, they showed that the lateral lesions were caused by inversion and strong dorsiflexion, whereas the medial lesions were caused by inversion, plantarflexion, and external rotation of the tibia on the talus. Berndt and Harty [2] classified the osteochondral lesions into four different stages of severity (Fig. 16.24).

Stage I   A small area of compression of subchondral bone.
Stage II   A partially detached osteochondral fragment.
Stage III   A completely detached osteochondral fragment remaining in the crater.
Stage IV   A displaced osteochondral fragment.

Berndt and Harty [2] observed better results with operative than nonoperative treatment. Davidson et al. [15] agreed that early operative intervention produced superior results and prevented arthrosis of the ankle. Mukherjee and Young [34], however, reported satisfactory results in ten patients with small nondisplaced lesions treated by nonoperative methods. They recommended, however, that small displaced fragments be treated by excision and that large displaced fractures be treated by open reduction and internal fixation wherever possible.

Fig. 16.24. The four stages of osteochondritis dissecans of the talus [2]. See text for details. Reprinted with permission from Canale ST, Belding RH: Osteochondral lesions of the talus. J Bone Joint Surg 62A:97, 1980.

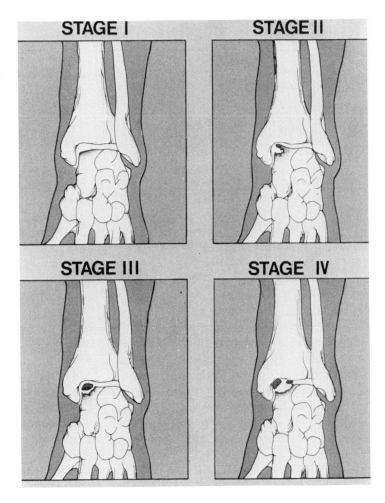

Kenny [24] described two instances in which the osteochondral fragment had inverted upon itself. At operation, the articular surface of the fragment was found to be embedded in the crater, making union virtually impossible. Kenny suggested obtaining tomograms if an inverted lesion is suspected.

At the Campbell Clinic, we reviewed 31 cases of osteochrondritis dissecans treated since 1940 [9]. There were 14 medial lesions, 15 lateral lesions, and two central lesions. Symptoms were noted in the second and third decade of life in the majority of patients. Twenty-five of the 31 lesions were associated with a history of significant trauma. It appeared from our study that most lateral lesions were caused by trauma, as were the majority of medial lesions. We were unable, however, to attribute six of the medial lesions to trauma. Four of these occurred in two females with bilateral involvement.

As suggested by Berndt and Harty [2], strong inversion associated with dorsiflexion of the ankle causes the lateral portion of the talus to impinge against the fibula, resulting in osteochondral fracture at this site. The fragment is prone to displacement, especially if the injury is associated with rupture of the lateral ankle ligaments. Medial lesions similarly occur in conjunction with an inversion injury, as strong plantarflexion and lateral rotation of the tibia on the talus result in a powerful impaction and grinding of the talar border.

In our experience, the lateral lesions were consistently wafer-shaped, resembling an osteochondral fracture, and as a result were more likely to become displaced into the ankle joint. The medial lesions were deeper, cup-shaped, and less likely to become displaced (Fig. 16.25).

From our experience [9] and that of Berndt and Harty [2], we make the following recommen-

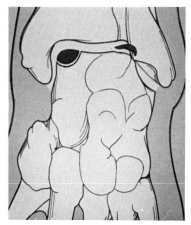

Fig. 16.25. Schematic illustration of typical cup-shaped medial and wafer-shaped lateral lesions.

dations concerning treatment: Stage I and stage II lesions, regardless of location, should be treated with nonoperative measures, such as immobilization in plaster, patellar tendon–bearing brace, ankle corset, or arch support. Stage III medial lesions should be treated by similar conservative measures with anticipation of good clinical results and delayed, if any, development of arthrosis; if symptoms persist after such treatment, then surgical excision and curettage of the lesion should be performed. Lateral stage III and both medial and lateral stage IV lesions should be treated by excision of the fragment and curettage of the underlying subchondral bed before the development of degenerative arthritis.

We have had no experience with pinning of fragments, but if the fragment is exceptionally large, this should certainly be considered. Small pins can be used to traverse the fracture site; however, breakage or loosening of the pins in the joint is a real possibility. The fragment can be pinned across the joint, but this too can be complicated by pin breakage. We agree with Berndt and Harty that defects will frequently fill in with fibrocartilage after excision and curettage, and we would not presently recommend pinning unless the fragment constitutes a significant percentage of the articular surface. One of us (S.T.C) has recently reviewed a case of Dr. J. Böhler [4] in which a "fibrinogen glue" was used to internally fix a detached fragment in its crater (Fig. 16.26) and, in short-term follow-up, the result appears excellent.

A fragment inverted upon itself is an indication for immediate operative treatment. This configuration places the cartilaginous face of the fragment in the depth of the crater adjacent to bone, and nonunion is almost certain under these circumstances. If the fragment appears radiologically to be floating in the crater, inversion should be seriously considered (Fig. 16.27). Conventional tomography is frequently helpful in this regard.

Lateral lesions can usually be approached without difficulty through an anterolateral incision (Chapter 2), since the lesion is usually located adjacent or anterior to the fibula. Osteotomy of the medial malleolus, however, is

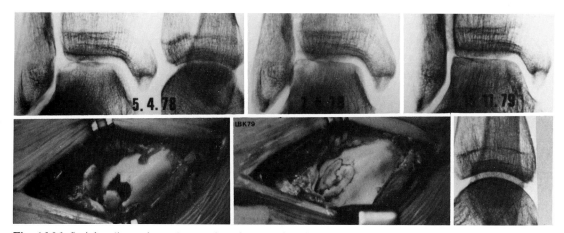

Fig. 16.26. Serial radiographs and operative photographs of a large lateral osteochondral fragment internally fixed with "fibrinogen glue" (courtesy of Dr. J. Bohler).

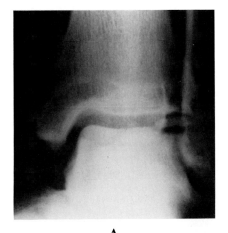

A

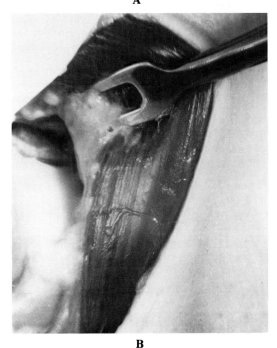

B

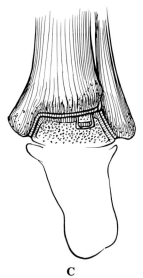

C

Fig. 16.27. **A** Radiograph of a lateral stage III lesion. Because of the elevated position of the fragment and the radiolucent area in the depth of the crater, an inverted fragment should be suspected. **B** An inverted fragment will give the radiographic appearance of a lucent zone between the fragment and the depth of the crater because of interposed articular cartilage. **C** Operative photograph of an inverted fragment revealing subchondral bone on the superior surface and articular cartilage on the inferior surface. If an inverted lesion is present, spontaneous healing will not occur.

occasionally necessary to obtain adequate exposure of a posteromedial lesion.

In summary, lateral lesions are associated with trauma and caused by inversion or inversion-dorsiflexion. These lesions are generally shallow, likely to be associated with persistent symptoms, and more likely to become displaced into the ankle joint. Medial lesions, on the other hand, may be traumatic or atraumatic in origin. They tend to be morphologically deep but are less likely to produce symptoms. We recommend that advanced stage III lateral lesions and all stage IV lesions (medial or lateral) be treated by early operation.

References

1. Anderson HG: Medical and Surgical Aspects of Aviation. London, Oxford Medical, 1919.
2. Berndt AL, Harty, M: Transchondral fractures (osteochondritis dissecans) of the talus. J Bone Joint Surg 41A:988, 1959.
3. Blair HC: Comminuted fractures and fracture dislocations of the body of the astragalus: Opera-

tive treatment. Am J Surg 59:37, 1943.

4. Böhler J: Personal communication, 1980.
5. Boyd HB: Personal communication, 1976.
6. Boyd HB, Knight RA: Fractures of the astragalus. South Med J 35:160, 1942.
7. Buckingham WW Jr: Subtalar dislocations of the foot. J Trauma 13:753, 1973.
8. Cabot H, Binney H: Fractures of the os calcis and astragalus. Ann Surg 45:51, 1818.
9. Canale ST, Belding RH: Osteochondral lesions of the talus. J Bone Joint Surg 62A:97, 1980.
10. Canale ST, Kelly FB Jr: Fractures of the neck of the talus. Long-term evaluation of 71 cases. J Bone Joint Surg 60A:143, 1978.
11. Canale ST, Shelton WR: Avascular lesions of bones and joints. In: Practice of Surgery. Hagerstown, Md., Harper & Row, 1979.
12. Christensen SB, Lorentzen JE, Krogsoe O, Sneppen O: Subtalar dislocation. Acta Orthop Scand 48:707, 1977.
13. Coltart WD: Aviator's astragalus. J Bone Joint Surg 34B:545, 1952.
14. Cooper A: Treatise on Dislocations and on Fractures of the Joints. Boston, Wells and Lilly, 1818.
15. Davidson AM, Steele HD, MacKenzie DA, Penny JA: A review of 21 cases of transchondral fracture of the talus. J Trauma 7:378, 1967.
16. Edmonson AS, Crenshaw AH (eds.): Campbell's Operative Orthopaedics, 6th ed. St. Louis, Mosby, 1980.
17. Fabricius H: Observatio LXVII (letter to Dr. Philibertos). Observationum et Curationum Chirurgic arum Centuriae. 1608, p. 140.
18. Garcia A, Parkes JC: Fractures of the foot. In Giannestras NJ (ed): Foot Disorders. Medical and Surgical Management, 2nd ed. Philadelphia, Lea & Febiger, 1973.
19. Gray H: Anatomy of the Human Body, 28th ed. Edited by C.M. Goss. Philadelphia, Lea & Febiger, 1966.
20. Haliburton RA, Barber JR, Fraser RL: Further experience with peritalar dislocation. Canad J Surg 10:322, 1967.
21. Haliburton RA, Sullivan R, Kelly PJ, Peterson LFA: The extra-osseous and intra-osseous blood supply of the talus. J Bone Joint Surg 40A:1115, 1958.
22. Hawkins LG: Fractures of the neck of the talus. J Bone Joint Surg 52A:991, 1970.
23. Kappis M: Weitere Beiträge zur traumatisch-mechanischen Entstehung der "spontanen" Knorpelablösungen (sogen. Osteochondritis Dissecans). Dtsch Z Chir 171:13, 1922.
24. Kenny CH: Inverted osteochondral fracture of the talus diagnosed by tomography. J Bone Joint Surg 63A:1020, 1981.
25. Kenwright J, Taylor RG: Major injuries of the talus. J Bone Joint Surg 52B:36, 1970.
26. Kleiger B: Fractures of the talus. J Bone Joint Surg 30A:735, 1948.
27. König: Über freie Körper in den Gelenken. Dtsch Z Chir 27:90, 1888.
28. Leitner B: Obstacles to reduction in subtalar dislocations. J Bone Joint Surg 36A:299, 1954.
29. Marks KL: Flake fracture of the talus progressing to osteochondritis dissecans. J Bone Joint Surg 34B:90, 1952.
30. McKeever FM: Fracture of the neck of the astragalus. Arch Surg 46:720, 1943.
31. McKeever FM: Treatment of complications of fractures and dislocations of the talus. Clin Orthop 30:45, 1963.
32. Miller OL, Baker LD: Fracture and fracture-dislocation of the astragalus. South Med J 32:125, 1939.
33. Mindell ER, Cisek EE, Kartalian G, Dziob JM: Late results of injuries to the talus. Analysis of 40 cases. J Bone Joint Surg 45A:221, 1963.
34. Mukherjee SK, Young AB: Dome fractures of the talus. A report of 10 cases. J Bone Joint Surg 55B:319, 1973.
35. Mulfinger GL, Trueta J: The blood supply of the talus. J Bone Joint Surg 52B:160, 1970.
36. Mulroy RD: The tibialis posterior tendon as an obstacle to reduction of a lateral anterior subtalar dislocation. J Bone Joint Surg 37A:859, 1955.
37. Pennall GF: Fractures of the talus. Clin Orthop 30:53, 1963.
38. Rendu A: Fracture intra-articulaire parcellaire de la poulie astraglienne. Lyon Med 150:220, 1932.
39. Roden S, Tillegard P, Unander-Scharin L: Osteochondritis dissecans and similar lesions of the talus. Report of 55 cases with special reference to etiology and treatment. Acta Orthop Scand 23:51, 1953.
40. Schrock RD, Johnson WF, Waters CH Jr: Fractures and fracture-dislocations of the talus. J Bone Joint Surg 24:560, 1942.
41. Shands AR Jr: The incidence of subastragaloid dislocation of foot, with report of one case of inward type. J Bone Joint Surg 10:306, 1928.
42. Smith H: Subastragalar dislocation. A report of seven cases. J Bone Joint Surg 19:373, 1937.
43. Stealy JH: Fracture of the astragalus. Surg Gynecol Obstet 8:36, 1909.
44. Wendel: Uber Luxatio pedis sub talo. Dtsch Z Chir 80:251, 1905.
45. Wildenauer E: Die Blutversorgung des Talus. Z Anat 115:32, 1950.
46. Yvars MF: Osteochondral fractures of the dome of the talus. Clin Orthop 114:185, 1976.

Chapter 17 Arthrodesis and Arthroplasty

Robert P. Good

Historically, arthrodesis has been considered the treatment of choice for posttraumatic degenerative arthritis of the tibiotalar joint [10]. Today, it still represents the standard with which all other procedures must be compared. Arthrodesis is indicated when arthritic symptoms of pain, deformity, and loss of useful function are no longer manageable by conservative measures.

In the preoperative evaluation it is important to assess the status of the talocalcaneal joint. The presence of arthritis there may jeopardize the success of tibiotalar fusion [9,17,39,41,55]. If the subtalar joint is already significantly involved, primary fusion of both tibiotalar and talocalcaneal joints should be considered [39].

In 1974 White [74] summarized 22 different techniques that had been developed to obtain fusion of the ankle. Since then, additional methods have been described [12,13,33,71]. The number of different techniques is testimony to the fact that no single procedure is uniformly applicable.

Technical Considerations

Removal of Articular Cartilage

Many arthrodesis techniques include removal of all articular cartilage as an integral part of the procedure (Fig. 17.1) [1,11,15,28,29,71,72]. This carpentry of bone is quite useful when there is a need to correct deformity. Removal of articular cartilage also has the theoretical advantage of opposing broad surfaces of cancellous bone to facilitate early union. Several authors [8, 12,25,30,33,34,37,41,55,57,70,74], however, have demonstrated that the complete removal of all cartilage is not necessary to obtain osseous union (Fig. 17.2). Gallie [25] believed that once ar-

throdesis was achieved any remaining articular cartilage eventually ossified. Procedures which do not necessitate removal of all articular carti-

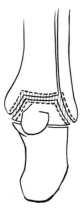

Fig. 17.1. Most arthrodesing techniques employ removal of articular cartilage as an integral part of the procedure.

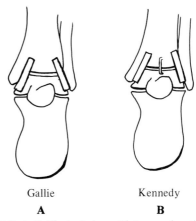

Gallie   Kennedy

A   **B**

Fig. 17.2. A Gallie technique. Slots crossing the joint are prepared to receive bone graft. Weight-bearing articular cartilage is not disturbed. **B** Kennedy modified the technique by the addition of a staple for fixation. He also advocated removal of articular cartilage to achieve correction of varus or valgus deformity. Results of both techniques are comparable.

lage have the advantage of requiring less extensive dissection and of preserving stability of the talus within the mortise.

Compression

In 1951 Charnley [14] demonstrated the value of compression in achieving fusion of the ankle. Since then, others have documented the benefit of this measure [3,13,39,45,58,69,71]. Compression offers effective immobilization, maintains contact during necrosis and viscoelastic creep, and promotes early union [15,40]. Compression, however, should be considered an adjunct to the various arthrodesing procedures and not as a substitute for careful, meticulous handling of the bony surfaces. It adds somewhat to the complexity of the procedure but should be considered in those cases where difficulty in obtaining union is anticipated, i.e., following infection or a failed previous arthrodesis attempt.

Bone Crafting

The use of autogenous bone graft has been advocated by many authors (Fig. 17.3). Campbell [13] obtained an osteoperiosteal graft from the distal tibia and placed this over the anterior aspect of the denuded ankle joint. This was augmented posteriorly by raising flaps of bone from the os calcis and distal tibia as additional graft material. Many authors [5,8,11,28,32,44,50–52,63,64,68,70,72] have recommended the use of a corticocancellous tibial strut graft across the ankle joint to provide bony contact and lend some degree of immediate stability. Disadvantages include the unpredictability of cortical bone and the possibility of fracture through the graft or the donor site.

The use of the iliac crest as a source of graft material has many proponents. Chuinard [16] described the interposition of a full thickness iliac graft between the distal tibia and talus. This technique is quite useful in children because the distal tibial epiphyseal plate is not violated (Fig. 17.4). White [74] reported the use of two horseshoe-shaped tricortical crest grafts inserted through a posterior exposure. Campbell et al. [12] have obtained excellent results using vertically placed iliac crest grafts (Fig. 17.5). We have had no

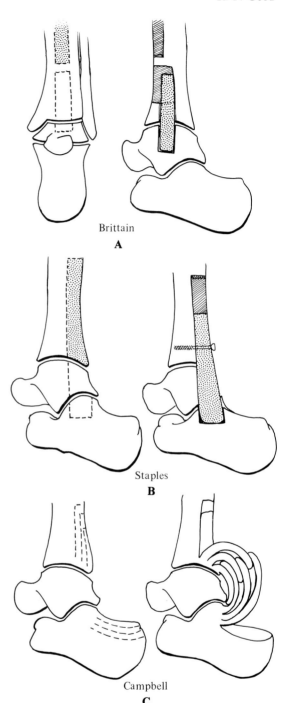

Fig. 17.3. Examples of techniques which employ local autogenous bone graft. **A** Brittain, 1942 [11]. **B** Staples, 1956 [64]. **C** Campbell, 1929 [13].

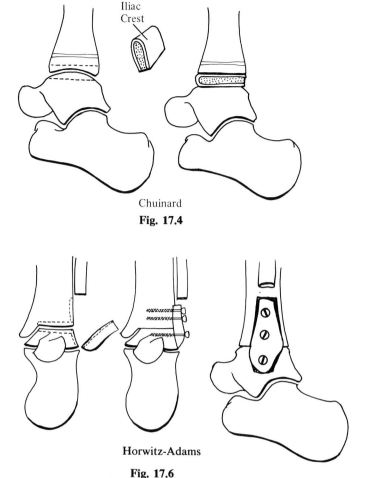

Chuinard

Fig. 17.4

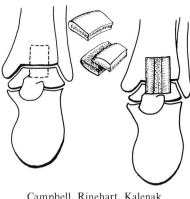

Campbell, Rinehart, Kalenak

Fig. 17.5

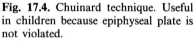

Horwitz-Adams

Fig. 17.6

Fig. 17.4. Chuinard technique. Useful in children because epiphyseal plate is not violated.

Fig. 17.5. Use of iliac crest graft as described by Campbell et al. [12].

Fig. 17.6. Transfibular approach for arthrodesis as described by Horwitz [35] and Adams [1].

experience with this procedure but are intrigued with the dual advantages of abundant cancellous surface and cortical stability. Using the iliac crest as a source of graft material has the disadvantage of requiring an additional incision with resultant increase in morbidity.

Fibular Osteotomy

Goldthwait [29] advocated osteotomy of the fibula to permit better apposition of the denuded talus within the ankle mortise. In 1942, Horwitz [35] utilized the lateral approach of Gatellier [27] and applied the longitudinally split fibula as a bone graft. Variations of this technique have been described by Adams [1], Wilson [75], and others [71] (Fig. 17.6). Fibular osteotomy provides wide

exposure of the ankle joint and facilitates removal of articular cartilage [4,71]. Recently, however, some authors [47,49] have reported less than ideal results with the transfibular approach because of an association with nonunion, and because of difficulties in correcting varus and valgus deformity. The fibula has also been used as a dowel graft placed either transversely [30,55] or vertically (Fig. 17.7) [7].

The particular approach to the ankle, whether anterior, posterior, medial, and/or lateral, should be determined by the condition of overlying skin, the specific pathologic anatomy, the presence or absence of deformity, and the surgeon's individual bias and experience.

One of the following three techniques can be applied to most of the clinical situations encountered.

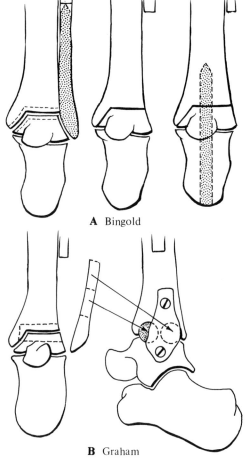

A Bingold

B Graham

Fig. 17.7. Fibula used as dowel graft. **A** Bingold, 1956 [7]. **B** Graham, 1970 [30].

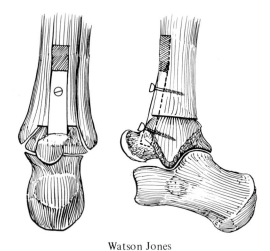

Watson Jones

Fig. 17.8. Arthrodesis employing anterior sliding tibial strut graft (after Watson-Jones [72]). See text for details.

Anterior Sliding Graft Technique

The patient is positioned supine and a tourniquet is applied to the proximal thigh. The ankle joint is approached through an anterior longitudinal incision placed lateral to the extensor hallucis longus tendon, as described in Chapter 3. Using an osteotome or oscillating saw, a rectangular section of cortical bone, 2 cm × 6 cm, is removed from the anterior aspect of the distal tibia (Fig. 17.8). This step improves visualization of the joint surfaces and facilitates removal of the articular cartilage and subchondral bone. Care should be taken to fashion the surfaces so that deformity is corrected and maximal bony contact is provided with the ankle in the corrected position. Next, if necessary, a threaded Steinmann pin can

be inserted through the os calcis and the talus into the tibia to maintain the ankle in proper alignment during the remainder of the procedure.

A hole is created in the neck and body of the talus to receive the tibial graft. The graft should be placed well into the depth of the talus to ensure stability and adequate bony contact. Screws may be placed through the graft into the tibia and/or talus to help maintain position. Care must be taken that the graft does not distract the raw bony surfaces. If a transarticular Steinmann pin has been employed, it is removed at this stage. Cancellous bone obtained from the bed of the donor site in the distal tibia is then placed around the ankle joint anteriorly. The wound is approximated and a well-molded long leg cast is applied. At 6 weeks this is converted to a short leg cast and weight bearing is permitted. Immobilization should be maintained until there is evidence of osseous union (Fig. 17.9).

Compression Arthrodesis

Compression arthrodesis can be accomplished through a variety of surgical approaches. Charnley's original description [14] utilized a transverse incision with transection of the tendons and neurovascular bundle. Although Charnley [15], as well as Ratliff [58], reported few complications

Fig. 17.9. Appearance of ankle 4 years following anterior arthrodesis utilizing tibial strut graft.

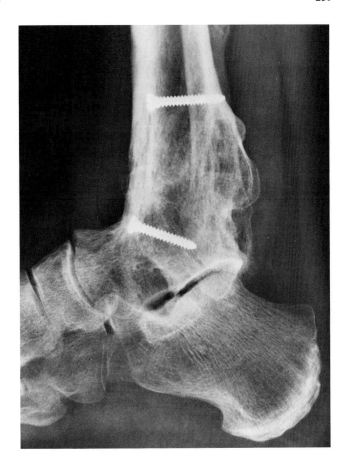

with this method, it has obvious theoretical disadvantages.

Technique (Modified Charnley)

The medial and lateral incision exposure described by Anderson [4] provides excellent visualization of the ankle joint. Both malleoli are osteotomized and the articular surface of the distal tibia is removed, so that a flat bed of cancellous bone is created (Fig. 17.10). This should be oriented in a plane perpendicular to the long axis of the tibial shaft. The foot is brought into proper position and the dome of the talus is similarly prepared so as to ensure maximum bony contact. Pins are then placed in the distal tibia and the talus, and an external fixator is applied to provide compression (Fig. 17.11). The talus must not be displaced forward because this will reduce the prominence of the heel, creating an objectionable cosmetic appearance. It also shortens the posterior lever arm, placing the foot at a mechanical disadvantage. Provided adequate fixation can be

obtained, the use of a cast is optional. At 4 to 6 weeks the external fixator is removed, and the patient maintained in a short leg walking cast until there is clinical and roentgenographic evidence of union.

Posterior Approach

The posterior approach is quite useful when there has been previous injury or surgery to the anterior aspect of the ankle. There is the added theoretical advantage that the blood supply to the talus is minimally violated through this exposure. This method can also be utilized in children since the distal epiphyseal plate is not disturbed.

Technique (White) [74]

The patient is placed in the prone position and a pneumatic tourniquet is applied to the proximal

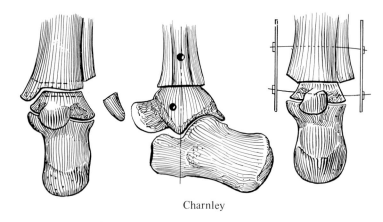

Fig. 17.10. Modified Charnley compression technique using a two-pin fixator. Charnley specified that the talar pin be positioned slightly anterior to the axis of ankle flexion/extension so as to resist the equinus pull of the Achilles tendon.

Charnley

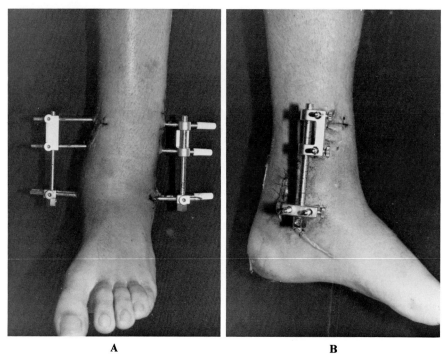

A   B

Fig. 17.11. Compression arthrodesis using a four-pin fixator. Pin placement is much less critical than with the Charnley two-pin device.

thigh [74]. A posterolateral incision (Chapter 3) is employed with care to avoid injuring the sural nerve, which lies in the subcutaneous tissue of the lateral flap. The Achilles tendon is sectioned in such a manner as to allow Z-plasty at closure. The plantaris tendon is transsected and the flexor hallucis longus muscle is retracted medially after its origin on the distal fibula has been detached. This reveals the posterior capsule which is then incised to expose the tibiotalar joint. Transverse parallel cuts are made through the talus and distal tibia to remove the corresponding articular surfaces. Two tricortical horseshoe-shaped grafts, obtained from the posterior iliac crest, are tapped into the prepared bed (Fig. 17.12). This provides immediate stability and apposition of cancellous surfaces. The Achilles tendon is repaired and the wound is closed. Aftercare is the same as that described for the anterior sliding graft technique.

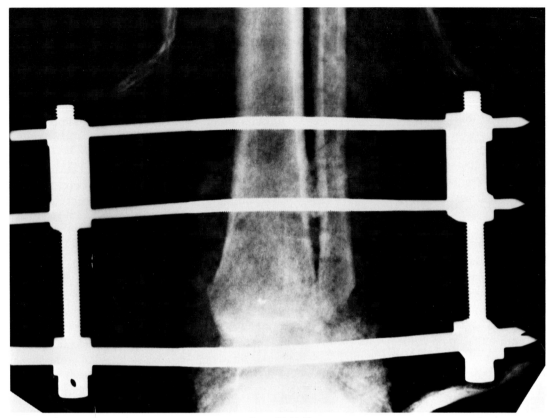

Fig. 17.11 C

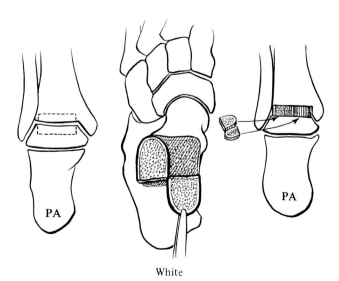

Fig. 17.12. Posterior approach for arthrodesis as described by White [74]. See text for details.

White

Position of Fusion and Gait

In 1955 Watson-Jones [72] stated that the ideal position for ankle fusion was at approximately 15° of equinus. He, and others [6,13,28,31], believed that equinus was necessary to facilitate walking and to accommodate the heel height of common footwear. For similar reasons some authors [6,28] believed that females should be fused in a greater degree of equinus than males. Recently, however, the position of fusion and its affect on gait have been studied in greater detail [22,43,48,59,62]. Stauffer et al. [67] determined that the range of motion in a normal ankle during walking was approximately 10° of dorsiflexion and 14° of plantarflexion, for a total arc of 24°. Maximum plantarflexion apparently occurs after heel strike, with gradual dorsiflexion occurring through the gait cycle until just before heel-off. In a fused ankle, the total tibio-pedal motion has been found to be 11–18°, with most of this occurring at the talonavicular joint [22,43,62]. Almost all of the motion through the mid-foot is in the direction of further plantarflexion (Fig. 17.13) [43,49]. When an ankle is fused in the neutral position, the tibiopedal plantarflexion will closely approximate the 14° of plantarflexion normally occurring at the ankle. Therefore, the ankle fused in neutral position lacks only 10° of dorsiflexion compared with the normal side. When the ankle is fused in a position of equinus, there develops a greater discrepancy in dorsiflexion without any added benefit from the plantarflexed position. It was formerly believed that compensatory hypermobility developed at the mid-foot following arthrodesis of the ankle [41,42,60], but recently this has been questioned [38].

Patients fused with the ankle in neutral position can be expected to walk with little or no limp while barefoot, and are able to accommodate most normal footwear [43,62]. Individuals whose ankle is fused in more than 10° of equinus tend to have a vaulting type of gait when barefoot, problems related to hyperextension of the knee, a greater incidence of pain in the mid-foot and metatarsal areas, and a tendency toward secondary arthritic changes in the remaining tarsal joints [24,36,41,43,62]. On the basis of clinical studies and gait analysis, it would seem that the optimum position of ankle fusion is within a few

degrees in either direction of neutral. Furthermore, this position need not be significantly altered because of the patient's gender.

Although the talocalcaneal joint is not included in the fusion, its motion is usually diminished following ankle arthrodesis [23,38,49, 59,62]. The reasons for this remain unclear. Authors uniformly agree that deviation in the direction of either varus or valgus should be avoided [23,44,49]. Deviation of more than 5° has been associated with less satisfactory clinical results. The rotational alignment should be determined according to the uninvolved extremity [71].

Complications

Satisfactory results can be expected following ankle arthrodesis in 75–90% of patients [42,44, 49,59,62]. The procedure, however, is not without complications. Postoperative infection, osteomyelitis, and even below-knee amputation has been reported [9,19,44,49,52]. Meticulous technique is essential and prophylactic antibiotic coverage should be seriously considered [17].

Care must be employed to avoid impingement upon or violation of the talocalcaneal joint (Fig. 17.14). This can result in a failed procedure because of persistent pain.

Malunion

Operative revision for malposition has been required in up to 10% of patients [26]. Excessive equinus or dorsiflexion is undesirable as it will likely disturb the patient's gait. The incidence of malunion can be reduced to a minimum if meticulous technique is employed and intraoperative roentgenograms are obtained [47]. When mild malposition occurs, shoe modifications can often improve the patient's gait.

Nonunion

Failure to achieve osseous union has been reported in up to 23% of patients [2,9,46]. No single procedure has been demonstrated to be particularly infallible in this regard. The use of autogenous bone graft, malleolar osteotomy, in-

Fig. 17.13. Lateral roentgenograms demonstrating tibiopedal motion following ankle arthrodesis.

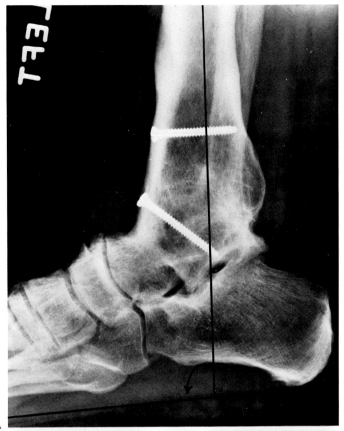

A

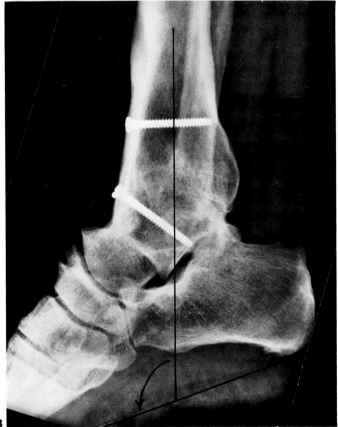

B

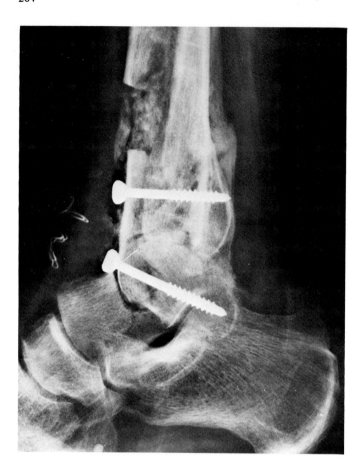

Fig. 17.14. Lateral roentgenogram demonstrating screw penetrating talo-calcaneal joint.

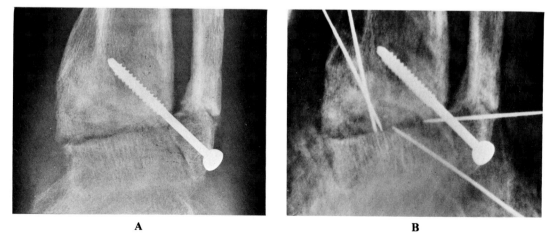

A   B

Fig. 17.15. Use of electrical stimulation. **A** Painful nonunion following attempted arthrodesis. **B** Electrodes in place. **C** Appearance 6 months following initiation of electrical stimulation.

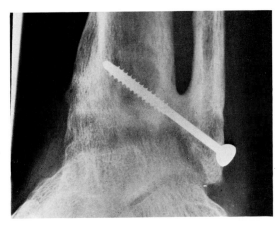

Fig. 17.15. C

ternal fixation, and compression techniques are helpful but have not been shown to statistically affect the ultimate fusion rate. Fibrous union is not necessarily symptomatic [14,31]. The decision for further treatment must be made on the basis of a clinical rather than a purely radiographic evaluation.

The treatment of a failed ankle fusion has traditionally consisted of reexploration with the addition of bone graft. The success of electric stimulation in effecting union at fracture sites has been most encouraging and may eventually represent the treatment of choice for nonunion when the ankle is in good alignment and there is no synovial pseudoarthrosis (Fig. 17.15) [20]. The use of electric stimulation as an adjunct to primary arthrodesis is not presently recommended but may prove to be beneficial in the future.

Total Ankle Arthroplasty

Due to the success with prosthetic replacement of other joints, an interest in replacement arthroplasty of the ankle has emerged. Uniaxial and multiaxial prostheses have been developed and employed in instances of posttraumatic degenerative arthritis [21,53,54,56,61,65,66,73]. Although the initial results were optimistic, recent reports presenting longer follow-up are somewhat discouraging. DeMottaz et al. [18] observed that 81% of their patients continued to have pain postoperatively; 89% demonstrated a radiolucent line at 1 year; and 10% developed clinical loosen-

ing. Murray et al. [53] found that 58% of their patients with a follow-up of 1–5 years had persistent pain. Total ankle arthroplasty may hold promise in the future but until further experience has been gained and more favorable results recorded, ankle arthrodesis remains the procedure of choice for patients with posttraumatic degenerative arthritis [18].

References

1. Adams JC: Arthrodesis of the ankle joint. Experiences with the transfibular approach. J Bone Joint Surg 30B:506, 1948.
2. Ahlberg A, Henricson AS: Late results of ankle fusion. Acta Orthop Scand 52:103, 1981.
3. Altcheck M: Charnley ankle arthrodesis. J Bone Joint Surg 50A:1255, 1968.
4. Anderson R: Concentric arthrodesis of the ankle joint. A transmalleolar approach. J Bone Joint Surg 27:37, 1945.
5. Ansart MB: Pan-arthrodesis for paralytic flail foot. J Bone Joint Surg 33B:503, 1951.
6. Barr JS, Record EE: Arthrodesis of the ankle joint. Indication, operative technique and clinical experience. N Engl J Med 248:53, 1953.
7. Bingold AC: Ankle and subtalar fusion by a transarticular graft. J Bone Joint Surg 38B:862, 1956.
8. Blair HC: Comminuted fractures and fracture dislocations of the body of the astragalus. Am J Surg 59:37, 1943.
9. Boobbyer GN: The long-term results of ankle arthrodesis. Acta Orthop Scand 52:107, 1981.
10. Boyd HB: Indication for fusion of the ankle. Orthop Clin North Am 5:191, 1974.
11. Brittain HA: Arthrodesis of the ankle. In: Architectural Principles in Arthrodesis. Baltimore, Williams & Wilkins, 1942, pp. 58–63.
12. Campbell CJ, Rinehart WT, Kalenak A: Arthrodesis of the ankle. Deep autogenous inlay graft with maximum cancellous bone apposition. J Bone Joint Surg 56A:63, 1974.
13. Campbell WC: An operation for the induction of osseous fusion in the ankle joint. Am J Surg 6:588, 1929.
14. Charnley J: Compression arthrodesis of the ankle and shoulder. J Bone Joint Surg 33B:180, 1951.
15. Charnley J: Compression arthrodesis of the ankle. In: Compression Arthrodesis. Edinburgh, Livingston, 1953, pp. 133–156.
16. Chuinard EG, Peterson RE: Distraction-compression bone-graft arthrodesis of the ankle. A method especially applicable in children. J Bone Joint Surg 45A:481, 1963.
17. Davis RJ, Millis MB: Ankle arthrodesis in the management of traumatic ankle arthrosis: A long-term retrospective study. J Trauma 20:674, 1980.

18. DeMottaz JD, Mazur JM, Thomas WH, Sledge CB, Simon SR: Clinical study of total ankle replacement with gait analysis. A preliminary report. J Bone Joint Surg 61A:976, 1979.

19. Detwiler CK, Frenette JP, Chiroff RT: Ankle arthrodesis. Fifteen year's experience. NY State J Med 76:1803, 1976.

20. Esterhai JL Jr: Personal communication, 1982.

21. Evanski PM, Waugh TR: Management of arthritis of the ankle. An alternative of arthrodesis. Clin Orthop 122:110, 1977.

22. Evanski PM, Waugh TR: Tibiopedal motion after ankle fusion and arthroplasty. In Bateman JE, Trott AW (eds): The Foot and Ankle. New York, Thieme-Stratton, 1980, pp. 36–39.

23. Fjermeros H, Hagen R: Post-traumatic arthrosis in the ankle and foot treated with arthrodesis. Acta Chir Scand 133:527, 1967.

24. Fuller J, Rostrup O, Huckell JR: Ankle arthrodesis. A clinical review. J Bone Joint Surg 56B:587, 1974.

25. Gallie WE: Arthrodesis of the ankle joint. J Bone Joint Surg 30B:619, 1948.

26. Gartland JJ: A goniometer for use at ankle fusion. J Bone Joint Surg 36A:884, 1954.

27. Gatellier J: The juxtaretroperoneal route in the operative treatment of fracture of the malleolus with posterior marginal fragment. Surg Gynecol Obstet 52:67, 1931.

28. Giberson RG, Janes JM: Tibiocalcaneal fusion: A surgical technique. Surg Gynecol Obstet 99:773, 1954.

29. Goldthwait JE: An operation for the stiffening of the ankle joint in infantile paralysis. Am J Orthop Surg 5:271, 1908.

30. Graham CE: A new method for arthrodesis of an ankle joint. Clin Orthop 68:75, 1970.

31. Hallock H: Arthrodesis of the ankle joint for old painful fractures. J Bone Joint Surg 27:49, 1945.

32. Hatt RN: The central bone graft in joint arthrodesis. J Bone Joint Surg 22:393, 1940.

33. Heining CF, DuPuy DN: Anterior dowel fusion of the ankle. In Bateman JE (ed): Foot Science. Philadelphia, Saunders, 1976, pp. 150–155.

34. Hone MR: Dowel fusion of the ankle joint. J Bone Joint Surg 50B:678, 1968.

35. Horwitz T: The use of the transfibular approach in arthrodesis of the ankle joint. Am J Surg 55:550, 1942.

36. Huckell JR, Fuller J: Arthrodesis of the ankle. In Bateman JE (ed): Foot Science. Philadelphia, Saunders, 1976, pp. 156–161.

37. Huggler AH: Technique of rearthrodesis in pseudarthrosis. In Chapchal G (ed): The Arthrodesis in the Restoration of Working Ability. New York, Thieme-Edition, 1975, pp. 137–138.

38. Jackson A: Tarsal hypermobility after ankle fusion—fact or fiction? J Bone Joint Surg 61B:470, 1979.

39. Jansen K: Arthrodesis of the ankle joint. Acta Orthop Scand 32:476, 1962.

40. Johnson EW, Boseker EH: Arthrodesis of the ankle. Arch Surg 97:766, 1968.

41. Kennedy JC: Arthrodesis of the ankle with particular reference to the Gallie procedure. A review of 50 cases. J Bone Joint Surg 42A:1308, 1960.

42. Kimberley AG: Malunited fractures affecting the ankle joint. With special reference to 22 cases treated by arthrodesis. Surg Gynecol Obstet 62:79, 1968.

43. King HA, Watkins TB, Samuelson KM: Analysis of the foot position in ankle arthrodesis and its influence on gait. Foot and ankle 1:44, 1980.

44. Kivilaakso R, Langenskiold A, Salenius P: Arthrodesis of the ankle as a treatment for postfracture conditions. Acta Orthop Scand 37:409, 1966.

45. Koch F: Observations in 132 arthrodeses of the tibiotalar joint. In Chapchal G (ed): The Arthrodesis in the Restoration of Working Ability. New York, Thieme-Edition, 1975, pp. 146–148.

46. Lance EM, Pavel A, Fries I, Larsen I, Patterson RL: Arthrodesis of the ankle joint. A followup study. Clin Orthop 142:146, 1979.

47. Lance EM, Pavel A, Patterson RL, Fries I, Larsen IJ: Arthrodesis of the ankle. A follow-up study. J Bone Joint Surg 53A:1030, 1971.

48. Mazur JM, Schwartz E, Simon SR: Ankle arthrodesis. J Bone Joint Surg 61A:964, 1979.

49. Morrey BF, Wiedeman GP: Complications and long-term results of ankle arthrodesis following trauma. J Bone Joint Surg 62A:777, 1980.

50. Morris HD: Arthrodesis of the foot. Clin Orthop 16:164, 1960.

51. Morris HD, Hand WL, Dunn AW: The modified Blair fusion for fractures of the talus. J Bone Joint Surg 53A:1289, 1971.

52. Morris JD, Herrick RT: Ankle arthrodesis. In Bateman JE (ed): Foot Science. Philadelphia, Saunders, 1976, pp. 136–149.

53. Murray WR, Pfeffinger LL, Teasdale RD: Total ankle arthroplasty: A joint too far. J Bone Joint Surg 63B:459, 1981.

54. Newton St E III: Total ankle replacement arthroplasty. An alternative to ankle fusion. J Bone Joint Surg 57A:1003, 1975.

55. Ottolenghi CE, Animoso J, Burgo PH: Percutaneous arthrodesis of the ankle joint. Clin Orthop 68:72, 1970.

56. Pappas M, Buechel FF, DePalma AF: Cylindrical total ankle joint replacement. Surgical and biomechanical rationale. Clin Orthop 118:82, 1976.

57. Pridie KH: Arthrodesis of the ankle. J Bone Joint Surg 35B:152, 1953.

58. Ratliff AHC: Compression arthrodesis of the ankle. J Bone Joint Surg 41B:524, 1959.

59. Said E, Hunka L, Siller TN: Ankle fusions: A current study. In Bateman JE, Trott AW (eds): The Foot and Ankle. New York, Thieme-Stratton, 1980, pp. 131–136.

60. Said E, Hunka L, Siller TN: Where ankle fusion

stands today. J Bone Joint Surg 60B:211, 1978.

61. Scholz KC: Total ankle replacement arthroplasty. In Bateman JE (ed): Foot Science. Philadelphia, Saunders, 1976, pp. 106–135.

62. Simon SR, Mazur J: Ankle arthrodesis: Longterm follow-up with gait analysis. In Bateman JE, Trott AW (eds): The Foot and Ankle. New York, Thieme-Stratton, 1980, pp. 73–92.

63. Soren A: Safe inlay of bone graft in arthrodesis. Clin Orthop 58:147, 1968.

64. Staples OS: Posterior arthrodesis of the ankle and subtalar joints. J Bone Joint Surg 38A:50, 1956.

65. Stauffer RN: Total ankle joint replacement as an alternative to arthrodesis. Geriatrics 31:79, 1976.

66. Stauffer RN: Total ankle joint replacement. Arch Surg 112:1105, 1977.

67. Stauffer RN, Chao EYS, Brewster RC: Force and motion analysis of the normal, diseased, and prosthetic ankle joint. Clin Orthop 127:189, 1977.

68. Stewart M: Arthrodesis. In Edmonson AS, Crenshaw AH (eds): Campbell's Operative Orthopaedics, Vol. 1. St. Louis, Mosby, 1980, pp. 1100–1141.

69. Thomas FB: Arthrodesis of the ankle. J Bone Joint Surg 51B:53, 1969.

70. VanGorder GW, Chen C-M: The central-graft operation for fusion of tuberculous knees, ankles, and elbows. J Bone Joint Surg 41A:1029, 1959.

71. Verhelst MP, Mulier JC, Hoogmartens MJ, Spaas F: Arthrodesis of the ankle joint with complete removal of the distal part of the fibula. Clin Orthop 118:93, 1976.

72. Watson-Jones R: Injuries of the ankle. In: Fractures and Joint Injuries. Baltimore, Williams & Wilkins, 1955, pp. 853–857.

73. Waugh TR, Evanski PM, McMaster WC: Irvine ankle arthroplasty: Design, operative technique and preliminary results. J Bone Joint Surg 58A:729, 1976.

74. White AA III: A precision posterior ankle fusion. Clin Orthop 98:239, 1974.

75. Wilson HJ: Arthrodesis of the ankle. A technique using bilateral hemimalleolar onlay grafts with screw fixation. J Bone Joint Surg 51A:775, 1969.

Chapter 18 Ankle Injuries in the Child

PETER D. PIZZUTILLO

Injury of the child's ankle deserves special consideration because of possible effects on the highly specialized cartilage cells of the physis. Many anatomic differences exist between the immature ankle and that of the adult, but the essential difference involves the physis but its growth potential. Nonunion, incongruity of joint surface, and degenerative changes are potential sequelae at any age, but interference with growth in the child may also create problems of leg-length discrepancy, progressive angular deformity, and progressive joint surface incongruity.

The physes of long bones have a constant architecture that develops as the result of a continuum of cellular differentiation (Fig. 18.1). Adjacent to the epiphysis is a layer of resting germinative cells that evolve to a more active proliferating layer. Epiphyseal vessels divide to create a diffuse network to the resting cells and may provide undifferentiated cells to this zone for later development. The proliferating zone consists of actively dividing chondrocytes oriented in longitudinal columns that are separated by strands of collagen. These cells enlarge and may undergo vascular invasion and degeneration, or may persist as osteoblasts. The intercellular matrix exhibits progressive calcification with invasion by sinusoidal vessels from the metaphyseal arterial system. Osteoid deposition and mineralization result in ossification at the metaphyseal border of the physis that is responsible for longitudinal growth [3].

The growth zone at each end of a long bone has been characterized as a weakened area by Foucher [24] and Poland [42]. Using animal models, Vogt [23], Leser [23], Jahn [23], and Retzius [23] produced growth disturbance by surgical trauma to the physis; they observed that more significant deformity occurred when areas of active mitosis were traumatized.

Haas [23,24] reported that a constant plane of separation could be produced by manual pressure on the epiphysis after the perichondrium around the epiphyseal plate had been sharply incised. He demonstrated that the epiphyseal plate displaced with the epiphyseal fragment. Mi-

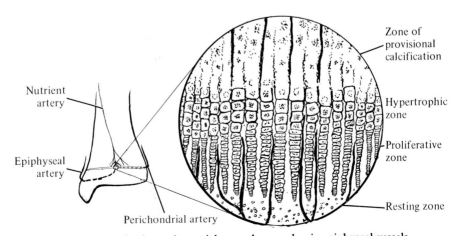

Nutrient artery

Epiphyseal artery

Perichondrial artery

Zone of provisional calcification

Hypertrophic zone

Proliferative zone

Resting zone

Fig. 18.1. Specialized cartilage cells of the physis receive a rich vascular supply via epiphyseal vessels.

croscopic study not only confirmed his impression but also demonstrated a constant cleavage plane "in the region of large vesicular cells, a thin layer of which adheres to the metaphysis." Haas used the reproducible cleavage plane in the immature dog as a model to study the effects of surgical trauma on the metaphysis, the juxtaepiphyseal column of cartilage cells, and the growth plate as a whole. From detailed gross and microscopic observation, he concluded that the most important area for longitudinal growth was the zone of cartilage columns adjacent to the epiphysis. This was the first documented localization of growth within the epiphyseal plate of long bones. Haas's model of epiphyseal separation did not result in significant interruption of longitudinal growth and he concluded that direct trauma to the cartilage cell columns was necessary to alter growth.

Kaplan [28] emphasized that most injuries to the immature ankle were caused by indirect forces. He observed that the zone of calcification and early ossification in the epiphyseal plate no longer possessed the elasticity of cartilage and had not yet attained the strength of bone. Thus, it was more vulnerable to trauma. Furthermore, the distal tibial and fibular epiphyseal plates are extracapsular structures with ligamentous and capsular attachments directly to their epiphyseal segment (Fig. 18.2). Indirect forces transmitted through these insertions have a direct effect on

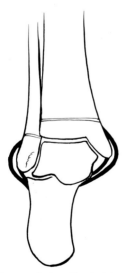

Fig. 18.2. The physes of the distal tibia and fibula are extracapsular with ligamentous and capsular attachments directly to their epiphyses.

the epiphyseal plate. Kaplan observed that epiphyseal separation resulted in either mild shortening or overgrowth of the involved bone; when the severity of injury was sufficient to destroy physeal cells, significant growth inhibition developed.

Leg-Length Discrepancy

When the germinative and proliferative cells have been destroyed through most of the distal tibial physis, leg-length discrepancy will occur without deformity. The degree of discrepancy is dependent upon the remaining growth of the uninvolved limb. In the 5- to 7-year-old child, a clinically significant discrepancy can be expected because of the growth potential, whereas in the 11- to 13-year-old child, no difference should develop. It is fortunate that ankle injury most commonly involves the latter group of patients.

Angular Deformity

When only a portion of the distal tibial physis has been destroyed, no further growth will occur at the involved area, but continued growth of the remaining physis will result in deformity of variable degree, depending on the remaining expected growth. The more immature the bone, the greater the potential angular deformity. Longitudinal growth will also be mildly retarded. In severe adduction injuries of the ankle, the medial half of the distal tibial physis is traumatized. If growth ceases medially, the lateral portion of the distal tibial physis and the distal fibula continue to grow and a progressive varus deformity at the ankle develops (Fig. 18.3). Documented clinical examples of this problem have been reported by McFarland [36], Carothers and Crenshaw [12], Aitken [1], Elmslie [21], and Gill and Abbott [22].

Similar deformity may also develop after fractures that have propagated from the joint surface, through the epiphysis, and into the physeal plane [37]. The continuity of the germinative and proliferative cell layers is disrupted and bony union between disorganized layers will result. If a significant degree of growth potential exists at the

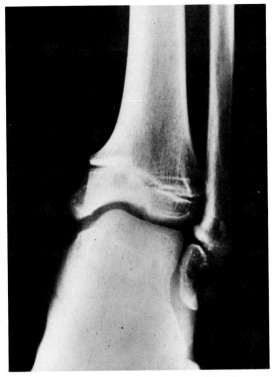

Fig. 18.3. The growth arrest line at the lateral aspect of the distal tibia and the elongation of the distal fibula indicate increased growth at these areas in relation to the closing physis at the medial portion of the distal tibia.

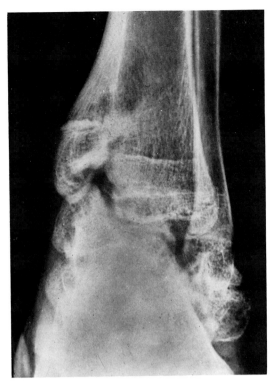

Fig. 18.4. Progressive joint surface incongruity may develop if significant growth potential exists at the time of injury.

time of injury, progressive deformity as well as joint surface incongruity will develop (Fig. 18.4).

Vascular Disturbance

In addition to direct injury of the physeal cells, compromise of the epiphyseal blood supply may occur, with resultant avascular necrosis of the distal tibial epiphysis [45,49]. Interference with bone growth and joint surface disruption may also result. The major vessels to the epiphysis, physis, and metaphysis have been precisely demonstrated by Dale and Harris [17]. Two major patterns of vascular supply exist, depending on the degree of epiphyseal coverage by hyaline cartilage. Those epiphyses that are entirely covered by hyaline cartilage, such as the proximal femoral epiphysis, are vascularized by nutrient vessels that pass through the perichondrium at the epiphyseal plate. Those epiphyses that are only

partially covered by hyaline cartilage, such as the distal tibial and fibular epiphyses, have direct blood supply that enters at a distance from the epiphyseal plate (Fig. 18.1). The epiphysis that is totally covered with hyaline cartilage will sustain immediate interruption of its vascular supply with physeal separation, whereas the epiphysis that is partially covered by hyaline cartilage may sustain physeal separation without intrinsic damage to its vascular supply. The uninjured germinative and proliferative cells separate with the epiphysis, maintain a blood supply from the epiphyseal vessels, and thus continue to grow.

Clinical Evaluation

Although fractures may result from direct trauma or compressive forces, indirect trauma is the most common mechanism of ankle injury in childhood. The history obtained from a child, like the adult, is frequently unreliable, but careful clinical examination and radiographic findings will usually elucidate the mechanism of injury. This information is helpful in planning reduction and definitive treatment and may suggest associated problems and potential complications. The Lauge-Hansen classification by mechanism of injury has been used by Dias and Tachdjian to classify most ankle fractures in children [19].

Initial clinical findings range from the swollen, deformed, and diffusely tender ankle to the normal-appearing ankle that is characterized by point tenderness along the physis. Ligamentous injury does occur in the child but is uncommon. Before the diagnosis of ankle sprain can be made with confidence, physeal injury must be excluded. Shear or compressive force may damage the distal tibial and fibular epiphyses without necessarily causing displacement. Even when epiphyseal displacement does occur, spontaneous reduction can make early diagnosis difficult [11].

Radiographic Evaluation

Radiographs of the involved ankle in the frontal and lateral views are mandatory for basic evalua-tion. Nondisplaced and displaced fractures with accompanying soft tissue changes are usually evident with these views. Interpretation may be difficult when centers of ossification have yet to appear, when nebulous changes are noted at the irregular physis, and when bony densities are seen at the tip of either malleolus. Mortise, oblique, and stress views of the involved ankle (Fig. 18.5) in addition to comparison radiographs of the opposite, uninvolved ankle will frequently clarify the findings.

One should not confuse accessory centers of ossification of the medial and lateral malleoli with fragments caused by trauma. Accessory centers at the tip of the medial malleolus have been observed in 17–24% of males and up to 47% of females [43,48]. Single or multiple ossicles are found bilaterally in two-thirds of cases (Fig. 18.6). At the medial malleolus, accessory centers of ossification become evident between 6 and 12 years of age and fuse approximately 18 months after they make their appearance. Occasionally, they remain unfused into adult life. Accessory centers at the tip of the lateral malleolus are seen much less frequently than at the medial malleolus.

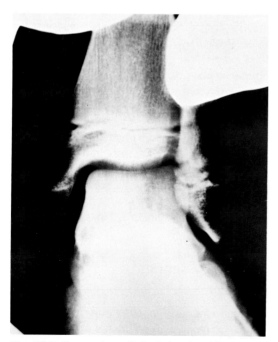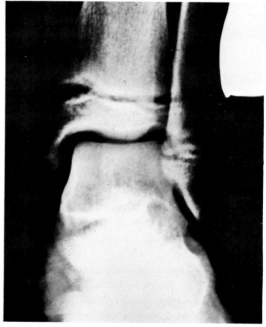

Fig. 18.5. Stress view of the injured ankle reveals medial gaping of the distal tibial physis in comparison with the normal side.

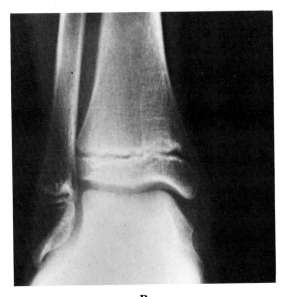 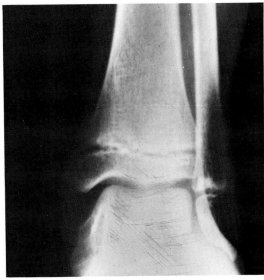

R   L

Fig. 18.6. Accessory center of ossification of the medial malleolus.

Types of Fracture

Shear force is responsible for the production of the Salter-Harris Type I and Type II fractures [46,47,54]. A line of separation develops at the zone of provisional calcification of the distal tibia and may remain entirely within the plane of the physis, a Salter I fracture (Fig. 18.7), or may propagate into the edge of the metaphysis, creating a Salter II fracture (Fig. 18.8). In both types, the germinative and proliferative layers of the physis as well as the epiphyseal blood supply displace with the epiphysis. Gentle force is all that is required for anatomic closed reduction. Following trauma, a transient slowing of growth will occur until metaphyseal blood vessels reestablish themselves. Permanent growth inhibition or angular deformity does not usually develop. Delayed manipulative reduction should be avoided in the young child because of the high risk of physeal damage. Mild angular deformity in the young child will frequently remodel. If satisfactory remodelling does not occur, osteotomy at a later date is a safer means of establishing normal alignment.

Bending and compression forces at the ankle result in Salter-Harris III and IV fractures [54]. The fracture line propagates across the epiphysis into the physis and results in malalignment of cellular layers (Figs. 18.9 and 18.10). With in-creasing force, crush injury of the physis may occur with cessation of growth in the area of involvement. Anatomic reduction by open methods is usually required to realign the physeal segments and to establish joint surface congruency. Internal fixation may be obtained with pins inserted parallel to the physis. Threaded pins should not traverse the physis for fear of causing premature physeal closure.

When severe compression force destroys the distal tibial physis in its entirety, progressive leg-length discrepancy will occur but angular deformity will not develop. The Salter-Harris V fracture initially presents with a normal radiograph but later exhibits growth retardation (Fig. 18.11) [5]. Recently, the existence of this fracture has been questioned, since no documented case has been reported to date [41]. Peterson has emphasized that premature closure may be the result of ischemia and immobilization [40] rather than direct trauma [25].

Tillaux Fracture

Kleiger [29,30] has reported that physiologic closure of the distal tibial physis begins at its midportion and progresses medially. Lateral closure occurs approximately 18 months later and has been observed between 14 and 18 years of age.

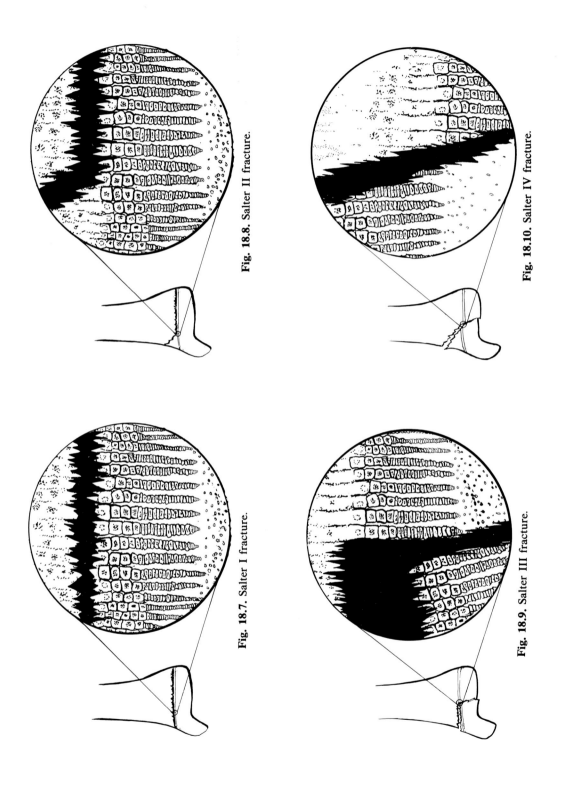

Fig. 18.8. Salter II fracture.

Fig. 18.10. Salter IV fracture.

Fig. 18.7. Salter I fracture.

Fig. 18.9. Salter III fracture.

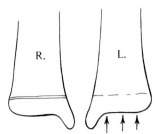

Fig. 18.11. Salter V fracture.

In the early phase of closure of the distal tibial physis, an external rotatory force at the ankle may result in isolated avulsion of the open lateral portion of the epiphysis (Fig. 18.12). The displaced lateral fragment is quadrilateral in the immature ankle and triangular in the adult, and has been referred to as a "Tillaux fracture." Although deformity is not expected because of the limited remaining growth potential, anatomic reduction must be obtained by closed or open means to restore the joint surface.

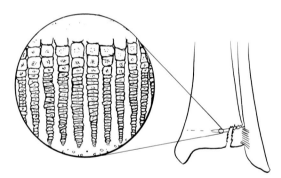

Fig. 18.12. Tillaux fracture.

Bosworth Rotational Fracture

In the younger child, severe external rotational forces may produce physeal separation characterized by external rotation of the distal tibial epiphysis on the metaphysis. This is associated with external rotation and displacement of the distal fibula, with or without fracture. Although part of the interosseous ligament is usually ruptured, the anterior and posterior tibiofibular ligaments remain intact and bind the distal tibial epiphyses to the fibula (Fig. 18.13). This has been referred to as a "Bosworth rotational fracture

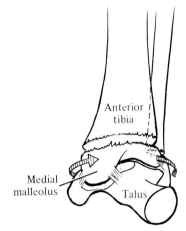

Fig. 18.13. Bosworth rotational fracture.

of the distal tibia" [10,33,38] because of its resemblance to the adult injury described by Bosworth. Clinical examination reveals fixed external rotation of the foot with a normal relationship of the foot to the medial and lateral malleoli. Radiographs are frequently interpreted as negative, but when carefully compared with radiographs of the normal ankle they will reveal irregularity of the physis and, occasionally, a small metaphyseal fragment. Reduction is usually accompanied by a sudden jerk that is indicative of restoration of the distal fibula into the fibular incisura of the distal tibia. Growth retardation has not been associated with this injury.

Triplane Fracture

The triplane fracture of the distal tibia is an uncommon injury. Johnson and Fahl [27] reported a plantarflexion injury with epiphyseal displacement that in retrospect is highly suggestive of this fracture. Marmor [35] and subsequently others [34,39,52] described the injury more specifically. Cooperman et al. [15] reported their experience with triplane fractures in 15 patients with an average age of 13 years and 5 months. The age of injury indicates that closure of the medial half of the distal tibial physis had occurred. On an anteroposterior radiograph, the fracture plane is sagittally directed into the midportion of the distal tibial epiphysis and is propagated horizontally through the lateral half of the physis (Fig.

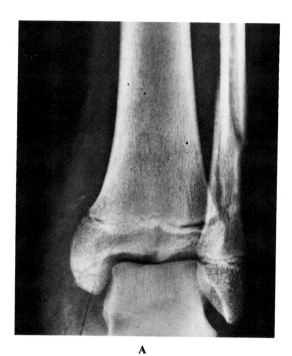
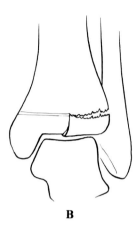

A

B

Fig. 18.14. Triplane fracture—anteroposterior radiograph (**A**) and schematic (**B**).

18.14). The lateral radiograph reveals a fracture in the coronal plane extending proximally from the physis into the posterior metaphysis (Fig. 18.15); posterior displacement of this dorsal fragment may be present. Experience to date suggests that two or three fragments may be present in the triplane fracture. Anatomic reduction is required and may frequently be obtained by closed methods and maintained by casting. If satisfactory reduction is not obtained by closed means, open restoration of rotational alignment and joint surface integrity is necessary. Although premature physeal closure does occur, it is of little clinical significance because of the limited growth potential in this age group.

Complications

When adequate reduction is not obtained in fractures that disrupt the physis, a central bone bridge is likely to develop (Fig. 18.16). In the child with remaining growth potential, further inhibition of growth and additional angular deformity can be avoided by resection of the bone bridge and implantation of a mechanical barrier to reossification such as fat or silicone [8,9,31,32].

The success of this procedure depends both on the size of the bone bridge and on completeness of resection. If more than half of the cross-sectional area of the physis is involved in the bridge, successful reinitiation of growth by the remaining open portion of the physis is much less likely. This procedure will arrest progressive deformity but cannot be relied upon to correct deformity that is already evident.

If a large area of distal tibial physis ceases growing, as in adduction injuries of the ankle, subsequent deformity can also be minimized by epiphysiodesis of the remaining physis and of the distal fibular physis. Staged epiphysiodesis of the contralateral distal tibial and fibular physes may be needed if a significant leg-length discrepancy is anticipated.

Summary

Interference with the growth potential of the immature ankle may create problems of leg-length discrepancy, progressive angular deformity, and progressive joint surface incongruity. The final results of epiphyseal trauma will depend on the

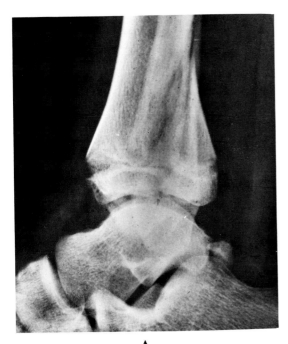
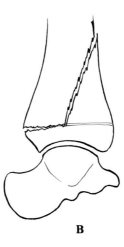

B

A

Fig. 18.15. Triplane fracture—lateral radiograph **(A)** and schematic **(B)**.

presence and degree of direct injury to the germinative and proliferative cells of the physis, the type of vascular supply to the epiphysis, the remaining growth potential of the involved physis, the degree of joint surface disruption, and the quality of reduction.

Emphasis should be placed on prompt treatment to include gentle reduction by closed or occasionally open means. The child should be

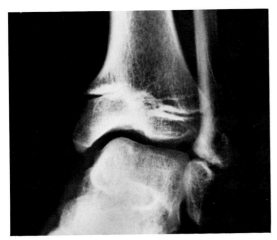

Fig. 18.16. Bony bridge across central distal tibial physis.

followed regularly until growth is completed to permit early detection of growth disturbance.

References

1. Aitken AP: The end results of a fractured distal tibial epiphysis. J Bone Joint Surg 18:685, 1936.
2. Aitken AP, Magill HK: Fractures involving the distal femoral epiphyseal cartilage. J Bone Joint Surg 34A:96, 1952.
3. Albright JA, Brand RA: The Scientific Basis of Orthopaedics. New York, Appleton, 1979.
4. Barash ES, Siffert RS: The potential for growth of experimentally produced hemiepiphyses. J Bone Joint Surg 48A:1548, 1966.
5. Bishop HA: Fractures and epiphyseal separation fractures of the ankle. Am J Roentgenol 28:49, 1932.
6. Blount WP: Fractures in Children. Baltimore, Williams & Wilkins, 1955, pp. 183–194.
7. Boissevain ACH, Raaymakers ELFB: Traumatic injury of the distal tibial epiphysis. Reconstr Surg Trauma 17:40, 1979.
8. Bright RW: Surgical correction of partial epiphyseal plate closure in dogs by bone bridge resection and use of silicon rubber implants. J Bone Joint Surg 54A:1133, 1972.
9. Bright RW: Operative correction of partial epiphyseal plate closure by osseous-bridge resection and silicon rubber implant. J Bone Joint Surg 56A:655, 1974.

10. Broock GJ, Greer RB: Traumatic rotational displacements of the distal tibial growth plate. J Bone Joint Surg 52A:1666, 1970.

11. Cameron HU: A radiologic sign of lateral subluxation of the distal tibial epiphyses. J Trauma 15:1030, 1975.

12. Carothers CO, Crenshaw AH: Clinical significance of a classification of epiphyseal injuries at the ankle. Am J Surg 89:879, 1955.

13. Cassidy RH: Epiphyseal injuries of the lower extremity. Surg Clin North Am 38:1125, 1958.

14. Compere EL: Growth arrest in long bones as result of fractures that include the epiphysis. JAMA 105:2140, 1935.

15. Cooperman DR, Spiegel PG, Laros GS: Tibial fractures involving the ankle in children. J Bone Joint Surg 60A:1040, 1978.

16. Crenshaw AH: Injuries of the distal tibial epiphysis. Clin Orthop 41:98, 1965.

17. Dale GG, Harris WR: Prognosis of epiphyseal separation. J Bone Joint Surg 40B:116, 1958.

18. Danielsson LG: Avulsion fracture of the lateral malleolus in children. Injury 12:165, 1978.

19. Dias LS, Tachdjian MO: Physeal injuries of the ankle in children. Clin Orthop 136:230, 1978.

20. Eliason EL, Ferguson LK: Epiphyseal separation of the long bones. Surg Gynecol Obstet 58:85, 1934.

21. Elmslie RC: The relationship of fracture of the lower epiphysis of the tibia to arrest growth of the bone. J Orthop Surg 1:215, 1919.

22. Gill GG, Abbott LC: Varus deformity of ankle following injury to distal epiphyseal cartilage of tibia in growing children. Surg Gynecol Obstet 72:659, 1941.

23. Haas SL: A localization of the growing point in the epiphyseal cartilage plate of bones. Am J Orthop Surg 15:563, 1917.

24. Haas SL: The changes produced in the growing bone after injury to the epiphyseal cartilage plate. Am J Orthop Surg 1:67, 1919.

25. Hulten O: The influence of a fixation bandage on the peripheral blood vessels in the circulation. Acta Chir Scand 101:151, 1951.

26. Ireland J: Late results of separation of an epiphysis. Ann Surg 97:189, 1933.

27. Johnson EW Jr, Fahl JC: Fractures involving the distal epiphysis of the tibia and fibula in children. Am J Surg 93:778, 1957.

28. Kaplan L: Epiphyseal injuries in childhood. Surg Clin North Am 17:1637, 1937.

29. Kleiger B: Mechanisms of ankle injury. Orthop Clin North Am 5:127, 1974.

30. Kleiger B, Mankin HJ: Fracture of the lateral portion of the distal tibial epiphysis. J Bone Joint Surg 46A:25, 1964.

31. Langenskiold A: Traumatic premature closure of the distal tibial epiphyseal plate. Acta Orthop Scand 38:520, 1967.

32. Langenskiold A: An operation for partial closure of an epiphyseal plate in children and its experi-

mental basis. J Bone Joint Surg 57B:325, 1975.

33. Lovell ES: An unusual rotatory injury of the ankle. J Bone Joint Surg 50A:163, 1968.

34. Lynn MD: The triplane distal tibial epiphyseal fracture. Clin Orthop 86:187, 1972.

35. Marmor L: An unusual fracture of the tibial epiphysis. Clin Orthop 73:132, 1970.

36. McFarland B: Traumatic arrest of epiphyseal growth at the lower end of the tibia. Br J Surg 19:78, 1931.

37. Morris RH: Report of a case of vertical fracture through the lower tibial epiphysis during the period of bone growth and an operation for the correction of the resultant deformity. N Engl J Med 215:272, 1936.

38. Nevalos AB, Colton CL: Rotational displacement of the lower tibial epiphysis due to trauma. J Bone Joint Surg 59B:331, 1977.

39. Peiro A, Aracil J, Martos F, Mut T: Triplane distal tibial epiphyseal fracture. Clin Orthop 160:196, 1981.

40. Peterson CA, Peterson HA: Analysis of the incidence of injuries to the epiphyseal growth plate. J Trauma 12:275, 1972.

41. Peterson HA, Burkhart SS: Compression injury of the epiphyseal growth plate: fact or fiction? J Pediat Orthop 1:377, 1981.

42. Poland J: Traumatic Separation of the Epiphyses. London, Smith, Elder, 1898.

43. Powell HDW: Extra center of ossification for the medial malleolus in children. J Bone Joint Surg 43B:107, 1961.

44. Rang M: Children's Fractures. Philadelphia, Lippincott, 1974.

45. Robertson DE: Post-traumatic osteochondritis of the lower tibial epiphysis. J Bone Joint Surg 46B:212, 1964.

46. Salter RB: Injuries of the ankle in children. Orthop Clin North Am 5:147, 1974.

47. Salter RB, Harris WR: Injuries involving the epiphyseal plate. J Bone Joint Surg 45A:587, 1963.

48. Selby S: Separate centers of ossification of the tip of the internal malleolus. Am J Roentgenol 86:496, 1961.

49. Siffert RS, Arkin AM: Post-traumatic aseptic necrosis of the distal tibial epiphysis. J Bone Joint Surg 32A:691, 1950.

50. Smith MK: The prognosis in epiphyseal line fractures. Ann Surg 79:273, 1924.

51. Spiegel PG, Cooperman DR, Laros GS: Epiphyseal fractures of the distal ends of the tibia and fibula. J Bone Joint Surg 60A:1046, 1978.

52. Torg JS, Ruggiero RA: Comminuted epiphyseal fracture of the distal tibia. Clin Orthop 110:215, 1975.

53. Vahvanen V, Aalto K: Classification of ankle fractures in children. Arch Orthop Trauma Surg 97:1, 1980.

54. Weber BG, Brunner C, Freuler F: Treatment of Fractures in Children and Adolescents. Berlin, Springer-Verlag, 1980.

Index